Infectious Diseases in Geriatric Medicine

Editors

THOMAS T. YOSHIKAWA
DEAN C. NORMAN

CLINICS IN
GERIATRIC MEDICINE

www.geriatric.theclinics.com

August 2016 • Volume 32 • Number 3

ELSEVIER

1600 John F. Kennedy Boulevard • Suite 1800 • Philadelphia, Pennsylvania, 19103-2899

http://www.theclinics.com

CLINICS IN GERIATRIC MEDICINE Volume 32, Number 3
August 2016 ISSN 0749–0690, ISBN-13: 978-0-323-45965-5

Editor: Jessica McCool
Developmental Editor: Colleen Viola

Clinics in Geriatric Medicine (ISSN 0749-0690) is published quarterly by Elsevier Inc., 360 Park Avenue South, New York, NY 10010-1710. Months of issue are February, May, August, and November. Business and Editorial Offices: 1600 John F. Kennedy Blvd., Suite 1800, Philadelphia, PA 191023-2899. Periodicals postage paid at New York, NY, and additional mailing offices. Subscription prices are $265.00 per year (US individuals), $557.00 per year (US institutions), $100.00 per year (US student/resident), $370.00 per year (Canadian individuals), $706.00 per year (Canadian institutions), $195.00 per year (Canadian student/resident), $390.00 per year (international individuals), $706.00 per year (international institutions), and $195.00 per year (international student/resident). Foreign air speed delivery is included in all *Clinics* subscription prices. All prices are subject to change without notice. POSTMASTER: Send address changes to *Clinics in Geriatric Medicine,* Elsevier Health Sciences Division, Subscription Customer Service, 3251 Riverport Lane, Maryland Heights, MO 63043. **Telephone: 1-800-654-2452 (U.S. and Canada); 314-447-8871 (outside U.S. and Canada). Fax: 314-447-8029. E-mail:** journalscustomerservice-usa@elsevier. com **(for print support) or** journalsonlinesupport-usa@elsevier.com **(for online support).**

Reprints. For copies of 100 or more, of articles in this publication, please contact the Commercial Reprints Department, Elsevier Inc., 360 Park Avenue South, New York, New York 10010-1710. Tel.: 212-633-3874; Fax: 212-633-3820, E-mail: reprints@elsevier.com.

Clinics in Geriatric Medicine is covered in *MEDLINE/PubMed (Index Medicus), EMBASE/Excerpta Medica, Current Contents/Clinical Medicine (CC/CM),* and the *Cumulative Index to Nursing & Allied Health Literature.*

Contributors

EDITORS

THOMAS T. YOSHIKAWA, MD
Department of Veterans Affairs Greater Los Angeles Healthcare System, David Geffen School of Medicine at the University of California at Los Angeles; Charles R. Drew University of Medicine and Science, Los Angeles, California

DEAN C. NORMAN, MD
Professor of Medicine and Geriatrics, Department of Veterans Affairs Greater Los Angeles Healthcare Center, David Geffen School of Medicine at the University of California at Los Angeles, Los Angeles, California

AUTHORS

THILINIE BANDARANAYAKE, MBBS
Clinical Fellow and Instructor in Medicine, Section of Infectious Diseases, Yale School of Medicine, New Haven, Connecticut

ANA BERLIN, MD, MPH
Assistant Professor, Department of Surgery, Rutgers New Jersey Medical School, Newark, New Jersey

REX BIEDENBENDER, MD, MPH
Jencare Neighborhood Medical Center, Virginia Beach, Virginia

SUZANNE F. BRADLEY, MD
Program Director, Infection Control, Veterans Affairs Ann Arbor Healthcare System; Professor of Internal Medicine, Division of Infectious Diseases, University of Michigan Medical School, Ann Arbor, Michigan

MARCO CASSONE, MD, PhD
Division of Geriatric and Palliative Care Medicine, University of Michigan Medical School, Ann Arbor, Michigan

HARLEY EDWARD DAVIDSON, PharmD, MPH
Department of Clinical Internal Medicine, Eastern Virginia Medical School, Insight Therapeutics, LLC, Norfolk, Virginia

PAUL K. EDWARDS, MD
Assistant Professor, Department of Orthopaedic Surgery, University of Arkansas for Medical Services, Little Rock, Arkansas

THOMAS M. FILE Jr, MD, MSc
Professor and Chair, Infectious Disease Section, Northeast Ohio Medical University, Rootstown, Ohio; Chair, Infectious Disease Division, Summa Health System, Akron, Ohio

GOWRISHANKAR GNANASEKARAN, MD, MPH
Department of Medicine-Geriatrics, University Hospitals, Case Medical Center, Case Western Reserve University, Cleveland, Ohio

MATTHEW BIDWELL GOETZ, MD
Chief, Infectious Diseases Section, Department of Medicine, VA Greater Los Angeles Healthcare System; Professor of Clinical Medicine, David Geffen School of Medicine at the University of California Los Angeles, Los Angeles, California

STEFAN GRAVENSTEIN, MD, MPH
Department of Medicine-Geriatrics, University Hospitals, Case Medical Center, Case Western Reserve University, Cleveland, Ohio; Health Services Policy and Practice, Warren Alpert Medical School, Brown University, Providence, Rhode Island

JASON MICHAEL JOHANNING, MD, MS
Department of Surgery, University of Nebraska Medical Center, Omaha, Nebraska

THOMAS J. MARRIE, MD, FRCPC
Professor, Department of Medicine, Dalhousie University, Halifax, Nova Scotia, Canada

SIMON C. MEARS, MD, PhD
Professor, Department of Orthopaedic Surgery, University of Arkansas for Medical Services, Little Rock, Arkansas

LONA MODY, MD, MSc
Professor of Internal Medicine, Division of Geriatric and Palliative Care Medicine, University of Michigan Medical School; Geriatrics Research Education and Clinical Center, VA Ann Arbor Healthcare System, Ann Arbor, Michigan

ANA MONTOYA, MD
Assistant Professor of Internal Medicine, Division of Geriatric and Palliative Care Medicine, University of Michigan Medical School, Ann Arbor, Michigan

LINDSAY E. NICOLLE, MD, FRCPC
Professor, Departments of Internal Medicine and Medical Microbiology, Health Sciences Centre, University of Manitoba, Winnipeg, Manitoba, Canada

DEAN C. NORMAN, MD
Professor of Medicine and Geriatrics, Department of Veterans Affairs Greater Los Angeles Healthcare Center, David Geffen School of Medicine at the University of California at Los Angeles, Los Angeles, California

SHOBITA RAJAGOPALAN, MD, MSCR, MPH
Los Angeles County Department of Public Health; Charles R. Drew University of Medicine and Science, Los Angeles, California

KENNETH SCHMADER, MD
Professor of Medicine; Chief, Division of Geriatrics, Center for the Study of Aging and Human Development, Duke University Medical Center; Director, Geriatric Research, Education and Clinical Center (GRECC), Durham Veterans Affairs Medical Center, Durham, North Carolina

JAKE SCOTT, MD
Fellow, Infectious Diseases Section, Department of Medicine, VA Greater Los Angeles Healthcare System, David Geffen School of Medicine at the University of California at Los Angeles, Los Angeles, California

ALBERT C. SHAW, MD, PhD
Associate Professor of Medicine, Section of Infectious Diseases, Yale School of Medicine, New Haven, Connecticut

MARY B. WHITE, MD
Department of Veterans Affairs, VA Greater Los Angeles Healthcare System, Los Angeles, California

THOMAS T. YOSHIKAWA, MD
Department of Veterans Affairs Greater Los Angeles Healthcare System, David Geffen School of Medicine at the University of California at Los Angeles; Charles R. Drew University of Medicine and Science, Los Angeles, California

Contents

Host Resistance and Immune Aging 415

Thilinie Bandaranayake and Albert C. Shaw

> Human immune system aging results in impaired responses to pathogens or vaccines. In the innate immune system, which mediates the earliest pro-inflammatory responses to immunologic challenge, processes ranging from Toll-like Receptor function to Neutrophil Extracellular Trap formation are generally diminished in older adults. Dysregulated, enhanced basal inflammation with age reflecting activation by endogenous damage-associated ligands contributes to impaired innate immune responses. In the adaptive immune system, T and B cell subsets and function alter with age. The control of cytomegalovirus infection, particularly in the T lineage, plays a dominant role in the differentiation and diversity of the T cell compartment.

Clinical Features of Infection in Older Adults 433

Dean C. Norman

> The impact of infectious diseases on older adults is far greater than on younger adults because of significantly higher morbidity and mortality caused by infection. The reasons for this greater impact include factors such as lower physiologic reserve due to age and chronic disease, age-related changes in host defenses, loss of mobility, higher risk for polypharmacy and adverse drug reactions, and being on drugs that increase the risk for infection (e.g., anticholinergic and other sedating medications increase the risk for pneumonia).

Principles of Antimicrobial Therapy in Older Adults 443

Suzanne F. Bradley

> Antibiotic use is common in older adults, and much of it is deemed unnecessary. Complications of antibiotic use may occur as a consequence of changes in age-related physiology and dosing with resulting drug toxicity and secondary infection. Knowing when it is appropriate to initiate antibiotics may help reduce unnecessary antibiotic use and prevent adverse drug events. Careful attention to antibiotic selection, dosing adjustments, and drug-drug interactions may also help prevent antibiotic-related adverse events.

Bacterial Pneumonia in Older Adults 459

Thomas J. Marrie and Thomas M. File Jr

> Community-acquired pneumonia is common in the elderly person; its presentation in this population is often confounded by multiple comorbid

illnesses, including those that result in confusion. Although severity-of-illness scoring systems might aid decision-making, clinical judgment following a careful assessment is key in deciding on the site of care and appropriate therapy.

women is benign and should not be treated. A diagnosis of symptomatic infection for elderly residents of long-term care facilities without catheters requires localizing genitourinary findings. Symptomatic urinary infection is overdiagnosed in elderly bacteriuric persons with nonlocalizing clinical presentations, with substantial inappropriate antimicrobial use. Residents with chronic indwelling catheters experience increased morbidity from urinary tract infection. Antimicrobial therapy is selected based on clinical presentation, patient tolerance, and urine culture results.

Herpes zoster causes significant suffering owing to acute and chronic pain or postherpetic neuralgia (PHN). Varicella-zoster virus–induced neuronal destruction and inflammation causes the principal problems of pain, interference with activities of daily living, and reduced quality of life in older adults. The optimal treatment of herpes zoster requires early antiviral therapy and careful pain management. For patients who have PHN, evidence-based pharmacotherapy using topical lidocaine patch, gabapentin, pregabalin, tricyclic antidepressants, or opiates can reduce pain burden. The live attenuated zoster vaccine is effective in reducing pain burden and preventing herpes zoster and PHN in older adults.

Bone and joint infections in the elderly patient include septic native joints, osteomyelitis, and prosthetic joint infection. Infections are difficult to treat and require a team approach. Surgical debridement and intravenous antibiotics are the keys to treatment. Prosthetic joint infections often need a two-stage approach to treatment. First the infected joint is removed and the infection treated, then a second prosthetic joint is placed. Prosthetic joint infection is becoming the most common complication after joint replacement surgery. Outcomes of treatment of bone and joint infections are related to the severity of the infection and condition of the host. Because the elderly are often frail, treatment is challenging.

Improved survival with combination antiretroviral therapy has led to a dramatic increase in the number of human immunodeficiency virus (HIV)–infected individuals 50 years of age or older such that by 2020 more than 50% of HIV-infected persons in the United States will be above this age. Recent studies confirm that antiretroviral therapy should be offered to all HIV-infected patients regardless of age, symptoms, CD4+ cell count, or HIV viral load. However, when compared with HIV-uninfected populations, even with suppression of measurable HIV replication, older individuals are at greater risk for cardiovascular disease, malignancies, liver disease, and other comorbidities.

CLINICS IN GERIATRIC MEDICINE

THE CLINICS ARE AVAILABLE ONLINE!
Access your subscription at:
www.theclinics.com

Preface

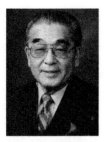 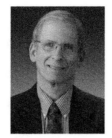

Thomas T. Yoshikawa, MD   Dean C. Norman, MD
Editors

Since 1992 when the topic of infectious diseases in older adults was first published in *Clinics in Geriatric Medicine*, there have been substantial progress and advances in the broad area of infections in older adults. These contributions have been made by geriatricians with interest and expertise in infections, infectious disease subspecialists with an interest in aging, and other medical and surgical specialist/subspecialists addressing infections in older patients in their practice. With the expanding aging population in both the United States and worldwide, health issues associated with aging are major personal and public health concerns. Although cardiovascular diseases, cancers, strokes, dementia, pulmonary disease, and diabetes mellitus are listed as major causes of death in older adults, in many instances the final cause of demise is complications associated with infections.

Over the nearly 25 years since the last *Clinics in Geriatric Medicine* on "geriatric infectious diseases," we have learned much about aging and infections, such that in this current issue of *Clinics in Geriatric Medicine* we will discuss only 13 infection-related topics compared to the 17 subjects we covered in the 1992 issue of *Clinics in Geriatric Medicine*. New topics covered in this issue include intra-abdominal infections, *Clostridium difficile* and Norovirus diarrheal diseases, bone and joint infections, human immunodeficiency virus infection, and herpes zoster infection. Updated concepts of aging and immunity are included in the article on Host Resistance and Immunology of Aging as well as current and new antibiotics recommended for common infections in older adults in the Principles of Antimicrobial Therapy article. The articles on Clinical Features of Infections, Bacterial Pneumonia, Tuberculosis, Urinary Tract Infection, Infections in Long-Term Care Setting and Vaccinations have all been revised to reflect the most current information on the diagnosis, treatment, and prevention of these infections.

We wish to thank all the authors for their outstanding contributions to this issue of *Clinics in Geriatric Medicine* and the Department of Veterans Affairs for

Clin Geriatr Med 32 (2016) xiii–xiv
http://dx.doi.org/10.1016/j.cger.2016.06.001
0749-0690/16/$ – see front matter © 2016 Published by Elsevier Inc.

geriatric.theclinics.com

their long and sustained support for their programs and services in geriatrics and long-term care.

Thomas T. Yoshikawa, MD
Department of Veterans Affairs
Greater Los Angeles Healthcare System
David Geffen School of Medicine
at the University of California at Los Angeles
11301 Wilshire Boulevard
Los Angeles, CA 90073, USA

Dean C. Norman, MD
Department of Veterans Affairs
Greater Los Angeles Healthcare Center
David Geffen School of Medicine
at the University of California at Los Angeles
11301 Wilshire Boulevard
Los Angeles, CA 90073, USA

E-mail addresses:
Toyoshikawa@cdrewu.edu (T.T. Yoshikawa)
Dnorman630@aol.com (D.C. Norman)

Host Resistance and Immune Aging

Thilinie Bandaranayake, MBBS, Albert C. Shaw, MD, PhD*

KEYWORDS

- Aging • Immunosenescence • Innate immunity • Inflammation • T cell • B cell

KEY POINTS

- Immunosenescence, describing age-associated changes in the immune system, generally results in impaired immune responses and contributes to the increased morbidity and mortality to infectious diseases and diminished vaccine responses found in older adults.
- A heightened pro-inflammatory environment, characterized by increased levels of proinflammatory and anti-inflammatory cytokines, acute phase reactants, and clotting factors, is found in older adults.
- Age-related chronic inflammation contributes to dysregulation of innate immune responses, potentially limiting or delaying further activation or contributing to inappropriate persistence of inflammation.
- B- and T-cell signal transduction and function in the adaptive immune system are both impaired in the context of aging. Chronic antigen stimulation throughout life, particularly in the control of cycles of cytomegalovirus reactivation, substantially diminishes the diversity of antigen receptors, particularly in the T-cell lineage.

INTRODUCTION

With age, immunologic function changes substantially, resulting in impaired responses to pathogens or vaccines. As a result, older adults are at increased risk for morbidity and mortality from infectious diseases and impaired responses to vaccination.[1] Clearly, nonimmunologic factors also contribute to these adverse outcomes; for example, age-related changes in chest wall mechanics and lung elasticity may affect respiratory mechanics and medications may affect cough—all potential contributors to respiratory infection risk.[2] However, it is evident that immunologic changes influence host defense against infection. The aging immune system is characterized by a variety

The authors' work was supported by the National Institutes of Health (HHS N272201100019C, U19 AI089992, K24 AG042489, and T32 AI007517) and was carried out in collaboration with the Yale Claude D. Pepper Older Americans Independence Center (P30AG21342). The authors regret being unable to include many important articles due to space and scope limitations.
Section of Infectious Diseases, Department of Internal Medicine, Yale School of Medicine, New Haven, CT 06520, USA
* Corresponding author.
E-mail address: albert.shaw@yale.edu

of alterations that encompass developmental impairment, diminished signaling, and the effects of antigen exposure history on chronic inflammation and antigen receptor repertoire diversity—all of which contribute to defects in immune activation in response to pathogens or vaccines. However, the aged innate immune system also shows substantial inflammatory dysregulation with a paradoxical heightened proinflammatory environment; this may arise in part from endogenous stimuli linked to cellular damage. Here an overview of age-related changes in human host defense is provided, with an emphasis on consequences for outcomes to pathogens or vaccines in older adults.

CHANGES IN INNATE IMMUNITY WITH AGING

The innate immune system is the first line of defense in mounting a host resistance response to antigens; it is responsible for the earliest responses to pathogens or vaccines.[3,4] Innate immune responses are mediated by a network of cell types that include neutrophils, monocytes/macrophages, dendritic cells (DCs), natural killer (NK) cells, eosinophils, and basophils; endothelial and epithelial cells may also play roles in innate immunity.[4] Innate immune responses are closely linked to the activation of inflammatory processes, including phagocytosis, intracellular killing, pathogen-induced proinflammatory cytokine production, and upregulation of costimulatory proteins on antigen-presenting cells (APCs), such as DCs, monocytes, or macrophages. Such costimulatory protein expression provides additional signals facilitating T-cell activation and thus links innate to adaptive (ie, mediated by antigen receptors on B and T cells) immune responses.

Age-related Dysregulation of Inflammation

Several lines of evidence indicate that chronic inflammation is a characteristic of the aging immune system in humans. In particular, levels of proinflammatory cytokines (particularly interleukin-6 [IL]-6, also tumor necrosis factor -α [TNF-α], IL-1β, and others), acute phase reactants such as C-reactive protein, and clotting factors (including D-dimer) are generally elevated in older compared with young adults.[5–10] Moreover, such increases in cytokine production have been correlated with all-cause mortality in several studies.[11–13] Basal elevation of proinflammatory cytokines and other products may affect the ability of the aged immune system to respond to new pathogens or vaccines; in this regard, both proinflammatory and anti-inflammatory cytokine production may be augmented, resulting in more complex patterns of age-related inflammatory dysregulation.[14] The cause underlying this heightened proinflammatory state (termed Inflamm-Aging[15,16]) remains incompletely understood, but may in part reflect the consequences of cellular damage and endogenous activators of the innate immune system, as described in later discussion.

Neutrophils

Neutrophils are short-lived cells that are among the first to migrate in response to an infectious agent. For example, chemotaxis, describing movement toward a gradient of a stimulus (such as a chemokine or cytokine), appears impaired in neutrophils from older compared with young adults.[17–19] Moreover, phagocytosis of pathogens, such as *Streptococcus pneumoniae* as well as intracellular killing, both appeared impaired in neutrophils from older versus young individuals.[20,21] In addition, the generation of neutrophil extracellular traps (NETs), extracellular scaffolds of extruded chromatin containing antimicrobial peptides and proteases, is also diminished in neutrophils from older adults—further affecting pathogen capture and killing.[22] Several age-related signal transduction defects have been reported in neutrophils; for example, diminished accuracy of neutrophil migration with age has been linked to increased Phosphoinositide-3 kinase neutrophil signal transduction.[18] Other alterations may influence neutrophil survival by affecting antiapoptotic pathways mediated by granulocyte macrophage colony stimulating factor[23,24]; moreover, Toll-like receptor-1 (TLR1)-dependent cytokine production, induction of activation markers, and glucose utilization were all diminished in neutrophils from older compared with young adults.[25] Although most of these studies indicate that neutrophil function is diminished with age, it should also be noted that defects in chemotaxis, for example, may result in both impaired trafficking to sites of infection and inappropriate persistence of neutrophils during the resolution of inflammation. Indeed, such delayed neutrophil egress from the lungs has been found in a murine model of burn injury[26]; such persistence, even of neutrophils with impaired function, could contribute to a heightened proinflammatory milieu in the context of aging.

Monocytes

Monocytes also contribute to innate immune responses as a source for cytokine and chemokine production. They are particularly adept at migrating from the circulation to sites of infection and inflammation, whereby they differentiate into macrophages and also to DCs.[27] Studies of monocyte function in the context of human aging have revealed evidence for both impaired function, and in some cases, a dysregulated, enhanced proinflammatory response. For example, studies of TLR function, a family of invariant membrane-associated receptors recognizing conserved portions of pathogens (so-called pathogen-associated molecular patterns), reveal an age-associated decrease in IL-6 and TNF-α production following stimulation of the TLR1/2 heterodimer with triacylated bacterial lipoproteins.[28,29] In addition, a generalized impairment in expression of costimulatory proteins (such as CD80) was found in monocytes from older compared with young adults following in vitro stimulation with a variety of TLR agonists[30]; such costimulatory proteins interact with ligands found on the T-cell surface, and together with the T-cell receptor for antigen, facilitate optimal T-cell activation and link innate to adaptive immune responses. These alterations in TLR-induced costimulatory protein expression could be expected to adversely affect innate and adaptive immunity, and indeed a significant association was found between TLR-induced costimulatory protein expression and antibody response to influenza vaccination.[30]

Other studies of monocyte function in the context of aging reveal further evidence of age-related dysregulation of inflammatory responses. For example, monocytes partially activated following isolation by adherence to plastic in vitro showed an age-associated increase in TLR5-induced cytokine production, using the TLR5 ligand flagellin[31]; interestingly, an increase in TLR5-induced cytokine production was also found in macrophages from aged mice,[32] suggesting a potential role for monocyte activation in augmenting some innate immune responses (and the possibility that preserved TLR5 function could be used for vaccine adjuvants in older adults).

Several studies suggest that the proportion of so-called inflammatory monocytes expressing high levels of both CD14 and CD16 on the cell surface (as compared with classical monocytes, which are CD14 + CD16− and nonclassical CD14lo CD16hi monocytes) is increased in older adults. Such inflammatory monocytes have been reported to be increased in adults with human immunodeficiency virus, sepsis, myocardial infarction, and other conditions associated with increased inflammation[27]; CD14 + CD16 + monocytes from older adults showed evidence of senescence and increased cytokine production in response to lipopolysaccharide (LPS) stimulation of TLR4 ex vivo.[28,33–35] The effects of aging on monocyte function, however, may be more complex, because studies of cytokine production in monocytes (using intracellular cytokine staining) following influenza vaccination in the absence of *ex vivo* stimulation revealed diminished production of IL-6 and TNF-α in both inflammatory (which were induced after vaccination) and classical monocytes from older compared with young adults. By contrast, basal levels of the anti-inflammatory cytokine IL-10 were markedly elevated in monocyte populations in older, but not young adults; an age-associated alteration in activation of a negative regulator of IL-10, dual specificity phosphatase (DUSP)-1 suggested a potential basis for impaired cytokine responses following vaccination or exposure to pathogens.[36] Interestingly, some studies have used CD14 + CD16 + monocytes as an indicator of age-related inflammation and have demonstrated that resistance exercise training in older adults resulted in diminished levels of such monocytes and decreased LPS-induced proinflammatory cytokine production[37,38]; these findings suggest that some changes associated with age-related inflammation may be reversible.

Dendritic Cells

DCs are professional APCs that also undergo age-related changes contributing to impaired host resistance. These cells may be broadly divided into myeloid DCs (mDCs), which express a variety of TLRs and are critical for production of IL-12 in Th1 responses, and plasmacytoid DCs (pDCs), which express a more narrow range of TLRs (such as TLR7 and TLR9) and are particularly adept at producing type I interferons in response to viral infections. TLR-induced cytokine production (including proinflammatory cytokines such as TNF-α, IL-6, and IL-12 in mDCs and type I interferons in pDCs) in both mDCs and pDCs appears diminished in cells from older compared with young adults in response to *ex vivo* activation of a broad range of TLRs, and the extent of TLR-induced cytokine production was strongly correlated with influenza vaccine antibody response.[39] Several additional studies indicate that pDCs and monocyte-derived DCs (which may be generated in vitro using growth factor stimulation and likely resemble DCs generated under inflammatory conditions) are defective in type I interferon production in response to stimulation by viruses such as West Nile and influenza virus,[40,41] and indeed, gene expression microarray analyses of monocyte-derived DCs have revealed decreased expression of interferon-stimulated genes.[42] At the same time, there is evidence for inflammatory dysregulation in DC populations as well. For example, LPS or self DNA-induced cytokine production was increased in monocyte-derived DCs from older compared with young adults, juxtaposed with in vitro impairment in migration (as assessed in vitro using a chemotaxis assay).[42–44] In addition, basal elevation in cytokine production has been found in pDCs, mDCs, and monocyte-derived DCs from older, but not young adults in the absence of ex vivo stimulation.[39,45] The findings of impaired type I interferon production but increased TLR-induced cytokine production in monocyte-derived DCs may reflect differences in signal transduction pathways mediating proinflammatory cytokine versus interferon production; alternatively, innate immune signaling pathways in addition to TLRs were likely induced in these monocyte-derived DC studies, which used viral stimulation that would also engage cytoplasmic innate immune receptors recognizing viral nucleic acids, such as Retinoic Acid Inducible Gene-I (RIG-I), Melanoma Differentiation Associated Gene-5, and others. Nonetheless, taken together, these studies provide evidence that DCs may reflect the aging-associated proinflammatory environment.

Natural Killer Cells

NK cells are the predominant class of innate immune lymphocytes[46] and function in cytokine production (identified as CD56bright CD16− NK cells) and cytotoxicity, particularly of virus-infected or cancer cells (CD56dim CD16+ cells). Cytotoxicity functions are regulated by a balance between activating receptors and receptors such as the killer immunoglobulin-like receptors that are inhibited by major histocompatibility complex (MHC) class I engagement. In general, NK cells in older adults show an increase in the CD56dim CD16+ cytotoxic population, which also represents a more differentiated population compared with CD56bright NK cells.[47–52] Expression of activating cytotoxicity receptors is also diminished with age,[53,54] with diminished cytotoxic function in older adults that has been linked to decreased mobilization of perforin to the NK cell immunologic synapse.[55] The consequences of age-related NK cell dysfunction remain incompletely understood, but it is worth noting that NK function has been associated with infection risk in at least one study of nursing home residents.[56]

Origins of Age-related Inflammation

The cause of so-called Inflamm-Aging remains incompletely understood, but is likely to reflect a combination of factors, not all of which originate in the immune system. For example, hormonal changes in the context of aging likely contribute; the loss of estrogen and testosterone production with age is associated with increased inflammatory markers in humans.[57,58] In addition, there is decreased production of dihydroepiandrosterone in older adults, a corticosteroid with immune enhancing properties (such as promoting Th1 cytokine production and decreasing LPS-induced TNF-α production).[59] Cells other than those typically associated with the immune system may also contribute to age-related inflammation, and indeed, a recent study of gene expression contributors to the age-related increase in IL-6 found a relatively limited contribution of elevated cytokine transcripts from leukocytes.[60] In this regard, evidence from animal models suggests that macrophages infiltrating adipose tissue shift to a proinflammatory profile with age.[61] Moreover, small studies of human adipose tissue revealed an age-related accumulation of fat cell progenitors that may contribute to age-related inflammation,[62] particularly in the context of the so-called senescence-associated secretory phenotype (SASP).[63] The SASP refers to the secretome of senescent cells (induced by replicative senescence or DNA damage for example), and in adipocytes could be inhibited by treatment with Jun-activated kinase inhibitors.[62] Recent studies in model systems have also identified the mammalian target of rapamycin (mTOR, which has pleiotropic effects in regulating the balance between anabolic and catabolic metabolism[64]) as another modulator of the SASP, wherein mTOR inhibition with rapamycin (clinically used in higher doses for transplant immunosuppression) also inhibited SASP proinflammatory cytokine production.[65,66] mTOR inhibition using rapamycin (clinically used for transplant immunosuppression in higher doses) has previously been shown to extend lifespan in mice and ameliorate inflammation associated with cerebral ischemia or heart failure.[67–69] Notably, low-dose rapamycin given before influenza vaccination in older adults resulted in a 20% increase in antibody titers compared with older adults given placebo.[70] As a result, there is considerable interest in developing mTOR inhibitors that can modulate immunosenescence-associated inflammation.

In addition to the SASP, the origins of chronic inflammation in older adults could reflect the presence of endogenous damage-associated molecular patterns that activate innate immune pattern recognition receptors. For example, levels of non-cell-associated DNA, presumably released from damaged or dying cells, are elevated in older adults[71–73]; mitochondrial DNA (mtDNA) in particular is increased in older compared with young adults and correlates with increased levels of proinflammatory cytokines at baseline and in trauma patients.[74,75] Notably, human monocytes treated with mtDNA develop endotoxin tolerance, in which they are refractory to sub-sequent TLR4 stimulation with LPS—a potential mechanism contributing to impaired innate immune responses in the setting of chronic inflammation.[76] The mechanisms by which mtDNA activates the innate immune system likely involve TLR9 recognition of DNA; consistent with this, mtDNA-induced NET formation in human neutrophils (with impaired NET formation in older adults) was reduced with TLR9 inhibition.[74] Oxidized mtDNA generated in the context of mitochondrial dysfunction and apoptosis activates the NOD-like receptor NLRP3, a cytoplasmic innate immune pattern recognition receptor.[77] NLRP3 activation results in the formation of the NLRP3 inflam-masome, a multiprotein scaffold containing NLRP3 and the adaptor protein apoptosis-inducing specklike protein containing a CARD (Caspase Activation and Recruitment Domain) domain (ASC).[78] When assembled, the NLRP3 inflammasome mediates the caspase 1–dependent processing of pro-IL-18 and pro-IL-1β to their activated, cleaved forms. In addition to oxidized mtDNA, NLRP3 is also engaged by necrotic cell damage[79–81]; in fact, the wide range of endogenous (uric acid, extracel-lular ATP, oxidized mtDNA, ceramide, β-amyloid), exogenous (silica, asbestos, alum), and infectious (influenza virus, bacterial pore-forming toxins, fungi) NLRP3 activators suggests that this receptor could contribute substantially to age-related inflammatory dysregulation.[78] Indeed, studies in NLRP3-deficient mice revealed a decrease in age-associated inflammation and improvements in bone loss and cognitive function[82]; in addition, recent findings in mice indicate that ASC aggregates from activated inflam-masomes can be released from dying cells into the extracellular space, where they may be taken up by other cells to activate new inflammasomes and amplify a proin-flammatory stimulus.[83,84] Taken together, these findings suggest NLRP3 as a potential target for therapeutic intervention to modulate inflammation in older adults. Changes in the innate immune system with age are depicted in **Fig. 1**.

CHANGES IN THE ADAPTIVE IMMUNE SYSTEM WITH AGING

Activation of the innate immune system facilitates the T- and B-cell-mediated adaptive immune response through the production of proinflammatory cytokines and expres-sion of costimulatory proteins on monocyte/macrophages or DCs. Such costimulatory proteins (eg, CD80, CD86, and others) interact with ligands on T cells (such as CD28) to provide critical second signals for optimal T-cell activation, in conjunction with T-cell receptor (TCR) recognition of a peptide from a pathogen or vaccine bound to a major histocompatibility antigen protein on the APC cell surface. As previously dis-cussed, this innate immune activation is dysregulated and generally impaired with aging; however, the function of the adaptive immune system is also disrupted in older adults, reflecting the effects of chronic antigenic stimulation and exposures and intrinsic alterations in B- and T-cell development and function. Here, a brief update is provided, emphasizing recent findings regarding adaptive immunosenescence in humans.

T-Cell Aging

Bone marrow progenitor cells migrate to the thymus, where T-cell development, or thymopoiesis, occurs. Thymopoiesis is notable for stages of proliferative expansion, and for positive selection (where T cells expressing a TCR that can recognize host MHC proteins on APCs are selected) and negative selection (where T cells recognizing autoreactive, or "self" antigens are deleted) processes. The thymus begins to involute during childhood and continues to involute at a rate of approximately 3% per year in adults.[85] Not surprisingly, thymic involution is accompanied by a decline in generation

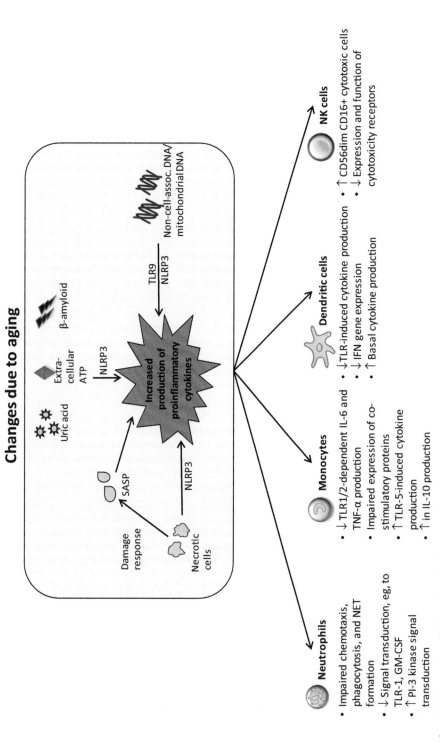

Fig. 1. Age-associated alterations in the innate immune system. Contributing factors to a heightened basal proinflammatory state and dysregulated responses in individual cell lineages are summarized. See text for details. GM-CSF, granulocyte macrophage colony stimulating factor; NLRP3, NOD-like receptor family, pyrin domain containing 3; NOD, nucleotide-binding oligomerization domain; PI-3, phosphoinositide-3.

of new (naïve) T cells. Although some studies have suggested that some degree of naïve T-cell generation continues in adulthood, one study using metabolic labeling and detection of T-cell receptor excision circles (the nonreplicating products of VDJ recombination at TCR loci that are associated with naïve T cells) has concluded that the vast majority (approximately 90% of CD4 T cells) of T cells in older adults are generated not from thymic activity but from division of cells in the existing T-lymphocyte pool.[86] Consequently, in older adults, most T cells appear to be antigen-experienced memory T cells. The effects of thymic involution on T-cell development were demonstrated in a study of young adults who had underwent thymectomy in the first month of life in the context of surgery for congenital heart disease. Numbers of CD4 and CD8 T cells were reduced in such adults, with diminished proportions of naïve T cells, compared with young adults who had not undergone thymectomy. Notably, a subset of young adults in the thymectomy group had T-cell parameters that were comparable to aged adults 75 years of age or older, including levels of nonmalignant oligoclonal T-cell expansions frequently found in older adults.[87] The occurrence of an aged T-cell profile in thymectomized young adults was strongly associated with seropositivity to cytomegalovirus (CMV), consistent with a substantial body of literature supporting the notion that control of CMV has a profound effect on the T-cell compartment in the context of aging.[88–92] CMV may reactivate throughout life without end-organ damage, such as in the setting of the stress of medical or surgical illness.[93] Notably, a recent study evaluating CMV seronegative and seropositive adults concluded that CMV appears to be the dominant factor in driving the increased proportion of effector memory T cells and likely also nonmalignant oligoclonal T-cell expansion seen in older adults.[94] Indeed, significant levels of CMV-specific, dysfunctional T cells can be detected in older adults,[91,95–98] and functional outcomes, such as mental status testing or ability to carry out activities of daily living, have been associated with CMV seropositivity or the presence of CMV-specific CD4 T cells.[99]

Analyses of TCR repertoire using high-throughput sequencing methods and peripheral blood mononuclear cells (PBMCs) as starting material revealed decreased diversity with age[100]; another analysis of purified naïve and memory T-cell populations revealed a more modest 3- to 5-fold decrease in diversity that may still be sufficient for adequate adaptive immune responses.[101] This last study was notable for analyzing multiple replicate libraries from purified T-cell subsets and used nonparametric statistical methods designed to address some of the challenges in measuring the immense potential range of T-cell diversity from relatively limited sample amounts.[102] It should be noted that CMV status of analyzed participants was unknown in the study showing a greater contraction in repertoire[100] and that CMV-seropositive subjects were excluded from the second study.[101] It seems likely that the effects of oligoclonal CMV-specific T cell expansion, if present, would result in substantial contraction in TCR diversity.

In addition to age-related decreases in T-cell generation, developmental and signaling alterations are found in cells from older adults, which contribute to functional deficits. For example, one of the most reliable age-related findings in the human T-cell compartment is the loss of CD28 expression on CD8 T cells.[103] CD28 interacts with cell-associated costimulatory protein ligands, such as CD80 and CD86, on APCs to provide a crucial second signal for T-cell activation (in conjunction with TCR recognition by peptide bound to host MHC proteins on APCs); the loss of CD28 expression in CD8 T cells is associated with alterations in T-cell activation in older individuals, and early studies indicated that reconstitution of CD28 expression in CD8+ CD28− human T cells restored IL-2 production.[104] In addition to loss of CD28, CD8 T cells express other markers of exhaustion, replicative senescence, or terminal differentiation in the context of aging (such as PD-1, CD57, or KLRG1) that limit the response to pathogens or vaccines.[105-107]

In contrast to aged mice, fewer studies have addressed signaling deficits in human T cells. However, in CD4 T cells from older compared with young adults, alterations in signaling have been found in naïve cells, whereby an increase in DUSP-6 protein expression was linked to a decline in expression of a specific micro-RNA (miR-181a)—resulting in decreased phosphorylation of the extracellular signal regulated kinase (ERK), a member of the mitogen activated protein (MAP) kinase family transducing TCR signals.[108] In memory CD4 T cells from older adults, increased gene expression of another MAP kinase phosphatase, DUSP4, also resulted in impaired ERK signaling.[109] In addition to alterations in signal transduction resulting in impaired TCR-dependent activation, recent studies have reported that the senescence phenotype (characterized by features such as inhibited telomerase expression and decreased proliferation and TCR signaling) in both CD8 effector memory and CD4 T cells (which lack CD28 expression) is strongly associated with aberrant signaling via the p38 MAP kinase; notably, p38 inhibition appeared to reverse the senescence phenotype.[110,111] Taken together, these findings provide evidence for both diminished activation (as in the ERK pathway) and inappropriate dysregulation (for p38) of signal transduction in T cells from older adults—mirroring the dysregulation and decreased responsiveness in the aged innate immune system.

B-Cell Aging

Like T cells, the B-cell lineage generates a highly diverse repertoire of rearranged antigen receptor genes, and there is evidence from analyses of complementarity determining region 3 in the immunoglobulin heavy chain variable region that diversity in bulk populations of B cells is substantially reduced with age and with changes in functional status such as the geriatric syndrome of frailty[112]; chronic infection with Epstein-Barr virus (which specifically infects B cells) or CMV influences B-cell repertoire, which may also be altered by the presence of nonmalignant oligoclonal B-cell expansion.[112,113] It should be noted, however, that some studies have shown relative preservation of diversity in tonsillar B cells.[114] Current use of next generation sequencing in purified B-cell populations has also revealed evidence for age-related repertoire changes, although as with studies of T cell repertoire, challenges remain in incorporating subject heterogeneity and variation into the analyses of the enormous amount of sequence information from studies of relatively few individuals.[115]

Mature B cells express a rearranged immunoglobulin antigen receptor on their cell surface and may undergo differentiation to plasma cells secreting immunoglobulin of the same specificity in defense against extracellular pathogens. Because many B-cell functions are dependent on T-cell help, the effects of aging on the B-cell lineage reflect both B-cell intrinsic changes and those resulting from altered T-B-cell interactions; an example of this would be impaired antibody response to influenza vaccine linked to impaired induction of antibody-producing plasmablasts.[116] However, intrinsic B-cell defects have been found in expression of activation-induced cytidine deaminase (AID), a protein that is essential for heavy chain class switching, in which the constant region exon (denoting the isotype and correlated with function, such as a μ constant region exon for IgM, γ1 constant region for immunoglobulin G1, and so on), encoding an expressed immunoglobulin heavy chain "switches" to a different exon, with deletion of the original exon and intervening DNA. AID is also required for another B-cell-specific process: somatic hypermutation, in which the variable region of an expressed immunoglobulin gene in mature B cells found in germinal centers of secondary lymphoid organs, such as lymph nodes, undergoes further mutation to enhance its affinity for a given antigen. The age-related impairment of AID expression was associated with a decreased proportion of B cells that had undergone class switching and with impaired influenza vaccine antibody responses.[117,118] Decreased AID expression was linked to decreased levels of the E47 transcription factor that regulates AID, and to upregulation in expression of specific microRNA species.[118,119] Notably, memory B cells from older adults were found to have increased gene expression of TNF-α, and the extent of basal TNF-α mRNA was negatively correlated with proliferative responses.[120] Finally, a history of CMV infection may also influence B-cell function; individuals with a positive CMV serology had increased intracellular levels of TNF-α in B cells and diminished AID gene expression and switched memory B-cell levels.[121] These findings in B cells reflect the dysregulated inflammatory responses found in cells of the innate immune system discussed above as well as the effects of CMV on T-cell function in older adults. A summary of age-associated alterations in B- and T-cell function is depicted in **Fig. 2**.

SYSTEMS ANALYSIS OF IMMUNE AGING

Several studies have used global analyses of cytokine production or gene expression to understand age-related alterations in immune response. In general, these studies have shown that immunologic challenge in older adults results in impaired responses when compared with young adults, but with evidence for dysregulated or delayed responses. Such a delayed and diminished gene expression signature of cytokine production in response to *in vitro* stimulation of TLR4, TLR7/8, and RIG-I (a cytoplasmic innate immune pattern recognition receptor RNA helicase that senses RNA, particularly in the setting of viral infection) was found in analyses of human PBMCs from older compared with young adults.[122] Transcriptomic analyses of PBMCs before and after influenza vaccination revealed altered kinetics for early induction of interferon-stimulated genes and for a day 7 postvaccine plasma cell gene expression

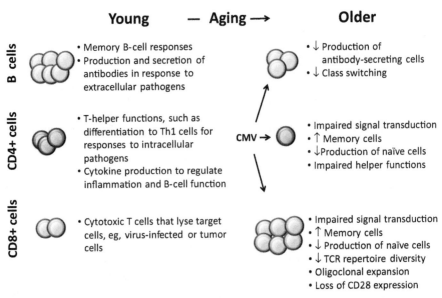

Young   — Aging →   Older

B cells
- Memory B-cell responses
- Production and secretion of antibodies in response to extracellular pathogens

- ↓ Production of antibody-secreting cells
- ↓ Class switching

CD4+ cells
- T-helper functions, such as differentiation to Th1 cells for responses to intracellular pathogens
- Cytokine production to regulate inflammation and B-cell function

CMV →

- Impaired signal transduction
- ↑ Memory cells
- ↓ Production of naïve cells
- Impaired helper functions

CD8+ cells
- Cytotoxic T cells that lyse target cells, eg, virus-infected or tumor cells

- Impaired signal transduction
- ↑ Memory cells
- ↓ Production of naïve cells
- ↓ TCR repertoire diversity
- Oligoclonal expansion
- Loss of CD28 expression

Fig. 2. Age-associated alterations in the adaptive immune system. Contrasts in function in B and T cells in young and older adults are summarized.

signature associated with a successful vaccine antibody response.[123] These studies also revealed age-related dysregulation of innate immune signaling pathways and a mitochondrial biogenesis gene expression signature that was associated with vaccine response in young and older adults, suggesting an intriguing link between metabolic activity and vaccine response. Other studies of influenza vaccination in older adults showed that prevaccine expression of apoptosis pathways was also correlated with vaccine response.[124] These studies have excluded neutrophils, which are not found in the PBMC compartment, but a recent study of neutrophil gene expression in patients with hemorrhagic shock revealed an impaired innate immune response in older compared with young adults.[125] Notably, older adults showed persistent gene expression signatures reflecting both inflammation and immunosuppressive states (such as impaired expression of antigen presentation or costimulatory proteins) at later time points when neutrophils from young adults had trended toward baseline—consistent with an emerging theme of impaired but dysregulated (and frequently delayed) response in the aged immune system.

FUTURE DIRECTIONS

Understanding the biology of altered immune response in the context of aging has obvious clinical impact, and future studies should incorporate the intrinsic heterogeneity in human cohorts (extending beyond gender and race to comorbid medical conditions, medication use, smoking, alcohol use, and other factors). In particular, the immunologic basis of alterations in functional status in older adults, such as frailty, remains incompletely understood. Examples of additional complexity include age-associated epigenetic effects, such as changes in methylation status, that strongly correlate with age and mortality.[126,127] Finally, studies of age-related changes in the intestinal microbiome are in early stages,[128] but it seems clear that engagement of innate and adaptive immunity by commensal organisms will influence immune responses to pathogens or vaccines. Integrating such complexity and heterogeneity into studies of the aging immune system will be challenging, particularly for large data sets arising from transcriptomic, microbiome, or other analyses, but will be essential to provide increasingly detailed insights for translation to pathways for therapeutic modulation and improvement of health in older adults.

REFERENCES

1. Yoshikawa TT. Epidemiology and unique aspects of aging and infectious diseases. Clin Infect Dis 2000;30:931–3.
2. Vaz Fragoso CA, Gill TM. Respiratory impairment and the aging lung: a novel paradigm for assessing pulmonary function. J Gerontol A Biol Sci Med Sci 2012;67:264–75.
3. Fulop T, Le Page A, Fortin C, et al. Cellular signaling in the aging immune system. Curr Opin Immunol 2014;29:105–11.
4. Shaw AC, Goldstein DR, Montgomery RR. Age-dependent dysregulation of innate immunity. Nat Rev Immunol 2013;13:875–87.
5. Bruunsgaard H, Andersen-Ranberg K, Jeune B, et al. A high plasma concentration of TNF-alpha is associated with dementia in centenarians. J Gerontol A Biol Sci Med Sci 1999;54:M357–64.
6. Fagiolo U, Cossarizza A, Scala E, et al. Increased cytokine production in mononuclear cells of healthy elderly people. Eur J Immunol 1993;23:2375–8.
7. Mari D, Mannucci PM, Coppola R, et al. Hypercoagulability in centenarians: the paradox of successful aging. Blood 1995;85:3144–9.

8. Paolisso G, Rizzo MR, Mazziotti G, et al. Advancing age and insulin resistance: role of plasma tumor necrosis factor-alpha. Am J Physiol 1998;275:E294–9.

9. Stowe RP, Peek MK, Cutchin MP, et al. Plasma cytokine levels in a population-based study: relation to age and ethnicity. J Gerontol A Biol Sci Med Sci 2010;65:429–33.

10. Wei J, Xu H, Davies JL, et al. Increase of plasma IL-6 concentration with age in healthy subjects. Life Sci 1992;51:1953–6.

11. Bruunsgaard H, Andersen-Ranberg K, Hjelmborg J, et al. Elevated levels of tumor necrosis factor alpha and mortality in centenarians. Am J Med 2003;115:278–83.

12. Harris TB, Ferrucci L, Tracy RP, et al. Associations of elevated interleukin-6 and C-reactive protein levels with mortality in the elderly. Am J Med 1999;106:506–12.

13. Reuben DB, Cheh AI, Harris TB, et al. Peripheral blood markers of inflammation predict mortality and functional decline in high-functioning community-dwelling older persons. J Am Geriatr Soc 2002;50:638–44.

14. Morrisette-Thomas V, Cohen AA, Fulop T, et al. Inflamm-aging does not simply reflect increases in pro-inflammatory markers. Mech Ageing Dev 2014;139:49–57.

15. Franceschi C, Bonafe M, Valensin S, et al. Inflamm-aging. An evolutionary perspective on immunosenescence. Ann N Y Acad Sci 2000;908:244–54.

16. Salvioli S, Monti D, Lanzarini C, et al. Immune system, cell senescence, aging and longevity–inflamm-aging reappraised. Curr Pharm Des 2013;19:1675–9.

17. Niwa Y, Kasama T, Miyachi Y, et al. Neutrophil chemotaxis, phagocytosis and parameters of reactive oxygen species in human aging: cross-sectional and longitudinal studies. Life Sci 1989;44:1655–64.

18. Sapey E, Greenwood H, Walton G, et al. Phosphoinositide 3-kinase inhibition restores neutrophil accuracy in the elderly: toward targeted treatments for immunosenescence. Blood 2014;123:239–48.

19. Wenisch C, Patruta S, Daxbock F, et al. Effect of age on human neutrophil function. J Leukoc Biol 2000;67:40–5.

20. Butcher SK, Chahal H, Nayak L, et al. Senescence in innate immune responses: reduced neutrophil phagocytic capacity and CD16 expression in elderly humans. J Leukoc Biol 2001;70:881–6.

21. Simell B, Vuorela A, Ekstrom N, et al. Aging reduces the functionality of anti-pneumococcal antibodies and the killing of streptococcus pneumoniae by neutrophil phagocytosis. Vaccine 2011;29:1929–34.

22. Hazeldine J, Harris P, Chapple IL, et al. Impaired neutrophil extracellular trap formation: a novel defect in the innate immune system of aged individuals. Aging Cell 2014;13:690–8.

23. Fortin CF, Larbi A, Dupuis G, et al. GM-CSF activates the JAK/STAT pathway to rescue polymorphonuclear neutrophils from spontaneous apoptosis in young but not elderly individuals. Biogerontology 2007;8:173–87.

24. Fortin CF, Larbi A, Lesur O, et al. Impairment of SHP-1 down-regulation in the lipid rafts of human neutrophils under GM-CSF stimulation contributes to their age-related, altered functions. J Leukoc Biol 2006;79:1061–72.

25. Qian F, Guo X, Wang X, et al. Reduced bioenergetics and Toll-like receptor 1 function in human polymorphonuclear leukocytes in aging. Aging (Albany NY) 2014;6:131–9.

26. Nomellini V, Brubaker AL, Mahbub S, et al. Dysregulation of neutrophil CXCR2 and pulmonary endothelial ICAM-1 promotes age-related pulmonary inflammation. Aging Dis 2012;3:234–47.

27. Wong KL, Yeap WH, Tai JJ, et al. The three human monocyte subsets: implications for health and disease. Immunol Res 2012;53:41–57.

28. Nyugen J, Agrawal S, Gollapudi S, et al. Impaired functions of peripheral blood monocyte subpopulations in aged humans. J Clin Immunol 2010;30:806–13.

29. van Duin D, Mohanty S, Thomas V, et al. Age-associated defect in human TLR-1/2 function. J Immunol 2007;178:970–5.

30. van Duin D, Allore HG, Mohanty S, et al. Prevaccine determination of the expression of costimulatory B7 molecules in activated monocytes predicts influenza vaccine responses in young and older adults. J Infect Dis 2007;195:1590–7.

31. Qian F, Wang X, Zhang L, et al. Age-associated elevation in TLR5 leads to increased inflammatory responses in the elderly. Aging Cell 2012;11:104–10.

32. Lim JS, Nguyen KC, Nguyen CT, et al. Flagellin-dependent TLR5/Caveolin-1 as a promising immune activator in immunosenescence. Aging Cell 2015;14:907–15.

33. Hearps AC, Martin GE, Angelovich TA, et al. Aging is associated with chronic innate immune activation and dysregulation of monocyte phenotype and function. Aging Cell 2012;11:867–75.

34. Merino A, Buendia P, Martin-Malo A, et al. Senescent CD14+CD16+ monocytes exhibit proinflammatory and proatherosclerotic activity. J Immunol 2011;186:1809–15.

35. Seidler S, Zimmermann HW, Bartneck M, et al. Age-dependent alterations of monocyte subsets and monocyte-related chemokine pathways in healthy adults. BMC Immunol 2010;11:30.

36. Mohanty S, Joshi SR, Ueda I, et al. Prolonged proinflammatory cytokine production in monocytes modulated by interleukin 10 after influenza vaccination in older adults. J Infect Dis 2015;211:1174–84.

37. Markofski MM, Flynn MG, Carrillo AE, et al. Resistance exercise training-induced decrease in circulating inflammatory CD14+CD16+ monocyte percentage without weight loss in older adults. Eur J Appl Physiol 2014;114:1737–48.

38. Timmerman KL, Flynn MG, Coen PM, et al. Exercise training-induced lowering of inflammatory (CD14+CD16+) monocytes: a role in the anti-inflammatory influence of exercise? J Leukoc Biol 2008;84:1271–8.

39. Panda A, Qian F, Mohanty S, et al. Age-associated decrease in TLR function in primary human dendritic cells predicts influenza vaccine response. J Immunol 2010;184:2518–27.

40. Prakash S, Agrawal S, Cao JN, et al. Impaired secretion of interferons by dendritic cells from aged subjects to influenza: role of histone modifications. Age (Dordr) 2013;35:1785–97.

41. Qian F, Wang X, Zhang L, et al. Impaired interferon signaling in dendritic cells from older donors infected in vitro with West Nile virus. J Infect Dis 2011;203:1415–24.

42. Cao JN, Agrawal A, Sharman E, et al. Alterations in gene array patterns in dendritic cells from aged humans. PLoS One 2014;9:e106471.

43. Agrawal A, Agrawal S, Cao JN, et al. Altered innate immune functioning of dendritic cells in elderly humans: a role of phosphoinositide 3-kinase-signaling pathway. J Immunol 2007;178:6912–22.

44. Agrawal A, Tay J, Ton S, et al. Increased reactivity of dendritic cells from aged subjects to self-antigen, the human DNA. J Immunol 2009;182:1138–45.

45. Prakash S, Agrawal S, Vahed H, et al. Dendritic cells from aged subjects contribute to chronic airway inflammation by activating bronchial epithelial cells under steady state. Mucosal Immunol 2014;7:1386–94.

46. Spits H, Artis D, Colonna M, et al. Innate lymphoid cells–a proposal for uniform nomenclature. Nat Rev Immunol 2013;13:145–9.

47. Campos C, Pera A, Lopez-Fernandez I, et al. Proinflammatory status influences NK cells subsets in the elderly. Immunol Lett 2014;162:298–302.

48. Campos C, Pera A, Sanchez-Correa B, et al. Effect of age and CMV on NK cell subpopulations. Exp Gerontol 2014;54:130–7.
49. Borrego F, Alonso MC, Galiani MD, et al. NK phenotypic markers and IL2 response in NK cells from elderly people. Exp Gerontol 1999;34:253–65.
50. Chidrawar SM, Khan N, Chan YL, et al. Ageing is associated with a decline in peripheral blood CD56bright NK cells. Immun Ageing 2006;3:10.
51. Hayhoe RP, Henson SM, Akbar AN, et al. Variation of human natural killer cell phenotypes with age: identification of a unique KLRG1-negative subset. Hum Immunol 2010;71:676–81.
52. Le Garff-Tavernier M, Beziat V, Decocq J, et al. Human NK cells display major phenotypic and functional changes over the life span. Aging Cell 2010;9: 527–35.
53. Solana R, Campos C, Pera A, et al. Shaping of NK cell subsets by aging. Curr Opin Immunol 2014;29:56–61.
54. Solana R, Tarazona R, Gayoso I, et al. Innate immunosenescence: effect of aging on cells and receptors of the innate immune system in humans. Semin Immunol 2012;24:331–41.
55. Hazeldine J, Hampson P, Lord JM. Reduced release and binding of perforin at the immunological synapse underlies the age-related decline in natural killer cell cytotoxicity. Aging Cell 2012;11:751–9.
56. Ogata K, An E, Shioi Y, et al. Association between natural killer cell activity and infection in immunologically normal elderly people. Clin Exp Immunol 2001;124: 392–7.
57. Abu-Taha M, Rius C, Hermenegildo C, et al. Menopause and ovariectomy cause a low grade of systemic inflammation that may be prevented by chronic treatment with low doses of estrogen or losartan. J Immunol 2009;183:1393–402.
58. Maggio M, Basaria S, Ble A, et al. Correlation between testosterone and the inflammatory marker soluble interleukin-6 receptor in older men. J Clin Endocrinol Metab 2006;91:345–7.
59. Hazeldine J, Arlt W, Lord JM. Dehydroepiandrosterone as a regulator of immune cell function. J Steroid Biochem Mol Biol 2010;120(2–3):127–36.
60. Pilling LC, Joehanes R, Melzer D, et al. Gene expression markers of age-related inflammation in two human cohorts. Exp Gerontol 2015;70:37–45.
61. Lumeng CN, Liu J, Geletka L, et al. Aging is associated with an increase in T cells and inflammatory macrophages in visceral adipose tissue. J Immunol 2011;187:6208–16.
62. Xu M, Tchkonia T, Ding H, et al. JAK inhibition alleviates the cellular senescence-associated secretory phenotype and frailty in old age. Proc Natl Acad Sci U S A 2015;112:E6301–10.
63. Tchkonia T, Zhu Y, van Deursen J, et al. Cellular senescence and the senescent secretory phenotype: therapeutic opportunities. J Clin Invest 2013;123:966–72.
64. Johnson SC, Rabinovitch PS, Kaeberlein M. mTOR is a key modulator of ageing and age-related disease. Nature 2013;493:338–45.
65. Herranz N, Gallage S, Mellone M, et al. mTOR regulates MAPKAPK2 translation to control the senescence-associated secretory phenotype. Nat Cell Biol 2015; 17:1205–17.
66. Laberge RM, Sun Y, Orjalo AV, et al. mTOR regulates the pro-tumorigenic senescence-associated secretory phenotype by promoting IL1a translation. Nat Cell Biol 2015;17:1049–61.
67. Flynn JM, O'Leary MN, Zambataro CA, et al. Late-life rapamycin treatment reverses age-related heart dysfunction. Aging Cell 2013;12:851–62.

68. Harrison DE, Strong R, Sharp ZD, et al. Rapamycin fed late in life extends life-span in genetically heterogeneous mice. Nature 2009;460:392–5.
69. Xie L, Sun F, Wang J, et al. mTOr signaling inhibition modulates macrophage/microglia-mediated neuroinflammation and secondary injury via regulatory T cells after focal ischemia. J Immunol 2014;192:6009–19.
70. Mannick JB, Del Giudice G, Lattanzi M, et al. mTOR inhibition improves immune function in the elderly. Sci Transl Med 2014;6:268ra179.
71. Jylhava J, Jylha M, Lehtimaki T, et al. Circulating cell-free DNA is associated with mortality and inflammatory markers in nonagenarians: the vitality 90+ study. Exp Gerontol 2012;47:372–8.
72. Jylhava J, Kotipelto T, Raitala A, et al. Aging is associated with quantitative and qualitative changes in circulating cell-free DNA: the vitality 90+ study. Mech Ageing Dev 2011;132:20–6.
73. Jylhava J, Nevalainen T, Marttila S, et al. Characterization of the role of distinct plasma cell-free DNA species in age-associated inflammation and frailty. Aging Cell 2013;12:388–97.
74. Itagaki K, Kaczmarek E, Lee YT, et al. Mitochondrial DNA released by trauma induces neutrophil extracellular traps. PLoS One 2015;10:e0120549.
75. Pinti M, Cevenini E, Nasi M, et al. Circulating mitochondrial DNA increases with age and is a familiar trait: implications for "inflamm-aging". Eur J Immunol 2014;44:1552–62.
76. Fernandez-Ruiz I, Arnalich F, Cubillos-Zapata C, et al. Mitochondrial DAMPS induce endotoxin tolerance in human monocytes: an observation in patients with myocardial infarction. PLoS One 2014;9:e95073.
77. Shimada K, Crother TR, Karlin J, et al. Oxidized mitochondrial DNA activates the NLRP3 inflammasome during apoptosis. Immunity 2012;36:401–14.
78. Elliott EI, Sutterwala FS. Initiation and perpetuation of nlrp3 inflammasome activation and assembly. Immunol Rev 2015;265:35–52.
79. Imaeda AB, Watanabe A, Sohail MA, et al. Acetaminophen-induced hepatotoxicity in mice is dependent on TLR9 and the NALP3 inflammasome. J Clin Invest 2009;119:305–14.
80. Iyer SS, Pulskens WP, Sadler JJ, et al. Necrotic cells trigger a sterile inflammatory response through the NLRP3 inflammasome. Proc Natl Acad Sci U S A 2009;106:20388–93.
81. Li H, Ambade A, Re F. Cutting edge: necrosis activates the NLRP3 inflammasome. J Immunol 2009;183:1528–32.
82. Youm YH, Grant RW, McCabe LR, et al. Canonical NLRP3 inflammasome links systemic low-grade inflammation to functional decline in aging. Cell Metab 2013;18:519–32.
83. Baroja-Mazo A, Martin-Sanchez F, Gomez AI, et al. The NLRP3 inflammasome is released as a particulate danger signal that amplifies the inflammatory response. Nat Immunol 2014;15:738–48.
84. Franklin BS, Bossaller L, De Nardo D, et al. The adaptor ASC has extracellular and 'prionoid' activities that propagate inflammation. Nat Immunol 2014;15:727–37.
85. Palmer DB. The effect of age on thymic function. Front Immunol 2013;4:316.
86. den Braber I, Mugwagwa T, Vrisekoop N, et al. Maintenance of peripheral naive T cells is sustained by thymus output in mice but not humans. Immunity 2012;36:288–97.
87. Sauce D, Larsen M, Fastenackels S, et al. Evidence of premature immune aging in patients thymectomized during early childhood. J Clin Invest 2009;119:3070–8.

88. Chidrawar S, Khan N, Wei W, et al. Cytomegalovirus-seropositivity has a profound influence on the magnitude of major lymphoid subsets within healthy individuals. Clin Exp Immunol 2009;155:423–32.
89. Litjens NH, de Wit EA, Betjes MG. Differential effects of age, cytomegalovirus-seropositivity and end-stage renal disease (ESRD) on circulating T lymphocyte subsets. Immun Ageing 2011;8:2.
90. Looney RJ, Falsey A, Campbell D, et al. Role of cytomegalovirus in the T cell changes seen in elderly individuals. Clin Immunol 1999;90:213–9.
91. Ouyang Q, Wagner WM, Voehringer D, et al. Age-associated accumulation of CMV-specific CD8+ T cells expressing the inhibitory killer cell lectin-like receptor g1 (KLRG1). Exp Gerontol 2003;38:911–20.
92. Wikby A, Johansson B, Olsson J, et al. Expansions of peripheral blood CD8 T-lymphocyte subpopulations and an association with cytomegalovirus seropositivity in the elderly: the Swedish NONA immune study. Exp Gerontol 2002;37:445–53.
93. Limaye AP, Kirby KA, Rubenfeld GD, et al. Cytomegalovirus reactivation in critically ill immunocompetent patients. JAMA 2008;300:413–22.
94. Wertheimer AM, Bennett MS, Park B, et al. Aging and cytomegalovirus infection differentially and jointly affect distinct circulating T cell subsets in humans. J Immunol 2014;192:2143–55.
95. Hadrup SR, Strindhall J, Kollgaard T, et al. Longitudinal studies of clonally expanded CD8 T cells reveal a repertoire shrinkage predicting mortality and an increased number of dysfunctional cytomegalovirus-specific T cells in the very elderly. J Immunol 2006;176:2645–53.
96. Khan N, Shariff N, Cobbold M, et al. Cytomegalovirus seropositivity drives the CD8 T cell repertoire toward greater clonality in healthy elderly individuals. J Immunol 2002;169:1984–92.
97. Ouyang Q, Wagner WM, Wikby A, et al. Large numbers of dysfunctional CD8+ T lymphocytes bearing receptors for a single dominant CMV epitope in the very old. J Clin Immunol 2003;23:247–57.
98. Ouyang Q, Wagner WM, Zheng W, et al. Dysfunctional CMV-specific CD8(+) T cells accumulate in the elderly. Exp Gerontol 2004;39:607–13.
99. Vescovini R, Biasini C, Telera AR, et al. Intense antiextracellular adaptive immune response to human cytomegalovirus in very old subjects with impaired health and cognitive and functional status. J Immunol 2010;184:3242–9.
100. Britanova OV, Putintseva EV, Shugay M, et al. Age-related decrease in TCR repertoire diversity measured with deep and normalized sequence profiling. J Immunol 2014;192:2689–98.
101. Qi Q, Liu Y, Cheng Y, et al. Diversity and clonal selection in the human T-cell repertoire. Proc Natl Acad Sci U S A 2014;111:13139–44.
102. Laydon DJ, Bangham CR, Asquith B. Estimating T-cell repertoire diversity: limitations of classical estimators and a new approach. Phil Trans R Soc B 2015;370:20140291.
103. Weng NP, Akbar AN, Goronzy J. CD28(-) T cells: their role in the age-associated decline of immune function. Trends Immunol 2009;30:306–12.
104. Topp MS, Riddell SR, Akatsuka Y, et al. Restoration of CD28 expression in CD28- CD8+ memory effector T cells reconstitutes antigen-induced IL-2 production. J Exp Med 2003;198:947–55.
105. Chou JP, Effros RB. T cell replicative senescence in human aging. Curr Pharm Des 2013;19:1680–98.

106. Dolfi DV, Mansfield KD, Polley AM, et al. Increased T-Bet is associated with senescence of influenza virus-specific CD8 T cells in aged humans. J Leukoc Biol 2013;93:825–36.

107. Henson SM, Akbar AN. KLRG1–more than a marker for T cell senescence. Age (Dordr) 2009;31:285–91.

108. Li G, Yu M, Lee WW, et al. Decline in miR-181a expression with age impairs T cell receptor sensitivity by increasing DUSP6 activity. Nat Med 2012;18: 1518–24.

109. Yu M, Li G, Lee WW, et al. Signal inhibition by the dual-specific phosphatase 4 impairs T cell-dependent B-cell responses with age. Proc Natl Acad Sci U S A 2012;109:E879–88.

110. Henson SM, Lanna A, Riddell NE, et al. P38 signaling inhibits mTORC1-independent autophagy in senescent human CD8(+) T cells. J Clin Invest 2014;124:4004–16.

111. Lanna A, Henson SM, Escors D, et al. The kinase p38 activated by the metabolic regulator AMPK and scaffold TAB1 drives the senescence of human T cells. Nat Immunol 2014;15:965–72.

112. Gibson KL, Wu YC, Barnett Y, et al. B-cell diversity decreases in old age and is correlated with poor health status. Aging Cell 2009;8:18–25.

113. Wang C, Liu Y, Xu LT, et al. Effects of aging, cytomegalovirus infection, and EBV infection on human B cell repertoires. J Immunol 2014;192:603–11.

114. Kolar GR, Mehta D, Wilson PC, et al. Diversity of the Ig repertoire is maintained with age in spite of reduced germinal centre cells in human tonsil lymphoid tissue. Scand J Immunol 2006;64:314–24.

115. Martin V, Bryan Wu YC, Kipling D, et al. Ageing of the B-cell repertoire. Phil Trans R Soc B 2015;370:20140237.

116. Sasaki S, Sullivan M, Narvaez CF, et al. Limited efficacy of inactivated influenza vaccine in elderly individuals is associated with decreased production of vaccine-specific antibodies. J Clin Invest 2011;121:3109–19.

117. Frasca D, Diaz A, Romero M, et al. Intrinsic defects in B cell response to seasonal influenza vaccination in elderly humans. Vaccine 2010;28:8077–84.

118. Frasca D, Landin AM, Lechner SC, et al. Aging down-regulates the transcription factor E2A, activation-induced cytidine deaminase, and Ig class switch in human B cells. J Immunol 2008;180:5283–90.

119. Frasca D, Diaz A, Romero M, et al. MicroRNAs miR-155 and miR-16 decrease AID and E47 in B cells from elderly individuals. J Immunol 2015;195:2134–40.

120. Frasca D, Diaz A, Romero M, et al. High TNF-alpha levels in resting B cells negatively correlate with their response. Exp Gerontol 2014;54:116–22.

121. Frasca D, Diaz A, Romero M, et al. Cytomegalovirus (CMV) seropositivity decreases B cell responses to the influenza vaccine. Vaccine 2015;33:1433–9.

122. Metcalf TU, Cubas RA, Ghneim K, et al. Global analyses revealed age-related alterations in innate immune responses after stimulation of pathogen recognition receptors. Aging Cell 2015;14:421–32.

123. Thakar J, Mohanty S, West AP, et al. Aging-dependent alterations in gene expression and a mitochondrial signature of responsiveness to human influenza vaccination. Aging (Albany NY) 2015;7:38–52.

124. Furman D, Jojic V, Kidd B, et al. Apoptosis and other immune biomarkers predict influenza vaccine responsiveness. Mol Syst Biol 2013;9:659.

125. Vanzant EL, Hilton RE, Lopez CM, et al. Advanced age is associated with worsened outcomes and a unique genomic response in severely injured patients with hemorrhagic shock. Crit Care 2015;19:77.

126. Jung M, Pfeifer GP. Aging and DNA methylation. BMC Biol 2015;13:7.
127. Marioni RE, Shah S, McRae AF, et al. DNA methylation age of blood predicts all-cause mortality in later life. Genome Biol 2015;16:25.
128. Zapata HJ, Quagliarello VJ. The microbiota and microbiome in aging: potential implications in health and age-related diseases. J Am Geriatr Soc 2015;63: 776–81.

Clinical Features of Infection in Older Adults

Dean C. Norman, MD

KEYWORDS

- Infectious diseases • Clinical Presentation • Fever

KEY POINTS

- The impact of infectious diseases is far greater on older persons than younger adults.
- Diagnostic delays may result from frequent nonclassical presentation of infectious disease in older adults.
- Fever, the cardinal sign of infection, may be blunted or absent in the aged.
- The absence of a robust fever in response to infection may impact host defenses.

OVERVIEW

The impact of infectious diseases on older adults is far greater than on younger adults because of significantly higher morbidities and mortalities caused by infection. The reasons for this greater impact include factors such as lower physiologic reserve due to age and chronic disease, age-related changes in host defenses, loss of mobility, higher risk for polypharmacy and adverse drug reactions, and being on drugs that increase risk for infection (eg, anticholinergic and other sedating medications increase the risk for pneumonia). Other factors contributing to disparate impact of infections on this age group include greater risk for hospitalization and therefore exposure to more virulent and difficult-to-treat nosocomial pathogens, undergoing invasive procedures, and receiving implants, all of which increase the risk of infection.

Unfortunately, failure to promptly diagnose a serious bacterial or viral infection in older patients increases the risk of complications and death. Clinicians should be aware that diagnostic delays may occur with infected older persons because infections may present in a nonclassical manner, and therefore, clinicians should be familiar with the various nonclassical manifestations of infections in this age group.

To help minimize risk of diagnostic delays, clinicians should first be aware that the types of infections encountered in the growing elderly population depend on both the clinical setting and the patient's functional status. Independent healthy older persons are more likely to develop respiratory infections, such as influenza and bacterial

Department of Medicine, UCLA David Geffen School of Medicine, 10833 Le Conte Avenue, Los Angeles, CA 90095, USA
E-mail address: dnorman630@aol.com

Clin Geriatr Med 32 (2016) 433–441
http://dx.doi.org/10.1016/j.cger.2016.02.005
0749-0690/16/$ – see front matter © 2016 Elsevier Inc. All rights reserved.

geriatric.theclinics.com

pneumonia, urinary tract infections not associated with indwelling bladder catheters, and intra-abdominal infections, such as cholecystitis and diverticulitis.

Pneumonia is the leading infection requiring transfer to an acute care hospital from a long-term care facility (LTCF). Infected institution-bound older persons are more likely to have pneumonia due to aspiration especially if they are receiving sedating medication or if neurovascular disease interfering with swallowing is present. Urinary tract infections are very common in long-term care residents, and the presence of a catheter, even a condom catheter, increases the risk of symptomatic and asymptomatic infection. Skin and soft tissue infections and, increasingly, gastrointestinal infections also occur frequently in residents of LTCFs.

In the acute care setting, hospitalized older persons are exposed to nosocomial pathogens, and nosocomial pneumonia risk per day of hospitalization is higher in this population than in the young. Intravenous catheter–associated bacteremia and sepsis as well as urosepsis from indwelling bladder catheters occur far too frequently in frail hospitalized elderly patients. Finally, clinicians should be aware that not all fevers encountered in acute care are due to infection. Common noninfectious causes of fever encountered in older persons in the acute care setting include acute myocardial infarction, cerebrovascular accident or hemorrhage, and drug fever.

Another important difference between infections occurring in the elderly and the young is that infectious diseases in the older age group are caused by a wider variety of pathogens compared with young adults. Thus, urinary tract infection in the elderly is more likely to be complicated and occur in men as well as women, and *Escherichia coli* is only one of several possible pathogens compared with the young, whereby most infections are cystitis, occur almost exclusively in women, and are overwhelmingly due to *E coli*. Thus, in contrast to the recommendations for treating routine cystitis in a young adult woman, a urine culture before initiating empiric antimicrobial therapy for symptomatic urinary tract infection in older adults is strongly recommended (see Nicolle LE: Urinary Tract Infections in the Older Adult, in this issue). Similarly, the pathogens responsible for most cases of community-acquired pneumonia (CAP) in the young adult include *Streptococcus pneumoniae*, *Mycoplasma pneumoniae*, and *Chlamydia pneumoniae*, while most cases of CAP in older persons are due to *S pneumoniae* with gram-negative bacilli causing a small but significant percentage of cases. Also a variety of other pathogens such as *Haemophilus influenzae* are possible[1–3] (see Marrie TJ: Bacterial Pneumonia in Older Adults, in this issue). Moreover, there are substantive differences between CAP and nursing home–acquired pneumonia (NHAP) pathogens.[4] Finally, meningitis in older adults is rarely due to viral infection, and most cases are caused by *S pneumoniae* and to a lesser extent by *Listeria monocytogenes*. Less commonly, other pathogens, such as gram-negative bacilli from bacteremia from a primary source or staphylococci introduced by surgery or trauma, cause meningitis in the elderly. In contrast, in young adults, *S pneumoniae* is less dominant and *Neisseria meningitidis* is a more important meningitis pathogen.[5]

PRESENTATION OF INFECTIOUS DISEASES IN OLD AGE

The nonclassical presentations of infection commonly observed in older adults occur especially in frail elderly and those with cognitive impairment. Acute changes in cognition, such as new onset confusion, lethargy and agitation, and other behavioral changes may be symptoms of infection. Similarly, falls and urinary and fecal incontinence may be the sole symptoms of infection at initial presentation. It is important to remember that serious bacterial and viral infections in older adults may not result in fever or other signs of inflammation. Bacteremia may also be afebrile and, like pneumonia, tachypnea or altered mental status may be the sole sign of infection. Thus, it is not surprising that in a recent large study of bacteremia, the oldest age groups much more often presented atypically (eg, reduced consciousness) than the younger patients.[6]

Older patients with pneumonia may not present with cough, chest discomfort, or sputum production. When 2569 hospitalized CAP patients versus 518 hospitalized NHAP patients were studied in a large German prospective multicenter study, it was determined that NHAP patients were more likely to present to the hospital without cough or purulent sputum production but were more likely to present with tachypnea and hypotension. More importantly, NHAP patients were far more likely to present with confusion compared with elderly CAP patients (49% vs 15%).[7]

Other examples of infection specific to nonclassical presentations in the older adult include meningitis, whereby diagnosis may be confounded by lack of stiff neck or the presence of severe cervical spine osteoarthritis. Another example is intra-abdominal infection, which may be present despite the absence of peritoneal findings. Before the widespread use of abdominal computed tomography, appendicitis had much higher morbidity and mortality compared with the young because the older appendix was often perforated by the time of surgery because of diagnostic delays from atypical presentation. Common nonclassical presentations of various intra-abdominal emergencies such as acute cholecystitis and appendicitis have been extensively reviewed.[8] Finally, symptomatic urinary tract infection may present without the classical symptoms of dysuria, urgency, and frequency, and flank tenderness may not be present even with upper tract infection.

Another important point to consider is that the presentation of infection or for that matter any acute illness in the elderly may not be proportional to the severity of the infection or illness. For example, one classic study demonstrated that pyelonephritis in elderly women despite presenting in a similar fashion to that of younger women resulted in bacteremia in half of the elderly patients versus none of the young.[9] In summary, any acute change in functional status in an older patient may herald the onset of an acute illness, and infection should be at the top or close to the top of any differential diagnosis in these cases (**Box 1**). There may be dissociation between the severity of symptoms and signs and the true severity of the acute illness.

SIGNIFICANCE OF BLUNTED FEBRILE RESPONSE IN OLDER PERSONS

Fever is the cardinal sign of infection, but its absence in older persons is common and may result in potentially damaging diagnostic delays. However, studies of bacteremia,[6,9,10] pneumonia,[7,11–14] endocarditis,[15–18] noscocomial febrile illness,[19] meningitis,[20] and intra-abdominal infection[8,21] demonstrate that a blunted fever response may be observed in up to one-third of infected elderly patients. In one study mentioned earlier, only 56% of CAP or NHAP patients presenting to an acute care hospital had a fever,[7] and another study of 320 patients hospitalized for infection ranging in age from 18 to 97 years found the average temperature on the first 3 days of infection to be lower by 0.15°C for each decade.[14]

Unfortunately, a blunted or absent febrile response to infection may have other negative implications besides interfering with timely diagnosis. There is evidence presented in the classic review of several hundred cases of bacteremia and fungemia by Weinstein and colleagues[22] that the more robust the fever response, the better chance for survival. Also, a prospective study of surgical patients with bloodstream infections demonstrated that those that achieved a robust fever defined as greater than or equal to 38.5°C had a mortality of 12.9% versus 27.7% for those that did not achieve this

---

Box 1
Nonclassical presentations of infection

Any infection

Change in cognition: (eg, confusion/agitation/lethargy)

Falls

Incontinence

Anorexia

"Failure to thrive"

Specific infection

Bacteremia
  May be afebrile
  Dyspnea, confusion, falls, hypotension, tachypnea

Pneumonia
  May be afebrile
  Cough, sputum production, and pleuritic chest pain may be absent

Intra-abdominal infection
  Peritoneal signs may be absent
  Anorexia

Meningitis
  Stiff neck may be absent
  Confusion, altered consciousness

Tuberculosis
  Weight loss, lethargy
  Failure to thrive

---

temperature. Moreover, the mean age of the febrile patients was significantly lower than the others, but older age was only slightly associated with increased risk of mortality.[23] These and other studies suggest that, for any age, the lack of a fever response to a serious infection may portend a poor prognosis. However, although fever may be in of itself an important host defense for certain species, the question of whether fever is an important host defense mechanism in humans remains controversial.

The best evidence that fever is an important adaptive host defense mechanism comes from animal models. The most compelling evidence is from experiments that showed infected poikilothermic (cold-blooded) animals migrate to warmer environments in order to raise body temperatures; this behavior improves survival. Two classic experiments confirmed the benefit of fever in of lizards and goldfish.[24,25] Desert iguana (*Dipsosaurus dorsalis*) and goldfish (*Carassius auratus*) were placed in terrariums and aquariums, respectively, which were kept at different temperatures. The body temperatures of these poikilothermic animals equilibrated with the environmental temperature of the terrarium or aquarium in which they were housed. Subsequently, the animals were infected: it turned out that those kept in the higher-temperature environments (thus higher body temperatures) had a much better chance of survival than those animals kept at lower temperatures. This effect was independent of any effect of temperature on the pathogen. Based on these and other animal data, including additional data generated from mammalian experiments, fever may be an important host defense mechanism in humans. The mechanisms by which fever may enhance host defenses in humans are not due to a direct effect on pathogens by physiologically achievable temperature elevations with few exceptions. *Treponema pallidum, N gonnorheae*, and certain strains of *S pneumoniae* growth may be inhibited at the upper limits of a normal febrile response to infection. Experimental data suggest that normal physiologically achievable elevations in body temperature may enhance immunity by enhancing production and activity of various cytokines (eg, interferon, interleukin-1, tumor necrosis factor-α) that in turn facilitate or enhance protective immune responses.

In order to determine the reasons for the observed blunted febrile response in older patients, it is necessary to understand the pathogenesis of fever. The current knowledge of the pathogenesis and clinical aspects of fever has been recently reviewed.[26,27] Although exogenous pyrogens including bacterial cell products such as endotoxin may cause fever independently from endogenous pyrogens (now referred to as pyrogenic cytokines), bacterial cell wall products such as endotoxin (lipopolysaccharide or LPS) are now known to bind to pattern recognition receptors known as Toll-like receptors (TLR) on macrophages and dendritic cells. TLR4 is the receptor that binds to LPS. TLR are a key host defense because stimulated TLR initiate the innate immune response to infection and are essential also for initiating the adaptive immune response. TLR signaling induces the inflammatory response, including the production of pyrogenic cytokines, such as tumor necrosis factor, interleukin-1, interleukin-6, interferon, and other cytokines. Exogenous pyrogens such as LPS and pyrogenic cytokines exert their effect by production of prostaglandin E2 in the periphery or by acting directly on the endothelium of the circumventricular organs of the preoptic area of the hypothalamus to initiate a complex biochemical cascade, including the central nervous system production of prostaglandin E2. Of note, some pyrogenic cytokines and LPS are able to affect the febrile response by directly acting on the brain, independent of prostaglandin E2 production. In any event, the resulting effect is an elevation of the "hypothalamic thermostat," that in turn results in shivering, vasoconstriction, and certain behavioral responses (eg, wrapping oneself in a blanket) to elevate core body temperature. When the infection subsides, the "thermostat" is reset to baseline; sweating and temperature-lowering behavior ensue, and normal temperature is restored. Aging in theory can affect any of the steps in these fever pathways. Aging appears to diminish TLR function, and it has been established that with aging there is diminished cytokine production. Reduced cytokine production in response to TLR stimulation has clinical consequences, including predicting failure to mount a protective antibody response to influenza vaccination.[28] Moreover, experiments in animal models of aging determined that an impaired fever response to endogenous pyrogens with normal aging[29-31] as well as diminished production of pyrogenic cytokines with age was a possible explanation for the reduced febrile response in aging humans.[28,32] Evidence from a mouse model presented evidence the aging brain may produce less prostaglandin E2 in response to direct exposure to LPS, suggesting another mechanism for reduced fever response with aging[33]; however, this was not found to be the case in aging rats. Evidence from another animal model suggests that the aging brain may respond normally to directly injected prostaglandin E2, implying that there may be a defect in pyrogenic cytokine initiation of prostaglandin synthesis in the brain.[34] Similarly, direct injection of interleukin-1 into the brain induced identical fever responses in old and young rodents, indicating blunted fever to infection in old rodents may be due in part to decreased pyrogenic cytokine production or the failure of pyrogenic cytokines produced in the periphery to reach the central nervous system.[35] Even if the biochemical cascade initiated by LPS or pyrogenic cytokines indirectly or directly in the brain did not change significantly with age, age-related changes in behavior, inability to initiate vasoconstriction and shivering, and changes in body fat with age may also play a role in the blunted febrile response.

BASELINE TEMPERATURE, SIGNIFICANCE OF FEVER, AND FEVER OF UNKNOWN ORIGIN

There are inherent inaccuracies in measuring temperature in individuals, and this is particularly true for older adults. Oral temperatures are affected by mouth breathing, patterns of respiration, ingestion of hot and cold liquids, and foods or smoking shortly before or during measurement. Other methods including tympanic membrane thermometers, disposable thermometers, and others that measure temporal artery or skin temperature hold promise, but it is not clear whether these newer methods are more accurate than traditional oral thermometry. Axillary temperatures are unreliable, and the much more accurate rectal temperatures are often impractical in debilitated, poorly cooperative patients. Diurnal temperature variation may also make temperature measurement results time dependent.

Nonetheless, for practical purposes, it can be assumed that baseline temperature declines significantly in the elderly. "The older the colder" is an expression that can help clinicians remember this point. This point has been especially affirmed for frail residents in LTCFs.[36–38] These studies further demonstrated that infections often resulted in normal increases in body temperature from baseline. However, because the baseline temperature was lower, the increase in temperature that accompanied infection often did not reach an oral temperature of 101°F, the level that clinicians in the past considered to be a definite fever. Taken together, these studies resulted in the Infectious Diseases Society of America recommending that fever in LTCF residents be defined as a single oral temperature greater than 100°F (or repeated oral temperatures greater than 99°F or an increase in temperature >2°F over baseline).[39] The later LTCF study of 12 LTCFs established 99.2°F as strongly suggestive of a fever (**Box 2**[38]). Even if no fever is detected, any decline in functional status, such as new onset confusion, loss of appetite, agitation, new onset of incontinence, or falling in residents of LTCF, should lead the clinician to consider the possibility of infection as the cause for the acute change.

A robust fever response in an older person has particular significance based on a large study of ambulatory patients; although younger patients who met the criterion of an oral temperature of 101°F were likely to have their fever to be caused by viral infection, the older patients who met this criterion were most likely to have a serious bacterial infection.[40] A subsequent study confirmed this finding as well as demonstrated a large percentage of elderly patients seen in the emergency department setting had no fever. It was further determined in this prospective evaluation of 221 patients aged 70 to 99 years that white blood cell counts in response to an infection were less in the aged when compared with the young.[41] The presence of fever, elevated white blood cell count, and bandemia (increase in number or percentage of "band" or early forms of neutrophils) in this study was highly associated with bacterial infection. Thus, it is strongly recommended that any older person with an oral temperature of 101°F or greater be evaluated for a serious bacterial or viral infection. Bandemia, when discovered even in the presence of a normal temperature and normal white blood cell count, was highly significant in a retrospective study of 365 bandemia

---

Box 2
Criterion for fever in older persons

Single oral temperature of 100°F or higher

Repeated oral temperatures of 99.2°F or higher

An increase of 2°F or more over baseline

patients compared with 407 controls. Blood cultures were positive in only 3.9% of controls but were seen in 18.1% of patients with moderate bandemia (11%–19% bands) and 25.9% of patients with high bandemia (greater than 20% bands).[42] Thus, bandemia in and of itself is an important finding.

Finally, the ultimate causes of fever of unknown origin (FUO) in older persons are similar to the young, and FUO is usually found to be caused by infection in most cases followed by rheumatologic disorders and malignancy. However, malignancy is more likely in the elderly compared with the young. Surprisingly, a cause for FUO in the elderly can be found in most cases (70%), and an FUO in an older person is well worth evaluating because a treatable condition is often found.[43–46]

REFERENCES

1. El-Solh AA, Sikka P, Ramadan F, et al. Etiology of pneumonia in the very elderly. Am J Respir Crit Care Med 2001;163:645–51.
2. El-Solh AA, Pietrantoni C, Bhat A, et al. Microbiology of severe aspiration pneumonia in institutionalized elderly. Am J Respir Crit Care Med 2003;167:1650–4.
3. Fernandez-Sabe N, Carratala J, Roson B, et al. Community-acquired pneumonia in very elderly patients: causative organisms, clinical characteristics and outcomes. Medicine 2003;82:159–69.
4. Liapikou A, Polverino E, Cilloniz C, et al. A worldwide perspective of nursing home-acquired pneumonia compared with community-acquired pneumonia. Respir Care 2014;59:1078–85.
5. Thigpen MC, Whitney CG, Messonnier NE, et al. Bacterial meningitis in the United States, 1998–2007. N Engl J Med 2011;364:2016–25.
6. Wester A, Dunlop O, Melby KK, et al. Age-related differences in symptoms, diagnosis and prognosis of bacteremia. BMC Infect Dis 2013;13:346.
7. Ewig S, Klapdor B, Pletz MW, et al. Nursing-home-acquired-pneumonia in Germany: an 8 year prospective. Thorax 2012;67:1332–8.
8. Ragsdale L, Southerland L. Acute abdominal pain in the older adult. Emerg Med Clin North Am 2011;29(2):429–48.
9. Gleckman R, Hibert D. Afebrile bacteremia. A phenomenon in geriatric patients. J Am Med Assoc 1982;248:1478–81.
10. Finkelstein M, Petkun WM, Freedman ML, et al. Pneumococcal bacteremia in adults: age-dependent differences in presentation and outcome. J Am Geriatr Soc 1983;31:19–27.
11. Bentley DW. Bacterial pneumonia in the elderly: clinical features, diagnosis, etiology and treatment. Gerontology 1984;30:297–307.
12. Marrie TS, Haldane EV, Faulkner RS, et al. Community-acquired pneumonia requiring hospitalization: is it different in the elderly? J Am Geriatr Soc 1985;33:671–80.
13. Metlay J, Schulz R, Li YH, et al. Influence of age on symptoms at presentation in patients with community-acquired pneumonia. Arch Intern Med 1997;157:1453–9.
14. Roghmann MC, Warner J, Mackowiak PA. The relationship between age and fever magnitude. Am J Med Sci 2001;322:68–70.
15. Terpenning MS, Buggy BO, Kauffman CA. Infective endocarditis: clinical features in young and elderly patients. Am J Med 1987;83:626–34.
16. Werner GS, Schulz R, Fuchs JB, et al. Infective endocarditis in the elderly in the era of transesophageal echocardiography: clinical features and prognosis compared with younger patients. Am J Med 1996;100:90–7.

17. Dhawan VK. Infective endocarditis in elderly patients. Clin Infect Dis 2002;34: 806–12.

18. Bassetti M, Venturini S, Crapis M, et al. Infective endocarditis in elderly: an Italian prospective multi-center observational study. Int J Cardiol 2014;177:636–8.

19. Trivalle C, Chassagne P, Bouaniche M, et al. Nosocomial febrile illness in the elderly: frequency, causes, and risk factors. Arch Intern Med 1998;158:1560–5.

20. Domingo P, Pomar V, de Benito N, et al. The spectrum of acute bacterial meningitis in elderly patients. BMC Infect Dis 2013;13:108–14.

21. Potts FE IV, Vukov LF. Utility of fever and leukocytosis in acute surgical abdomens in octogenarians and beyond. J Gerontol A Biol Sci Med Sci 1999;54A(2):M55–8.

22. Weinstein MP, Murphy JR, Reller RB. The clinical significance of positive blood cultures: a comprehensive analysis of 500 episodes of bacteremia and fungemia in adults. II. Clinical observations, with special reference to factors influencing prognosis. Rev Infect Dis 1983;5:54–70.

23. Swenson BR, Hedrick TL, Popovsky K, et al. Is fever protective in surgical patients with bloodstream infection? J Am Coll Surg 2007;204:815–21.

24. Kluger MJ, Ringler DM, Anver MR. Fever and survival. Science 1975;188:166–8.

25. Covert JB, Reynolds WM. Survival value of fever in fish. Nature 1977;267:43–5.

26. Sajadi MM, Mackowiak PA. Temperature regulation and the pathogenesis of fever. In: Mandell GL, Bennett JB, Dolin R, editors. Principles and practice of infectious diseases. 7th edition. London: Churchill Livingstone; 2014. p. 708–26 [Chapter 55]; (electronic edition updated 2014).

27. Blum FC, Biros MH. Fever in the adult patient. In: Mandell GL, Bennett JB, Dolin R, editors. Principles and practice of infectious diseases. 7th edition. London: Churchill Livingstone; 2014. p. 119–25 [Chapter 12].

28. Panda A, Qian F, Mohanty S, et al. Age-associated decrease in Toll-like receptor function in primary human dendritic cells predicts influenza vaccine response. J Immunol 2010;84:2518–27.

29. Norman DC, Yamamura RH, Yoshikawa TT. Fever response in old and young mice after injection of interleukin. J Gerontol 1988;43:M80–5.

30. Miller D, Yoshikawa TT, Castle SC, et al. Effect of age in fever response to recombinant tumor necrosis factor alpha in a murine model. J Gerontol 1991; 46:M176–9.

31. Miller DJ, Yoshikawa TT, Norman DC. Effect of age on fever response to recombinant interleukin-6 in a murine model. J Gerontol 1995;50A:M276–9.

32. Bradley SF, Vibhagool A, Kunkel SL, et al. Monokine secretion in aging and protein malnutrition. J Leukoc Biol 1989;45:510–4.

33. Grahn D, Norman DC, Yoshikawa TT. Fever and aging: central nervous system prostaglandin E2 in response to endotoxin. Exp Gerontol 1987;22:249–55.

34. Satinoff E, Peloso E, Plata-Salamn CR. Prostaglandin E2-induced fever in young and old Long-Evans rats. Physiol Behav 1999;67(1):149–52.

35. Plata-Salamán CR, Peloso E, Satinoff E. Interleukin-1β-induced fever in young and old Long-Evans rats. Am J Physiol 1998;275:R1633–8.

36. Castle SC, Norman DC, Yeh M, et al. Fever response in elderly nursing home residents: are the older truly colder? J Am Geriatr Soc 1981;39:853–7.

37. Castle SC, Yeh M, Toledo S, et al. Lowering the temperature criterion improves detection of infections in nursing home residents. Aging Immunol Infect Dis 1993;4:67–76.

38. Sloane PD, Kistler C, Mitchell M, et al. Role of body temperature in diagnosing bacterial infection in nursing home residents. J Am Geriatr Soc 2014;162:135–40.

39. High KP, Bradley SF, Gravenstein S, et al. Clinical practice guideline for the evaluation of fever and infection in older adult residents of long-term care facilities: 2008 update by the Infectious Diseases Society of America. Clin Infect Dis 2009;48:149–71.
40. Keating JH III, Klimek JJ, Levine DS, et al. Effect of aging on the clinical significance of fever in ambulatory adult patients. J Am Geriatr Soc 1984;32:282–7.
41. Wasserman M, Levenstein M, Keller E, et al. Utility of fever, white blood cells, and differential count in predicting bacterial infections in the elderly. J Am Geriatr Soc 1989;37:537–43.
42. Drees M, Kanapathippillai N, Zubrow MT. Bandemia with normal white blood cell counts associated with infection. Am J Med 2012;125:9–15.
43. Espositio AL, Gleckman RA. Fever of unknown origin in the elderly. J Am Geriatr Soc 1978;26:498–505.
44. Knockaert DC, Vanneste LJ, Bobbaers JH. Fever of unknown origin in elderly patients. J Am Geriatr Soc 1993;41:1187–92.
45. Ma JSX, Zhao S, Meng QQY. Fever of unknown origin in an older Chinese population. J Am Geriatr Soc 2012;60:169–70.
46. Hayakawa K, Ramasamy B, Chandrasekar PH. Fever of unknown origin: an evidence-based review. Am J Med Sci 2012;344:307–16.

Principles of Antimicrobial Therapy in Older Adults

Suzanne F. Bradley, MD

KEYWORDS

- Antibiotics • Pharmacokinetics • Aging • Long-term care
- Antimicrobial stewardship

KEY POINTS

- Antibiotic use is common in older adults; a significant proportion of this use is unnecessary, overly broad in spectrum, or the duration is too prolonged.
- Unnecessary antibiotic use contributes to complications, such as drug toxicity, other side effects, and alterations in normal flora that may result in secondary infections that may be difficult to treat.
- Understanding how body habitus, blood flow, and metabolism alter antibiotic distribution, levels, and dosing in the older adult can help minimize drug toxicity.
- Diagnosis of infection in older adults is challenging. Understanding what criteria are helpful for the diagnosis of infection and initiation of antibiotics in this population is helpful to minimize the unnecessary use of antibiotics.

INTRODUCTION

In general, older adults have more underlying conditions that predispose them to infection with more frequent complications and greater mortality. Recent studies of Medicare Part D data suggest that overall older adults receive more antibiotics than insured younger adults and children accounting for 1.10 versus 0.88 antibiotics per person per year, respectively.[1] In assisted living and nursing homes, antibiotic use increases to 2.53 to 4.56 versus 3 to 5 antibiotics per resident year.[2,3] Antibiotic use has also been shown to be particularly intensive at the end of life in frail dependent patients with severe irreversible dementia.[4] Less is known about prescription of antibiotics in the ambulatory care setting. In one national survey of ambulatory care visits in the United States from 2007 to 2009, 8% of adults aged 60 years and older received an antibiotic; the antibiotics prescribed were significantly more likely to be broader in spectrum than those prescribed for younger patients (**Box 1**).[5]

Conflicts of Interest: None.
Infectious Diseases Section 111i, Rm B804, Veterans Affairs Ann Arbor Healthcare System, 2215 Fuller Road, Ann Arbor, MI 48105, USA
E-mail address: sbradley@umich.edu

Clin Geriatr Med 32 (2016) 443–457
http://dx.doi.org/10.1016/j.cger.2016.02.009
0749-0690/16/$ – see front matter Published by Elsevier Inc.

> **Box 1**
> **Facts about antibiotic use in older adults**
>
> - Antibiotic use is common in older adults
>   - In assisted living facilities
>   - In long-term care facilities
>   - Who are functionally dependent with severe dementia
> - The antibiotics used to treat older adults tend to be broader in spectrum
> - Unnecessary antibiotic use may contribute to
>   - Drug toxicities
>   - Hypersensitivity reactions
>   - Secondary infections
>   - Antibiotic resistance

IMPACT OF ANTIBIOTIC USE IN OLDER ADULTS

More antibiotic use in older adults does not necessarily confer more benefit. A significant proportion of older adults receive antibiotics for inappropriate indications or the duration of therapy is too long. Inappropriate prescribing for adults ranges from 26% in residents of assisted living facilities to 25% to 75% of nursing home residents.[6,7]

Furthermore, older adults who receive an antibiotic are also significantly more likely to have a complication of antibiotic use, such as an adverse drug event. Older adults aged 65 years and older accounted for 13.5% of adverse events related to antibiotics that required emergency room care in the United States from 2004 to 2006.[8] The use of nitrofurantoin, a drug on the Beers Criteria list of "always inappropriate" drugs, was the third most common cause of medication-related adverse events in addition to trimethoprim-sulfamethoxazole and levofloxacin.[9] Older adults who receive antibiotics are also more likely to have an adverse drug event than those who do not receive treatment.[10] Although adverse events from antibiotics are half-again less likely than high-risk drugs, such as warfarin, insulin, and digoxin, the impact is not trivial.[9,10] Adverse events, such as allergic and drug-drug interactions, other side effects, and drug toxicities may occur. In addition, antibiotics alter the patient's normal flora (microbiome) and may contribute to secondary infections with *Clostridium difficile* or emergence of multidrug-resistant bacteria, such as methicillin-resistant *Staphylococcus aureus*, vancomycin-resistant enterococci, extended-spectrum β-lactamase, or carbapenemase-producing gram-negative bacilli (GNB).[11,12] Anticipating drug interactions, using appropriate doses, and minimizing the unnecessary use of antibiotics may help prevent adverse events in the elderly person and the emergence of antibiotic resistance.

AGING AND ANTIBIOTIC PHARMACOKINETICS

Aging influences the pharmacokinetics of antibiotics at multiple levels through its impact on the absorption, distribution, and elimination of these drugs. Absorption of antibiotics, which follows ingestion by oral or enteric routes, may be diminished by an increase in gastric pH and gastric emptying, atrophy of mucosal surfaces, and reduced intestinal motility, sphincter activity, and splanchnic blood flow with aging. Resulting reduced gastric acidity can slow the dissolution of tablets, impede drug release, and alter solubility of some drugs. Reduced gastrointestinal motility may facilitate the degradation of some drugs before they are absorbed (**Table 1**).[13–15]

Once absorbed, the systemic distribution of antibiotics within various tissues is influenced by changes in drug solubility, intravascular protein concentration, alterations in body composition, and reduced cardiac output and organ blood flow.

Table 1
Age-related changes in pharmacokinetics and impact on ATB dosing

Problem	Result	Impact on ATB	How to Alter ATB Dosing
↓ Stomach emptying ↓ GI blood flow	↓ Absorption	All oral ATB	Increase oral dose or give intravenously
↓ Serum albumin	↓ Protein binding	β-lactams	Monitor closely toxicity and drug interactions
↓ Renal blood flow	↓ Renal clearance	β-Lactams	Increase dosing intervals and/or reduce dose
		Quinolones	Monitor for toxicity and drug interactions
		Aminoglycosides	—
↓ Hepatic blood flow	↓ Hepatic clearance	Clindamycin β-Lactams	Reduce dosing especially if renal and liver failure
↑ Fluid volume	↑ Volume of distribution	Aminoglycosides β-Lactams	Increase dosing and measure levels if available
Obesity	Volume of distribution overestimated	Quinolones β-Lactams Vancomycin	Use lean/ideal body weight for dosing

Abbreviations: ATB, antibiotic; GI, gastrointestinal.

Adapted from McKinnon PS, Davis SL. Pharmacokinetic and pharmacodynamics issues in the treatment of bacterial infectious diseases. Eur J Clin Microbiol Infect Dis 2004;23:277; with permission.

Many antibiotics are highly water-soluble and protein bound; their levels are highest in tissues that receive greater blood flow versus those with little blood flow, such as fat. The resulting decline in serum proteins, such as albumin, increasing fat, decreased lean body mass, and reduction in body water lead to a reduction in the volume of distribution in the older adult. Given the smaller volume of distribution with increasing age, higher serum levels of water-soluble antibiotics are achieved with standard dosing. For lipid-soluble antibiotics, the approximately 40% increase in body fat with increasing age, coupled with declines in lean muscle mass and total body water allows for a wider distribution of drug, and these drug levels may be too low (see **Table 1**).[13–16] Given the changes in body composition in aging, it is important to measure drug levels frequently if they are available (**Box 2**).

Finally, antibiotics and their metabolites are eliminated from the body through hepatobiliary and renal metabolism. After absorption from the gastrointestinal tract, antibiotics must first pass through the liver where clearance of protein bound/water-soluble antibiotics is influenced by hepatic portal vein and arterial blood flow and metabolism by hepatic enzymes. Declines in liver size and reduction in hepatic blood by approximately 30% to 50% occur with increasing age, so antibiotic levels and their metabolites may accumulate leading to high levels in older adults. Additional factors seen in the elderly population, such as age-related changes in cytochrome P-450 enzymes, underlying liver disease, genetic factors, frailty, and other drugs, can also influence antibiotic metabolism.[13,14,17]

Water-soluble antibiotics or their metabolites are predominantly excreted via the kidneys. These drugs are eliminated as a function of glomerular filtration and tubular secretion and absorption. In the aged, renal function declines as a result of reduced renal blood flow and parenchymal mass (10% per decade) and loss of functional glomeruli.[13,14,18] Between ages 20 and 90 years, glomerular filtration may decline by

---

Box 2
Estimation of creatinine clearance in older adults

Cockcroft and Gault Equation

$$\text{Men} = \frac{(140 - \text{Age}) \,(\text{Lean Body Weight kg}^a)}{72 \times \text{serum Cr}}$$

Women = male value × 0.85
Lean body weight (men) = 50 kg + 2.3 kg (inches >60)
Lean body weight (women) = 45.5 + 2.3 kg (inches >60)

Abbreviation: Cr, creatinine.
a Use actual body weight if the patient weight is less than calculated lean body weight.

35% to 50%.[13] On that basis, a significant proportion of older adults will have a glomerular filtrate rate less than 60 mL/min (stage 3 kidney disease).[18] The doses of most renally excreted antibiotics should be reduced if the patient has a creatinine clearance of 50 mL/min or less.[13]

Because of changes in hepatic and renal functions with aging, the rate of elimination of antibiotics typically declines in older adults. Adjustment of antibiotic doses and dosing intervals may be necessary depending on the cause and severity of the underlying infection and the mechanism of elimination of the antibiotic. Antibiotics that are eliminated by renal metabolism should have dosage adjustments made using estimates of creatinine clearance (see **Box 2**).[14,18] Actual body weight should be used to calculate creatinine clearance for underweight individuals and lean body weight for obese patients.[18] Unfortunately, there is no simple method to estimate the degree of hepatic impairment; adjustments based on serum levels may be helpful if available.[13,14,17] The few common antibiotics that are eliminated primarily by hepatic metabolism are listed in **Table 2**.[15]

Table 2
Common antimicrobial agents that are eliminated primarily by hepatic metabolism

Drug	Route	Reduction for Renal Dysfunction?
Penicillins		
Naficillin/oxacillin	Hepatic	No
Cephalosporins		
Cefotaxime	Hepatic/renal	Yes
Ceftriaxone	Hepatic	No
Quinolones		
Ciprofloxacin	Hepatic/renal	Yes
Levofloxacin	Hepatic/renal	Yes
Moxifloxacin	Hepatic	No
Tetracyclines		
Doxycycline	Hepatic	No
Minocycline	Hepatic	No
Macrolides		
Azithromycin	Hepatic	No
Clarithromycin	Hepatic/renal	Yes
Erythromycin	Hepatic	—

INITIAL APPROACH TO PRESUMPTIVE INFECTION

Although the clinical presentation may be atypical in older adults, it is important to focus initial therapeutic choices on the most likely causes of infection.[19,20] The clinician must determine what symptoms and signs are present and the infectious and noninfectious etiologies that might cause these findings. If the illness is not severe and the patient is clinically stable, the clinician may elect to wait for diagnostic testing to confirm if there is an infection, the site of infection, the cause of infection, and drug susceptibilities; empirical antibiotic therapy may be started if there is concern for severe infection (**Box 3**). The Loeb Criteria were developed to help clinicians decide what minimum patient symptoms and signs would justify the initiation of empirical antibiotics versus awaiting results of diagnostic testing (**Table 3**).[21]

If patients only have systemic symptoms and signs suggestive of infection (eg, fever) but physical findings fail to yield an obvious focus of infection, then the clinician may have to base empirical treatment on the place of acquisition and the most common etiologies found in those locations.[21] With some exception, whether the infection was acquired in the community, acute care hospital, or in the long-term care setting, the most common clinical infectious syndromes are generally the same in the older adult: infections of the urinary tract, respiratory tract, skin and soft tissue, and gastrointestinal tracts.[12,19] However, empirical antimicrobial therapeutic choices given for these conditions change because of differences in microbial etiologies and antimicrobial susceptibility patterns in those locations.

Fortunately, many illnesses are self-limited. Brief courses of empirical antimicrobial therapy are often given because it is perceived as simple, the patient and family demand it, and the consequences seem few. Unfortunately, in an era where *C difficile* infection is increasingly virulent and community-associated and untreatable antibiotic-resistant infections are on the rise, one can no longer take comfort that empirical use of antibiotics is easy and without consequences. It is important, therefore, that if the patient does not respond to initial treatment, the physician carefully reassesses the diagnosis rather than changing antibiotics alone.

Box 3
How to choose initial antibiotic therapy

- Identify the most likely location where the patient acquired the infection (community, nursing home, hospital)
- Identify the most likely site of infection
- Know the most common organisms that inhabit that/those sites
- Know local antibiotic resistance patterns in the locations where the infection was acquired
- Choose antibiotics
  - To which the most common and likely organisms are susceptible
  - That penetrate the likely site of infection (eg, central nervous system)
  - That are bactericidal (cell-wall active) for severe infection
  - That are bacteriostatic antibiotics for intracellular bacteria or those that lack cell walls
  - That minimize drug-drug interactions and have few drug toxicities
- Choose intravenous antibiotics if
  - The infection is severe, life-threatening, and intravenous therapy is allowable per advanced directives
  - Absorption by the gastrointestinal tract is not reliable
  - Effective drug levels cannot be achieved by oral administration

Table 3
Empirical treatment of presumed infection in older adults: when to begin

	Categories	Minimum Criteria
Urinary tract infection		
Fever[a]	No catheter	*One or more*: new or worsening urgency, frequency, suprapubic pain, gross hematuria, CVA tenderness, urinary incontinence
Fever	Chronic indwelling catheter	New CVA tenderness *and* rigors without cause *or* new-onset delirium[b]
Respiratory tract infection		
High fever	>102°F (>38.9°C)	Respiratory rate >25 breaths/min *or* productive cough
Fever	≤102°F (≤38.9°C)	Cough *plus one* of the following: tachycardia >100 beats/min, delirium, rigors, respiratory rate >25 breaths/min
Afebrile	COPD	New or increased cough and purulent sputum production
Afebrile	No COPD	New cough with purulent sputum and one of the following: respiratory rate >25 breaths/min *or* delirium
Skin/soft tissue infection		
Applies to intact skin, devices, or ulcers	—	Fever or new or increasing redness, tenderness, warmth, or swelling at the affected site[c]
Fever/focus unknown		
—	—	Fever *and one* of the following: new onset delirium *or* rigors

Abbreviations: COPD, chronic obstructive pulmonary disease; CVA, costovertebral angle.
  [a] Fever is defined as a single temperature of greater than 100°F (>37.9°C) or >2.4°F (>1.5°C) unless otherwise stated.
  [b] Delirium is defined by Diagnostic and Statistical Manual of Mental Disorder, 4th edition.
  [c] Does not include nonbacterial infections (herpes), deep tissue or bone infection. Noninfectious causes, such as burns, thromboembolic disease, and gout, can be mistaken for skin/soft tissue infection.
  Adapted from Loeb M, Bentley DW, Bradley S, et al. Development of minimum criteria for the initiation of antibiotics in residents of long-term-care facilities: results of a consensus conference. Infect Control Hosp Epidemiol 2001;22:121–3; with permission.

WHAT ANTIBIOTICS TO PRESCRIBE

Discussion of optimal antibiotic therapy for each clinical infectious syndrome is beyond the scope of this article. The reader should refer to the appropriate article for further discussion of the causes of various clinical infectious syndromes and their treatment. Knowledge of local antimicrobial susceptibility and resistance patterns through facility antibiograms or public health information networks is invaluable in informing the clinician in making the best decisions possible for their patient.

Some generalizations can be made about the antimicrobial susceptibilities of the various antibiotic classes and other unique characteristics (**Table 4**). For example, most penicillins and carbapenems have reliable activity against susceptible enterococci and oral anaerobes (streptococci), but not methicillin-susceptible *S aureus* (MSSA) or enteric anaerobes, such as *Bacteroides fragilis*. Addition of β-lactamase

Table 4
Choosing β-lactam antibiotics: some generalizations about differences in antimicrobial susceptibilities

Antibiotic/ Bacteria	Streptococci	PSSA	MSSA	MRSA	PCNS-Ent	PCNR-Ent	Haemophilus influenzae β-Lactam (−)	Haemophilus influenzae β-Lactam (+)	Escherichia coli	Proteus	Klebsiella	Serratia	Enterobacter	Pseudomonas	Oral Anaerobes	Bacteroides fragilis
Penicillins/ carbapenems																
Penicillin	+	+	−	−	+	−	−	−	−	−	−	−	−	−	+	−
Dicloxacillin/ nafcillin	+	+	+	−	−	−	−	−	−	−	−	−	−	−	−	−
Ampicillin/ amoxacillin	+	+	−	−	+	−	+	−	+/−	+/−	−	−	−	−	+	−
Ampicillin/ sulbactam	+	+	+	−	+	−	+	+	+	+	+/−	+/−	−	−	+	+
Piperacillin	+	+	−	−	+	−	+	+	+	+	+	+	+	+	+	−
Piperacillin/ tazobactam	+	+	+	−	+	−	+	+	+	+	+	+	+	+	+	+
Ertapenem	+	+	+	−	−	−	+	+	+	+	+	+	+	−	+	+
Imipenem/ meropenem	+	+	+	−	+	−	+	+	+	+	+	+	+	+	+	+
Cephalosporins																
Cephalexin/ cefazolin	+	+	+	−	−	−	−	−	+	+	+/−	−	−	−	−	−
Cefuroxime	+	+	+	−	−	−	+	+	+	+	+/−	−	−	−	−	−
Ceftriaxone	+	+	+/−	−	−	−	+	+	+	+	+	+	+	−	−	−
Ceftazidime	+	+/−	−	−	−	−	+	+	+	+	+	+	+	+	−	−
Ceftazidime/ avibactam	+	+/−	−	−	−	−	+	+	+	+	+	+	+	+	−	−
Cefepime	+	+	+	−	−	−	+	+	+	+	+	+	+	+	−	−
Ceftaroline	+	+	+	+	−	−	+	+	−	−	−	−	−	−	−	−

Abbreviations: MRSA, methicillin-resistant *Staphylococcus aureus*; MSSA, methicillin-susceptible *S aureus*; PCNR-ENT, penicillin-resistant enterococci; PCNS-ENT, penicillin-susceptible enterococci; PSSA, penicillin-susceptible *S aureus*.

inhibitors, such as clavulanate, tazobactam, or sulbactam, in combination with a penicillin (ampicillin or piperacillin) results in activity against MSSA and improved activity against intrinsically resistant aerobic GNB and *B fragilis*.[20,22]

In contrast, most cephalosporins do not have substantial activity against enterococci or anaerobes. Activity against MSSA is greatest among the first-generation cephalosporins (cephalexin or cefazolin) and declines as activity against GNB, particularly *Pseudomonas aeruginosa*, increases. Addition of newer β-lactamase inhibitors, such as avibactam, to ceftazidime or ceftolozane increases activity against β-lactamase-producing GNB, but it does not change their activity against MSSA or anaerobes. Only a few cephalosporins, such as cefuroxime (second-generation) or the third- and fourth-generation cephalosporins (ceftriaxone, ceftazidime, cefepime) are able to penetrate the blood-brain barrier and achieve sufficient levels to treat the central nervous system.[20,22–24]

Bactericidal antibiotics that act against bacterial cell walls and rapidly kill bacteria, such as the β-lactams, glycopeptides, and cyclic lipopeptides (daptomycin), are recommended for treatment of severe illness. Ceftaroline, unlike other β-lactam antibiotics, is able to avidly bind to cell wall penicillin-binding protein 2a, resulting in activity against methicillin-resistant *S aureus*.[22] Bactericidal antibiotics are not always the best choices to treat certain infections. Cell-wall active antibiotics have minimal activity against bacteria that are not replicating and are metabolically inactive; these bacteria are typically present within biofilms associated with device-related infections. Cell-wall active antibiotics also do not penetrate well into human cells, so they are not effective against intracellular infections, such as *Legionella pneumophila*. Bacteriostatic antibiotics, such as the macrolides, tetracyclines, and quinolones, are the treatments of choice for many intracellular infections.

Finally, antibiotic resistance continues to be a major issue. β-lactamases, such as penicillinases, extended-spectrum β-lactamases, and carbapenemases that inactivate cell-wall active antibiotics, have become increasingly common mediators of antibiotic resistance particularly among GNB. β-lactam-resistant bacteria also harbor resistance to many other antibiotic classes. Therefore, it is critical to obtain cultures and antimicrobial susceptibilities particularly if resistance to antibiotics is common in the facility or community, and if the patient is not responding to empirical treatment as expected.

CHOOSING THE ROUTE OF ANTIBIOTIC ADMINISTRATION

Choosing the route of administration of an antimicrobial agent depends on the severity of illness, the ability of the patient to take an oral agent, bioavailability of the drug, goals of care, and the ability to give parenteral antibiotics in a given setting. Topical antimicrobial agents may be appropriate for superficial infections involving the superficial skin and mucosal surfaces. Administration of oral antibiotics may be appropriate for infections of varying severity. The patient must be able to swallow reliably or have enteral access by a nasogastric tube or enteral feeding tube. Knowledge of which antibiotics are available in liquid formulations or readily dissolve into solution is helpful to facilitate administration by the enteral route when drugs in pill form cannot be swallowed or crushed.

The patient's gastrointestinal tract must also be capable of absorbing the drug. Some antibiotics (linezolid, quinolones, fluconazole, voriconazole) are highly bioavailable meaning that high serum levels can be achieved after oral administration that approach or equal levels obtained when given intravenously. When treating infections with oral agents, it is important to ensure that other drugs that inactivate the antibiotic are not given or are administered at least 2 hours apart from each other. Coadministration of divalent cations, such as calcium, aluminum, and iron, may bind with tetracyclines and quinolones and inhibit their absorption.

For some patients, the goals of care preclude administration of intravenous (IV) antibiotics or transfer to settings where resources are available to give these drugs. In this instance, oral antibiotics to treat severe infections that normally would be treated with IV antibiotics may be appropriate. Although it is not clear that antibiotics contribute to the comfort of patients at the end of life, it is known that the most intensive use of IV antibiotics occurs within the last 2 weeks of life in frail functionally dependent nursing home residents with advanced dementia. Oral antibiotics have been used in the care of patients at the end of life in other countries with similar outcomes.[4]

IV antibiotics may be necessary if the infection is particularly severe, it is located in an anatomic location where drug penetration is difficult (central nervous system infection or endocarditis), there are no oral agents to which the organisms are susceptible, and the goals of care are compatible with this approach. Where the IV antibiotics should be administered should be based on the acuity of the illness, the stability of the patient, and the need for monitoring and care by nursing staff and other personnel. The choice of IV catheter depends on the anticipated duration of therapy; the need for other therapies, such as transfusion, chemotherapy, or hyperalimentation; the frequency of administration of the antibiotic; and the likelihood that the drug will cause phlebitis. β-lactam antibiotics may be given by shorter midline catheters for 2 to 4 weeks. For drugs that can cause phlebitis (vancomycin) or if longer therapy is needed a peripherally inserted central catheter and temporary or semipermanent central venous catheter can be considered.[25]

If the patient is clinically stable, the infection is defined, a specific treatment plan is in place, and appropriate follow-up is arranged then transfer to a chronic care facility or outpatient antimicrobial parenteral therapy (OPAT) can be considered.[26] The treatment plan should include how often the monitoring of drug effects and the patient's response to therapy should be performed; who should receive those results; what is the anticipated duration of therapy; and who is responsible for deciding when to stop therapy, remove the catheter, and provide posttreatment follow-up (**Box 4**). For OPAT, the patient or their caretakers must be able to follow directions regarding the appropriate care of their catheter and have transportation to appointments for follow-up clinical evaluation and diagnostic testing. Patients should not be referred for OPAT if the home situation is in doubt regarding hygienic care of the catheter and subsequent refusal of home care visits is likely with unreliable clinical and diagnostic follow-up.[26]

Box 4	
Monitors for the patient's response to treatment and antibiotic side effects	
Monitor	**Subjective/Objective Parameters**
Physical findings	Improvement of fever and focal signs and symptoms
Diagnostic findings	Improvement of diagnostic findings
Inflammatory markers	Improvement in anemia
	Improvement in leukocytosis, neutrophilia, bands, or thrombocytosis
	Decline in erythrocyte sedimentation rate, C-reactive protein
Drug side effects	New mucocutaneous findings on examination
	Complete blood count and differential (eosinophils)
	Blood urea nitrogen, creatinine
	Liver function tests
	Antibiotic levels

COMMON SIDE EFFECTS OF ANTIMICROBIAL AGENTS

Antibiotics may cause of variety of adverse drug reactions that can involve virtually every organ system (**Table 5**). Antibiotics may cause side effects that are predictable (type A) and relate to their pharmacologic properties, such as dose-related drug

Table 5
Antibiotic side effects by organ system

Organ System/Symptom or Sign	Drugs
Auditory/vestibular	Macrolides, streptomycin, gentamicin, minocycline
Cardiac	
Prolonged QT interval, torsade de pointes	Quinolones, macrolides, oxazolidinones, azoles
Central nervous system	
Confusion/delirium	Quinolones, mefloquine
Meningitis, encephalitis	Trimethoprim-sulfamethoxazole, metronidazole
Seizures	Carbapenems, β-lactams, metronidazole
Serotonin syndrome	Oxazolidinones
Peripheral neuropathy	Isoniazid, metronidazole
Hematopoietic	
Aplastic anemia	Trimethoprim sulfamethoxazole
Autoimmune anemia	Rifampin
Agranulocytosis	Trimethoprim sulfamethoxazole
Neutropenia	Metronidazole, β-lactams, vancomycin
Thrombocytopenia	Rifampin, oxazolidinones, β-lactams, vancomycin
Hepatobiliary	
Hepatitis	Azoles, trimethoprim sulfamethoxazole, rifampin, isoniazid, tetracycline
Cholestasis	Ceftriaxone
Mucocutaneous (see **Box 4**)	
Phototoxicity	Tetracyclines, quinolones, voriconazole
Musculoskeletal	
Rhabdomyolysis	Daptomycin, azoles
Tendonitis/arthritis	Quinolones
Ocular	
Optic neuritis	Oxazolidinones, ethambutol
Scotoma	Voriconazole
Pancreatic	
Hypoglycemia	Quinolones, oxazolidinones, trimethoprim
Pancreatitis	Metronidazole
Pulmonary	
Pneumonitis	Nitrofurantoin, daptomycin
Renal	
Acute tubular necrosis	Aminoglycosides, vancomycin
Acute interstitial nephritis	Nafcillin, β-lactams
Fanconi syndrome	Tetracyclines
Hyperkalemia	Trimethoprim sulfamethoxazole

toxicities.[27] Depending on the antibiotic and its metabolites, direct toxic effects may involve a variety of organs including cardiac, renal, hematopoietic, mucocutaneous, and central nervous systems. Unpredictable reactions (type B) include immunologic drug reactions, drug intolerances, and idiosyncratic reactions (**Box 5**). Most antibiotic-related emergency room visits in the United States are caused by allergic reactions (~80%). Even so, nonallergic events including gastrointestinal and neuro-psychiatric disturbances are common.[8]

Penicillins, sulfonamides, and nitrofurantoin are the most common antibiotics (>2%) that account for allergic reactions followed by cephalosporins, carbapenems, quino-lones, and minocycline (0.1%–2%). With the exception of red man syndrome and maculopapular rash (type IVb), prior exposure of 1 to 2 weeks duration is required for most allergic manifestations to occur.

ANTIBIOTICS AND INTERACTIONS WITH COMMON DRUGS USED BY OLDER ADULTS

Polypharmacy is common among older adults, so it is understandable that interac-tions between antibiotics and other drugs may contribute to adverse events. It is important to review the patient's medication list for potential drug interactions partic-ularly if the clinician is not familiar with the antibiotic being used. Some common drug interactions that may have deadly consequences are discussed next.

Trimethoprim, frequently combined with sulfamethoxazole, inhibits the secretion of potassium in the distal renal tubule resulting in hyperkalemia. A seven-fold increased risk of hospitalization caused by hyperkalemia has been reported when this antibiotic has been used.[28,29] This antibiotic should be used with caution in conjunction with angiotensin-converting enzyme inhibitors, spironolactone, and other potassium-sparing diuretics that are common among older adults with such diseases as diabetes mellitus, hypertension, and liver disease.[28] Phenytoin toxicity also is increased as trimethoprim-sulfamethoxazole inhibits the metabolism of the antiseizure medication by cytochrome 2C9 and cytochrome 2C8.[29] Trimethoprim-sulfamethoxazole may

Box 5		
Immunologic reactions to antibiotics		
Reaction Type	**Manifestation**	**Common Antibiotics**
I (IgE)	Anaphylaxis, angioedema, urticaria, bronchospasm	β-lactams, sulfonamides
II (IgG + complement)	Hemolytic anemia, thrombocytopenia, neutropenia	Penicillins, cephalosporins, sulfonamides
III (IgG + AgAb complexes)	Serum sickness, fever, vasculitis	Penicillins, cephalosporins, sulfonamides
IVa (TH1 lymphocytes)	Allergic contact dermatitis	Penicillins, neomycin, sulfonamides
IVb (TH2 lymphocytes)	Maculopapular rash	Amoxicillin, ampicillin, sulfonamides
IVc (CTL)	Stevens-Johnson syndrome, hepatitis bullous exanthems, toxic epidermal necrolysis	Sulfonamides, penicillins, macrolides
Nonimmunologic	Red man syndrome	Vancomycin

Abbreviations: AgAb, antigen-antibody complexes; CTL, cytotoxic T lymphocytes; TH, T helper.
Adapted from Akinyemi D'J, Celik GE, Adkinson NF. Hypersensitivity to antibiotics. In: Schlossberg D, editor. Clinical infectious disease. New York: Cambridge University press; 2014. p. 1372; with permission.

contribute to hypoglycemia in patients treated with sulfonylureas by similar mechanisms.[29]

Many antibiotics inhibit the growth of bacteria and vitamin K production in the gastrointestinal tract, a pathway that is also inhibited by warfarin.[29] Antibiotic use in older adults who take warfarin can lead to a significant increase in international normalized ratio with possible bleeding particularly if the patient is clinically unstable; chronically ill; and trimethoprim-sulfamethoxazole, quinolones, fluconazole, or amoxicillin have been concurrently prescribed.[29–31]

Azoles are commonly used to treat candidosis, onychomycosis, and other fungal infections in older adults. Azoles (fluconazole, itraconazole, voriconazole, posaconazole) can cause serious adverse events when taken with a wide variety of drugs. The drug interactions vary with the azole given. In general, most azoles cause toxic levels when given with the following drug classes: statins, warfarin, oral hypoglycemics, transplant medications, antiarrhythmics, and antiseizure medications. It is therefore critically important to carefully assess the patient's list of medications and review potential adverse drug reactions before beginning treatment with any azole.[32]

Oxazolidinones (linezolid, tedizolid) are associated with serotonin syndrome. These antibiotics inhibit monomine oxidase, an enzyme that metabolizes and blocks the reuptake of serotonin. Fever, agitation, confusion, headache, tachycardia, hypertension, and other symptoms can result when oxazolidinones are used in conjunction with drugs that are known to cause serotonin syndrome. Serotonin-reuptake inhibitors, other antidepressants, and meperidine should be avoided when using this antibiotic class.[33]

Torsades de pointes and sudden death may result in patients with long QT syndrome. Increasing numbers of antibiotics have been associated with prolongation of the QT interval including azoles, macrolides, oxazolidinones, and quinolones.[34] Patients with a history of a QT interval of 500 milliseconds or greater and those on antiarrythmics are at greatest risk of torsades de pointes. A 12-lead electrocardiogram should be obtained to evaluate the QT interval before starting these antibiotics.

Interactions with calcium channel blockers and clarithromycin and erythromycin that cause effects on the vascular system have also been reported. Hypotension or shock may ensue if metabolism of calcium channel blockers is blocked by these macrolides that inhibit their metabolism via cytochrome 3A4.[29] Azithromycin has no effect on this cytochrome. Clarithromycin has also been associated with significantly increased risk of hospitalization with digoxin toxicity when compared with erythromycin and azithromycin.[29]

ANTIMICROBIAL STEWARDSHIP

Antibiotic use among older adults is high particularly in hospitals and long-term care facilities where they are the predominant patient population. The impact of unnecessary antibiotic use on this age group is significant in terms of adverse events and infections caused by C difficile and antibiotic-resistant pathogens. Recent efforts have been made to establish formal antimicrobial stewardship programs to improve the use of antibiotics.[35,36] The White House recently released a National Action Plan that included establishment of antimicrobial stewardship programs in health care facilities, including long-term care facilities.[37] The optimal approach in long-term care remains to be determined. Use of guidelines, treatment algorithms, educational programs, and consultative services has been evaluated.[35] Interventions have focused on individual problems, such as treatment of asymptomatic bacteriuria, use of antibiotic prophylaxis for urinary tract infections, pneumonia, and the impact of the program on C *difficile* rates. More frequent use of narrow-spectrum antibiotics and shorter durations of treatment have also been emphasized.

SUMMARY/DISCUSSION

Older adults are at great risk of infection and the appropriate use of antibiotics can be life-saving. Antibiotics can also pose a threat to the elderly patient if they are given inappropriately or when they are not carefully dosed and monitored. National and international efforts are focusing on ways to preserve the remaining antibiotics and develop new ones. In the interim, although the diagnosis of infection is difficult in the older adult, it is vitally important to try to establish if infection is present, if antibiotic treatment is warranted, and what clinical syndromes and pathogens are likely to be present based on the evidence and resources available. Defining the problem as carefully as possible can help in the decision to treat and selection of empirical antibiotics. Treatment based on culture and susceptibilities, rather than reliance on empiricism, can help narrow the spectrum of antibiotics further, minimize the impact of those drugs on the patient's normal flora, and preserve therapeutic options.

REFERENCES

1. Zhang Y, Steinman MA, Kaplan CM. Geographic variation in outpatient antibiotic prescribing among older adults. Arch Intern Med 2012;127:1465–71.
2. Sloane PD, Zimmerman S, Reed D, et al. Antibiotic prescribing in 4 assisted-living communities: incidence and potential for improvement. Infect Control Hosp Epidemiol 2014;35:S62–8.
3. Pakyz AL, Dwyer LL. Prevalence of antimicrobial use among United States nursing home residents: results of a national survey. Infect Control Hosp Epidemiol 2010;31:661–2.
4. D'Agata E, Mitchell SL. Patterns of antimicrobial use among nursing home residents with advanced dementia. Arch Intern Med 2008;168:357–62.
5. Shapiro DJ, Hicks LA, Pavia AT, et al. Antibiotic prescribing for adults in ambulatory care in the USA, 2007–09. J Antimicrob Chemother 2014;69(1):234–40.
6. Nicolle LE, Bentley DW, Garibaldi R, et al. Antimicrobial use in long-term-care facilities. Infect Control Hosp Epidemiol 2000;21:537–45.
7. Loeb M. Antibiotic use in long-term-care facilities: many unanswered questions. Infect Control Hosp Epidemiol 2000;21:680–3.
8. Shehab N, Patel PR, Srinivasan A, et al. Emergency department visits for antibiotic-associated adverse events. Clin Infect Dis 2008;47:735–43.
9. Budnitz DS, Shehab N, Kegler SR, et al. Medication use leading to emergency department visits for adverse drug events in older adults. Ann Intern Med 2007;147:755–65.
10. Field TS, Gurwitz JH, Harrold LR, et al. Risk factors for adverse drug events among older adults in the ambulatory setting. J Am Geriatr Soc 2004;52:1349–54.
11. Saraswati S, Sitaraman R. Aging and the human gut microbiota—from correlation to causality. Front Microbiol 2015;5:1–4.
12. Smith PW, Bennett G, Bradley S, et al. Infection prevention and control in the long-term-care facility. Infect Control Hosp Epidemiol 2008;29:785–814.
13. Miller SW. Therapeutic drug monitoring in the geriatric patient. In: Murphy JE, editor. Clinical pharmacokinetics. Bethesda (MD): American Society for Health-System Pharmacists; 2012. p. 45–71.

14. Hilmer SN, Ford GA. Chapter 8: general principles of pharmacology. In: Halter JB, Ouslander JG, Tinetti ME, et al, editors. Hazzard's geriatric medicine and gerontology. 6th edition. San Francisco (CA): McGraw Hill Medical; 2009.

15. Rho JP, Kim J. Pharmacology. In: Yoshikawa TT, Rajagopalan S, editors. Antibiotic therapy for geriatric patients. New York: Taylor & Francis; 2006. p. 67–76.

16. McKinnon PS, Davis SL. Pharmacokinetic and pharmacodynamics issues in the treatment of bacterial infectious diseases. Eur J Clin Microbiol Infect Dis 2004;23: 271–88.

17. McLachlan AJ, Pont LG. Drug metabolism in older people—a key consideration in achieving optimal outcomes with medicines. J Gerontol A Biol Sci Med Sci 2012;67(2):175–80.

18. Aymanns C, Keller F, Maus S, et al. Review on pharmacokinetics and pharmacodynamics and the aging kidney. Clin J Am Soc Nephrol 2010;5:314–27.

19. High KP, Bradley SF, Gravenstein S, et al. Clinical practice guideline for the evaluation of fever and infection in older adult residents of long-term care facilities: 2008 update by the Infectious Diseases Society of America. Clin Infect Dis 2009;48:149–71.

20. Bradley SF. Infectious disease. In: Ham RJ, Sloane PD, Warshaw GA, et al, editors. Primary care geriatrics: a case-based approach. 6th edition. Philadelphia: Saunders; 2014. p. 512–34.

21. Loeb M, Bentley DW, Bradley S, et al. Development of minimum criteria for the initiation of antibiotics in residents of long-term-care facilities: results of a consensus conference. Infect Control Hosp Epidemiol 2001;22:120–4.

22. Bradley SF. Staphylococcus. In: Schlossberg D, editor. Clinical infectious disease. New York: Cambridge University Press; 2014. p. 985–90.

23. Solomkin J, Hershberger E, Miller B, et al. Ceftolozane/tazobactam plus metronidazole for complicated intra-abdominal infections in an era of multidrug resistance: results from a randomized, double-blind, phase 3 trial (ASPECT-cIAI). Clin Infect Dis 2015;60:1462–71.

24. Zhanel GG, Lawson CD, Adam H, et al. Ceftazidime-avibactam: a novel cephalosporin/β-lactamase inhibitor combination. Drugs 2013;73:159–77.

25. Chopra V, Flanders SA, Sanjay S, et al. The Michigan appropriateness guide for intravenous catheters (MAGIC): results from a multispecialty panel using the RAND/UCLA appropriateness method. Ann Intern Med 2015;163:S1–40.

26. Tice AD, Rehm SJ, Dalovisio JR, et al. Practice guidelines for outpatient parenteral antimicrobial therapy. Clin Infect Dis 2004;38:1651–72.

27. Akinyemi DJ, Celik GE, Adkinson NF. Hypersensitivity to antibiotics. In: Schlossberg D, editor. Clinical infectious disease. New York: Cambridge University Press; 2014. p. 1371–82.

28. Antoniou T, Gomes T, Juurlink DN, et al. Trimethoprim-sulfamethoxazole-induced hyperkalemia in patients receiving inhibitors of the renin-angiotensin system: a population-based study. Arch Intern Med 2010;170:1045–9.

29. Hines LE, Murphy JE. Potentially harmful drug-drug interactions in the elderly: a review. Am J Geriatr Pharmacother 2011;9:364–77.

30. Ghaswalla PK, Harpe SE, Tassone D, et al. Warfarin-antibiotic interactions in older adults of an outpatient anticoagulation clinic. Am J Geriatr Pharmacother 2012; 10:352–60.

31. Clark NP, Delate T, Riggs CS, et al. Warfarin interactions with antibiotics in the ambulatory care setting. JAMA Intern Med 2014;174:409–16.

32. Kauffman CA. Antifungal drugs. In: Yoshikawa TT, Rajagopalan S, editors. Antibiotic therapy for geriatric patients. New York: Taylor & Francis; 2006. p. 337–51.

33. Narita M, Tsuji BT, Yu VL. Linezolid-associated peripheral and optic neuropathy, lactic acidosis, and serotonin syndrome. Pharmacotherapy 2007;27:1189–97.
34. Owens RC Jr, Nolin TD. Antimicrobial-associated QT interval prolongation: points of interest. Clin Infect Dis 2006;43:1603–11.
35. Dellit TH, Owens RC, McGowan JE Jr, et al. Infectious Diseases Society of America and the Society for Healthcare Epidemiology of America guidelines for developing an institutional program to enhance antimicrobial stewardship. Clin Infect Dis 2007;44:159–77.
36. Nicolle LE. Antimicrobial stewardship in long term care facilities: what is effective? Antimicrob Resist Infect Control 2014;3(1):6.
37. National action plan for combatting antibiotic-resistant bacteria. Available at: https://www.whitehouse.gov/sites/default/files/docs/national_action_plan_for_combating _antibotic-resistant_bacteria.pdf. Accessed September 25, 2015.

Bacterial Pneumonia in Older Adults

Thomas J. Marrie, MD, FRCPC[a],*, Thomas M. File Jr, MD, MSc[b,c]

KEYWORDS

- Pneumonia • Community-acquired • Elderly • Risk factors • Treatment • Etiology

KEY POINTS

- The incidence of pneumonia increases with increasing age.
- Risk factors for pneumonia include age, male sex, presence of chronic obstructive lung disease, congestive heart failure, smoking, and preceding viral infection. Use of inhaled corticosteroids, antipsychotic drugs, and anticholinergics seem to increase the risk of pneumonia, whereas angiotensin-converting enzyme inhibitors or angiotensin receptor blocking agents seem to be protective.
- Silent aspiration is common in elderly patients with pneumonia.
- Recent studies using multiplex polymerase chain reaction show a predominance of viruses, including rhinovirus, in studies of the cause of pneumonia. Bacterial and viral coinfection is frequent in elderly patients with pneumonia.
- Elderly persons with pneumonia, especially those who are residents of nursing homes, are less likely to report various symptoms of pneumonia as compared with younger patients. The presence of dementia, aphasia, or cognitive impairment contributes to such under reporting.
- In a patient with symptoms and signs of pneumonia, the absence of an opacity on chest radiography should not be construed to mean the patient does not have pneumonia. Instead the chest radiograph should be repeated in 24 hours or a computed tomography scan of the chest can be carried out. For elderly persons who are immobile, ultrasonography of the chest is probably the best diagnostic modality to determine if pneumonia is present.
- Severity-of-illness scoring systems and the use of biomarkers may help in deciding on the site of care, but there is no substitute for clinical judgment.
- Although dated, the guidelines from the Infectious Diseases Society of America and the American Thoracic Society are still used to determine empirical antimicrobial treatment of pneumonia.
- The use of glucocorticoids in severe pneumonia is an evolving area with little to no data in elderly patients.

Continued

Research Funding: Pfizer, Canada (T.J. Marrie).
[a] Department of Medicine, Dalhousie University, Halifax, Nova Scotia, Canada; [b] Infectious Disease Section, Northeast Ohio Medical University, Rootstown, OH, USA; [c] Infectious Disease Division, Summa Health System, 75 Arch Street, Suite 506, Akron, OH 44304, USA
* 59 Sprucebank Lane, RR1, Chester Basin, Nova Scotia B0J 1K0, Canada.
E-mail address: t.marrie@dal.ca

Clin Geriatr Med 32 (2016) 459–477
http://dx.doi.org/10.1016/j.cger.2016.02.012
0749-0690/16/$ – see front matter © 2016 Elsevier Inc. All rights reserved.

geriatric.theclinics.com

Continued

- Physiologic stability should be achieved before discharge.
- Pneumococcal pneumonia is often complicated by one or more cardiac events likely because of the ability of *Streptococcus pneumoniae* to damage the myocardium. Long-term mortality due to pneumonia may be more pronounced in young adults.

INTRODUCTION

Bacterial pneumonia is one of the most common infections in the elderly adult. Pneumonia is a disease of the alveoli and respiratory bronchioles caused by an infectious agent.[1] Pathologically, it is characterized by increased weight and replacement of the normal lung sponginess by induration (consolidation). This consolidation may involve most or all of a lobe or it may be patchy and localized around bronchi (bronchopneumonia). On microscopic examination, pneumonia caused by bacterial agents shows dense alveolar infiltration with polymorphonuclear leukocytes. Clinically, however, pneumonia is usually defined as a new opacity on chest radiograph and the presence of at least 2 of the following: fever, cough, sputum, pleurisy, temperature greater than 38°C, crackles, consolidation (dullness to percussion, bronchial breathing, egophony).[1]

The cause of the pneumonia is usually classified as definite, probable, or possible as modified from Marston and colleagues.[2] The pathogen is said to be the definite cause of pneumonia when it is isolated from blood or pleural fluid; there is a 4-fold increase in antibody titer to *Legionella pneumophila*, *Mycoplasma pneumoniae*, or *Chlamydophila pneumoniae*; it is probable when *Staphylococcus aureus*, *Streptococcus pneumoniae*, *Haemophilus influenzae*, or *Pseudomonas aeruginosa* is isolated from purulent sputum (sputum that has moderate or many neutrophils seen on gram stain) and possible when a pneumonia pathogen other than *Legionella* is isolated from purulent sputum in the absence of a compatible gram stain. We have now moved into the era of molecular diagnostics with multiplex polymerase chain reaction (PCR) as discussed later.

The pneumonia is also characterized as to the site of acquisition: community, nursing home, or hospital. The discussion in this article is confined to community-acquired pneumonia (CAP). Emphasis is placed on bacterial pneumonia in the elderly population.

EPIDEMIOLOGY

A considerable amount of data on the epidemiology of pneumonia has emerged in the last 3 decades. In Halifax County, Nova Scotia in the late 1980s, the rate of pneumonia requiring admission to the hospital was 1 per 1000 overall, for those 75 years of age or older it was 12 per 1000, and for the nursing home residents it was 33 per 1000.[3] In another study, the overall rate of pneumonia was low until 65 years of age when an abrupt increase occurred from 1 per 1000 to 60 per 1000 for those aged 90 years and older.[4] The percentage of patients presenting to the emergency department with pneumonia who were admitted to the hospital increased with increasing age from about 20% for those aged 20 to 24 years to 80% for those aged 80 years and older. The percentage of patients admitted to intensive care decreased with increasing age from 20% for those aged 20 years to 10% for those 80 years and older.[4] Rates of admission were higher for men than women from 70 years of age onward. There was a seasonal effect, with the overall rate of pneumonia doubling in the winter months.[4]

Jackson and colleagues[5] studied 46,237 seniors enrolled in Group Health in Seattle and followed them for 3 years. The overall rate of CAP was 18.2 per 1000 for those aged 65 to 69 years and 52.3 per 1000 for those aged 85 years or older; 59.3% were treated as outpatients. They calculated that, based on their data, there would be 915,900 cases of pneumonia among seniors in the United States each year and 1 in 20 aged 85 years or older will have a new episode of CAP each year. Peaks of pneumonia coincided with influenza virus circulation.[5]

Wortham and colleagues[6] used data from the National Ambulatory Medical Care survey from 1998 to 2009 to examine ambulatory patient encounters for pneumonia in the United States. Thirty-seven million visits occurred during the study period. Overall there were 12.6 to 15.7 visits per 1000 adults. For those older than 65 years, the number of visits decreased from 45 to 35 per 1000 over the study period.[6]

Risk Factors for Bacterial Pneumonia

In Jackson's study age, male sex, chronic obstructive pulmonary disease (COPD), asthma, diabetes mellitus, congestive heart failure, preceding viral infection, and smoking were risk factors for pneumonia.[5] Although increasing age is a risk factor for pneumonia, Baik and colleagues[7] were able to quantitate this risk. Compared with those aged 49 years or younger, those 60 to 64 years of age had a 2.75 times higher rate of pneumonia and those 70 years of age and older had a 4.17 times higher rate of pneumonia.[7] Koivula and colleagues[8] found that the following factors were associated with an increased risk of pneumonia: alcoholism (relative risk [RR] 9.0), asthma (RR 4.2), immunosuppression (RR 1.9), and being older than 70 years versus 60 to 69 years (RR 1.5). Some studies have determined the risk factors for pneumonia due to specific microorganisms. Thus, dementia, seizures, congestive heart failure, cerebrovascular disease, and chronic obstructive lung disease were particular risk factors for pneumococcal pneumonia.[9] In multiple studies cigarette smoking has been a risk factor for invasive pneumococcal infection. Nuorti and colleagues[10] best demonstrated this in a population-based study.

Among human immunodeficiency virus (HIV)–infected patients, the rate of pneumococcal pneumonia was 41.8 times higher than for those in the same age group who were not HIV infected.[11] Risk factors for legionnaires' disease include male sex, tobacco smoking, diabetes, hematologic malignancy, cancer, end-stage renal disease, and HIV infection.[12]

More recently, several studies have identified additional risk factors for bacterial pneumonia, especially among elderly adults. These risk factors include the use of inhaled corticosteroids[13] and the use of antipsychotic drugs.[14] The study by Gambassi and colleagues indicated that there will be one excess hospitalization for pneumonia for every 2 to 5 patients who have clinical improvement in their psychiatric symptoms.[14] Similarly, the use of anticholinergic medications has also been associated with increased pneumonia.[15] Interestingly, for those with dentures, wearing them during sleep doubles the risk of pneumonia.[16]

Well known as a risk for bacterial pneumonia is a preceding viral infection, especially influenza A. Indeed it was recognized during the influenza pandemic of 1918 that bacterial pneumonia either concomitantly or following the influenza played a major role in mortality.[17] Subsequently, preceding influenza has been recognized as a risk factor for Staphylococcus aureus pneumonia, both methicillin-sensitive and methicillin-resistant varieties.[18] An interaction has also been shown between respiratory syncytial virus and pneumococcal pneumonia in infants[19]; it is possible that the same relationship exists in adults.

The risk of pneumonia is decreased among patients who are taking angiotensin-converting enzyme inhibitors or angiotensin receptor blocking agents.[20] The basis for this is that improving cough and swallowing reflexes is mediated through increased levels of substance P and bradykinin, levels of which are increased by increasing angiotensin levels.

PATHOGENESIS

Pneumonia results when bacteria that gain access to the alveoli overwhelm host defenses. A detailed discussion of innate and acquired immunity as pertains to the lung is beyond the scope of this article. Quinton and Mizgerd[21] nicely summarize recent knowledge. Lung defense requires a careful balance between immune resistance and tissue resilience pathways shaped largely by nuclear factor kappa B (NF-kB) and signal transducer and activator of transcription 3 (STAT3). (NF-kB is a protein complex that controls cytokine production and plays a role in regulating the immune response; STAT3 is a cellular signaling system involved in regulating the immune response.) If there is too much, adult respiratory distress syndrome (ARDS), shock, and multiorgan failure can result; if there is too little, the infection is not contained.[21]

Combined decreases in both immune resistance and tissue resilience are responsible for the increased rate and severity of pneumonia in the elderly adult. However, the ways in which these vary over a lifetime are poorly understood.[21]

Colonization of the oropharynx by aerobic gram-negative rod bacteria is uncommon among healthy young adults, but 60% of this group will show such colonization during a viral illness.[22] Alcoholism, illness, and nursing home residence predispose to colonization of the upper airway with aerobic gram-negative bacteria.[23,24] Woods and colleagues[25,26] showed that trypsinization of normal buccal mucosal cells resulted in increased adhesion of P aeruginosa as a result of loss of fibronectin from the cell surface. They postulated that fibronectin loss during a variety of diseases accounted for colonization of the oropharynx by these bacteria.

There is a high incidence of silent aspiration in elderly patients with CAP. Kikuchi and colleagues[27] examined the role of silent aspiration during sleep in 14 elderly patients with CAP and 10 age-matched control subjects by applying a paste containing indium-111 wrapped in gauze and fixed to the teeth. Scanning of the thorax demonstrated that 71% of the study patients aspirated, compared with 10% of the control subjects.[27] Just more than 28% of patients with Alzheimer disease[28] and 51% of those who had had a stroke[29] aspirated, when assessed using videofluoroscopy. Croghan and colleagues[30] found that placement of a feeding tube in patients who had aspirated, as revealed by videofluoroscopy, was associated with a higher rate of pneumonia and death than for those who aspirated but did not receive such a tube.

The foregoing discussion raises the role of comorbid illnesses in the pathogenesis of pneumonia.[31] Most adults with pneumonia have one or more comorbidities, and one-third have multi-morbidity defined as 2 chronic conditions plus the pneumonia.[31] The comorbid illnesses among patients in the Pneumonia Patient Outcomes Research Team (PORT) study are given in **Box 1**.[32] This study was carefully done with research nurse interviews of all patients and all morbidities were defined. Noteworthy is that only 14.4% of these 1343 patients who required admission to the hospital had no comorbidities.[32]

Finally we arrive at the concept of frailty, which is "a state of vulnerability due to poor resolution of homoeostasis after a stressor event and is a consequence of cumulative decline in many physiologic systems during a lifetime."[33] Frailty can often explain why one 80 year old is vigorous and the other looks his or her age and is mostly bedridden.

CAUSE OF PNEUMONIA AND ETIOLOGIC DIAGNOSIS

Torres and colleagues[34] examined 3300 articles on the cause of CAP in adults in Western European countries from 2005 to 2012. Only 33 studies were suitable for inclusion

---

Box 1
Comorbid illnesses among 1343 patients hospitalized with pneumonia in the Pneumonia Patient Outcomes Research Team study

Comorbidity	Patients (%)
COPD	33.9
Coronary artery disease	26.0
Alcoholism or intravenous drug use	25.0
Cancer	17.8
Congestive heart failure	16.8
Neuromuscular disease	16.3
Diabetes mellitus	14.7
Immunosuppression	12.1
Renal disease	10.4
Dementia	10.0
Seizure disorder	5.6
None	14.4

Data from Fine MJ, Stone RA, Singer DE, et al. Processes and outcomes of care for patients with community-acquired pneumonia. Results from the Pneumonia Patient Outcomes Research Team (PORT) study. Arch Intern Med 1999;159:970–80.

---

in their review. The etiologic data from this study are summarized in **Table 1**. *S pneumoniae and H influenzae* were the most common pathogens; however, in everyday clinical practice an etiologic diagnosis is made in the minority of patients. In addition to knowing the most common pathogens that cause pneumonia, one must also know

---

Table 1
Cause of community-acquired pneumonia in Western European countries from 2005 to 2012

	Studies (N)	Range (%)
Gram-positive bacteria		
Streptococcus pneumoniae	19	12–85
Streptococcus viridians	1	1.7
Gram-negative bacilli		
Gram-negative enteric bacilli	10	0.6–42.9
Haemophilus influenzae	15	1.1–29.4
Pseudomonas aeruginosa	10	0.9–16
Pseudomonas spp	1	0.2–3.2
Klebsiella pneumoniae	5	0.3–5.0
Moraxella catarrhalis	5	0.3–2.3
Escherichia coli	3	0.6–2.1
Atypical bacteria		
Mycoplasma pneumoniae	10	0.7–61.3
Legionella pneumophila	12	1.7–20.1
Legionella spp	3	5.4–20
Chlamydophila pneumoniae	9	0.1–9.9
Coxiella burnetii	6	0.8–3.4
Virus	10	1.4–28.6

Adapted from Torres A, Blasi F, Peetermans WE, et al. The etiology and antibiotic management of community-acquired pneumonia in adults in Europe: a literature review. Eur J Clin Microbiol Infect Dis 2014;33:1072.

the likelihood that a pathogen will be resistant to the various antimicrobials. For example, in China 69% of isolates of *M pneumoniae* are resistant to macrolides.[35]

It is also important to be aware of risk factors for antibiotic-resistant pathogens. Such factors include residency in a nursing home or long-term care facility; hospitalization for 2 or more days in the previous 90 days; antibiotic therapy within the past 30 days; poor functional status; and presence of chronic lung disease.[36] Presence of 3 of these factors would indicate the need for coverage for drug-resistant pathogens; however, the presence of one methicillin-resistant *S aureus* (MRSA)–specific risk factor (prior MRSA infection or colonization; long-term hemodialysis; congestive heart failure) and another pneumonia-specific risk factor (hospitalization for $\geq$2 days during the previous 90 days; antibiotic use within the previous 90 days; nonambulatory status; tube feedings; immunocompromised state; use of gastric acid suppressive agents) may warrant MRSA coverage.[37]

The diagnostic yield from blood cultures is in the range of 10% to 15%, but this test should be done on all patients who are ill enough to require admission to hospital. However, it should be pointed out that this is no longer a quality measure for Centers for Medicare and Medicaid Services (CMS) pneumonia.[38] In a recent review, Prina and colleagues[35] stratified the microbiological evaluation according to the severity of the pneumonia. For those treated as outpatients, no evaluation is necessary; for those admitted with low-severity pneumonia, sputum culture is recommended; for moderate-severity pneumonia, blood and sputum culture is recommended; and urinary antigen testing is recommended for *S pneumoniae* and *Legionella*. Finally for those admitted to the intensive care unit (ICU), all of the foregoing plus sampling lower respiratory tract secretions by tracheobronchial aspirate or by bronchoalveolar lavage are indicated. In this setting, cultures should be done for fungi and *Mycobacterium tuberculosis* and also serology and multiplex PCR on respiratory secretions and occasionally lung biopsy.[35]

The availability of multiplex PCR allows nucleic acid amplification of several, usually 15, pathogens simultaneously.[39] What these studies have shown is that viruses are commonly present in the nasopharynx of patients with pneumonia and that 25% or more of patients have a mixed cause, that is, virus and bacteria coinfecting patients.[39–41] Indeed in the best study to date, Falsey and colleagues[42] showed that bacterial coinfection is associated with approximately 40% of viral respiratory tract infections requiring hospitalization.

CLINICAL FEATURES OF PNEUMONIA

A thorough history can often offer clues to the cause of the pneumonia. For example, recent travel followed by pneumonia suggests *Legionella* infection and also makes one think of pulmonary infarction as a possible mimic of the pneumonia. Exposure to a variety of animals can also result in pneumonia; for example, exposure to parturient cats in some areas is suggestive of *Coxiella burnetii* pneumonia. Immigration from a country where tuberculosis is endemic should suggest that diagnosis. The onset of the pneumonia can be abrupt with a shaking chill as for the classic, albeit infrequently, seen onset of pneumococcal pneumonia or it can be insidious with symptoms increasing over a few days. Cough that may or may not be productive is a cardinal symptom. Fever, chills, sweats, pleuritic chest pain, and dyspnea are all common; but usually all are not present in 100% of older patients with pneumonia. Fatigue, nausea, vomiting, diarrhea, delirium, anorexia, and abdominal pain can also occur.[32]

Particular attention should be paid to the vital signs during the physical examination. Temperatures of 40°C or greater are seen in only about 1% of patients,[32] whereas more than half of elderly patients are frequently afebrile.[43] In as study of 705,938 patients hospitalized in Germany from 2010 to 2012 with pneumonia, the investigators found that if a respiratory rate of 12 to 20 breaths per minute is taken as a baseline, patients with a respiratory rate of 27 to 33 per minute had an odds ratio of mortality of 1.72 and for those with a respiratory rate greater than 33 breaths per minute it was 2.55.[44] The risk of mortality is not associated with resting heart rate in patients with pneumonia, but it is in patients with COPD.[45] Among patients who are treated for pneumonia on an ambulatory basis, an oxygen saturation of 92% or less is associated with major adverse events.[46] Thus, patients with an oxygen saturation of 92% or less should be hospitalized. Daily assessment of vital signs gives important information for the discharge decision as discussed later.

In a study of 1812 patients with CAP categorized into 4 age groups (18–44 years, 43%; 45–64 years, 25%; 65–74 years, 17%; and 75 years and older, 15%), for 17 of the 18 symptoms recorded there were significant decreases in reported prevalence with increasing age. For example, cough was reported by 90% of those aged 18 to 44 years but only by 84% in the 75 years and older age group; dyspnea was reported in 75% and 61% and sputum production in 64% and 64% in these two age groups, respectively.[47]

Nursing home residents are less likely to experience chills, pleuritic chest pain, headache, anorexia, myalgias, and productive cough than similarly aged patients with CAP; only two-thirds of nursing home patients with pneumonia experience temperatures of greater than 100.4°F. The presence of congestive heart failure, COPD, or prior use of antibiotics may further complicate the diagnosis as do the presence of dementia, aphasia, and cognitive impairment.[48]

RADIOGRAPHIC ASSESSMENT OF PNEUMONIA

A pulmonary opacity on chest radiograph is the gold standard for the diagnosis of pneumonia. However, the gold standard is not without tarnish. It does lack sensitivity. In a study of 105 patients with a clinical diagnosis of CAP, 21% had a negative chest radiograph, 55% of whom developed a pulmonary infiltrate within 48 hours.[49] This finding was substantiated in a retrospective chart review of 1057 patients with pneumonia of whom 97 had both chest radiography and computed tomography (CT) of the chest done. There were 26 (27%) in whom the chest radiograph was either negative or nondiagnostic, and the CT scan was consistent with pneumonia.[50] Up to one-third of patients with suspected pneumonia and a negative chest radiograph have a lower respiratory tract infection. In a prospective cohort study of 2076 patients who were admitted to the hospital with suspected pneumonia, one-third had no pneumonia on the admission chest radiograph as read by a radiologist.[51] The nonpneumonia group was older and had higher pneumonia severity-of-illness scores. However, both groups had similar rates of positive sputum cultures (32% versus 30%) and positive blood cultures (8% in the pneumonia group and 6% in the nonpneumonia group). Approximately 64% of the isolates from blood in the patients with pneumonia were *S pneumoniae* compared with 5% in the nonpneumonia group.[51] The reverse occurred for aerobic gram-negative bacteria isolates, that is, 14% in pneumonia group and 40% in nonpneumonia group. The mortality rates were similar at 10% and 6%, respectively. The investigators concluded that the nonpneumonia group did have serious lower respiratory tract infection warranting therapy.[51]

There is also an issue of interobserver variability in the interpretation of chest radiographs in the clinical setting of suspected pneumonia. In one study, chest radiographs were done on day 3 for 247 ambulatory patients with suspected pneumonia. Two radiologists read the films. The kappa coefficient for interobserver agreement was 0.53 (moderate agreement). However, if chronic obstructive lung disease was present, kappa was much lower at 0.20; if *S pneumoniae* was the infecting agent, it was also low at 0.29.[52] Not infrequently, elderly patients with pneumonia have chest radiographs done using a mobile (portable) device. Four radiologists reviewed 40 mobile chest radiographs from residents of nursing homes who met a clinical definition of lower respiratory tract infection.[53] Only 6 of the 40 radiographs were judged to be of good to excellent quality and 16 were fair or poor. All 4 radiologists agreed on the interpretation of 21 of 37 radiographs: intraclass coefficient 0.54 (0.38–0.69).[53] What the foregoing means is that the chest radiograph has to be interpreted in conjunction with the clinical findings. It is also important to remember that many diseases can mimic pneumonia with identical clinical and radiographic findings. However, the subsequent clinical course of patients usually allows separation of pneumonia from the mimics.

Lung ultrasound has a sensitivity of 94% (92%–96%) and a specificity of 96% (94%–97%) for diagnosing pneumonia.[54] There is a learning curve, and operator dependency is an issue.[54] It would seem, however, that lung ultrasound has a role to play in the diagnosis of pneumonia in elderly patients, especially in those in whom portable radiographs are necessary.

Radiological imaging, including chest radiography, has a role to play in the ongoing management of patients with pneumonia. Four hundred and fifty-seven patients with CAP admitted to ICUs were classified into 4 groups: rapid radiographic spread of pulmonary infiltrates and bacteremia (n = 48), rapid radiographic spread without bacteremia (n = 183), bacteremia without rapid spread (n = 39), and neither rapid spread nor bacteremia (n = 187). Rapid radiographic spread was defined as an increase in size of the opacities by greater than 50% at 48 hours after presentation. The two groups with rapid spread had a greater risk of shock and death while in the ICU than the group with neither rapid spread nor bacteremia.[55] Empyema complicates about 1% of cases of CAP, and it is best confirmed by CT scanning.[56]

Radiographic resolution of pneumonia lags behind clinical improvement; in the elderly adult, it can take 12 to 14 weeks for the pneumonia to clear radiographically.[57]

At one time, a follow-up chest radiograph was recommended for almost all patients to ensure that the pneumonia had resolved because some cases of pneumonia are really pneumonia distal to an obstructed bronchus due to a carcinoma and such cases would be evident on follow-up. In a study of 3398 patients with pneumonia, 59% were 50 years of age or older and 17% were smokers. At 90 days 1.1% had a new lung cancer diagnosed, and this increased to 1.7% at 1 year and 2.3% at 5 years.[58] Follow-up chest radiographs are recommended for the those older than 50 years, especially if they are tobacco smokers, but not for all patients with CAP who are responding clinically.

SITE OF CARE DECISION

Once the diagnosis of pneumonia has been made, the next decision is whether to treat at home, in the hospital in a ward setting, or in the ICU. Such a decision involves determining the severity of the pneumonia. When asked why a patient with pneumonia was admitted to the hospital, her physician responded she looked sick. The problem with that is it is a subjective decision as evidenced by the almost 4-fold variation in admission rate for patients with pneumonia in 9 health care regions in Alberta.[59]

To combat this problem, severity-of-illness scoring systems were developed. The pneumonia severity index (PSI) is a comprehensive score made up of 20 demographic, physical, and laboratory findings.[60] It stratifies patients into 5 classes according to mortality risk. Designed to identify low-risk patients who could be managed in an ambulatory setting, the PSI lacks the ability to discriminate among sicker patients. Class IV and V patients both warrant hospital admission, but the PSI is not helpful in determining the need for ICU admission. Because age and comorbidities are the dominant drivers in the PSI, the severity of disease in young, previously healthy patients can easily be underestimated.[61] The CURB-65, developed by the British Thoracic Society, uses 5 pneumonia-specific criteria, each scoring one point, including acute confusion, blood urea nitrogen level greater than 7 mmol/L, respiratory rate greater than 30 breaths per minute, systolic blood pressure less than 90 mm Hg or diastolic blood pressure of 60 mm Hg or less, and 65 years of age or older.[62] The CURB-65 seems to be more discriminatory compared with the PSI among patients requiring hospital admission, with a score of 3 or greater denoting severe disease, which may warrant ICU admission. In contrast, the lack of comorbid disease burden in CURB-65 makes it easy to underestimate the mortality risk in elderly, frail patients who may decompensate significantly even with mild pneumonia. The Infectious Diseases Society of America and the American Thoracic Society proposed a scoring system to identify patients with severe pneumonia. Patients with one major or 3 minor criteria should be admitted to ICU.[63] Major criteria include the need for mechanical ventilation or the presence of septic shock. Minor criteria include $Pao_2:Fio_2$ ratio less than 250, respiratory rate greater than 30 breaths per minute, multi-lobar infiltrates, systolic blood pressure less than 90 mm Hg despite aggressive fluid resuscitation, blood urea nitrogen level greater than 20 mg/dL, leukopenia (<4000 cells per cubic millimeter), thrombocytopenia (<100,000 cells per cubic millimeter), and hypothermia (<36°C). Several studies support the use of these criteria.[64–66] A team from Australia developed SMART-COP to predict the need for intensive respiratory or vasopressor support in patients with CAP.[67] This list is only a partial list of the various severity scores that are available. In general they serve as a guide and are not a substitute for good clinical judgment, and they all suffer from being a static measurement in a dynamic situation. In other words, patients with pneumonia need frequent reassessment if they are ill enough to be admitted to the hospital. If the decision is to send patients home there should be instructions for patients or someone else to phone within 24 hours to report on progress.

The next stage in the assessment of the severity of pneumonia was to add biomarkers to the scoring systems discussed earlier. Espana and colleagues[68] evaluated C-reactive protein, procalcitonin and proadrenomedullin levels in combination with PSI, CURB-65, and severe CAP (SCAP) scores. A proadrenomedullin level of less than 0.5 nM/L with an SCAP score of 0 or 1 identified a subset of patients who were at low risk of pneumonia-related complications.[66]

In a population-based study in Edmonton, Alberta, 15% to 20% of those 60 years of age or younger with pneumonia were admitted to the ICU compared with 5% to 10% of those 75 years of age and older.[4] Clearly there are factors other than the severity of the pneumonia that have to be considered in the decision to admit to the ICU, especially in very elderly patients. A recent administrative database study of 1,112,394 Medicare Medicaid recipients aged 65 years and older hospitalized with pneumonia, 328,404 (29.5%) of whom were treated in an ICU showed that the ICU patients had a 5.7% lower mortality rate than those treated on the ward.[69] Clearly, advanced age is not a contraindication to ICU admission.

The most recent effort at predicting those who are at risk of a poor outcome from pneumonia has been to use genome-wide sequencing to identify genes that would indicate a high risk. Rautanen and colleagues[70] carried out a genome-wide association study in 3 cohorts of white adult patients admitted to ICUs with sepsis. Common variants in the *FER* gene were associated with survival. The *FER* gene encodes a nonreceptor protein tyrosine kinase that acts downstream of cell-surface receptors for growth factors and is ubiquitously expressed. It influences leukocyte chemotaxis and endothelial cell permeability.[70] Toll-like receptor 6 polymorphism is associated with a 5.83-fold increase risk of legionnaires' disease.[71]

Age alone should not determine who is admitted to the ICU for treatment of pneumonia.

ANTIBIOTIC THERAPY

Because the infecting pathogen is not known at the time of presentation (and often never), antibiotic therapy is chosen empirically based on severity of the pneumonia, presence of risk factors for drug-resistant pathogens, and knowledge of the local epidemiology. Many countries have used expert panels to develop guidelines for such empirical therapy. In general, North American guidelines differ from European ones. The North American guidelines are given in **Boxes 2** and **3**.

One of the major challenges with these guidelines is that they have never been validated in a randomized controlled trial. The closest we get to this is a recent study that tested the noninferiority of a β-lactam strategy to β-lactam-macrolide and fluoroquinolone strategies.[72] This trial was a cluster-randomized, crossover trial with strategies rotated in 4-month periods. It was carried out from February 2011 through August 2013 in 7 hospitals in the Netherlands. A total of 3325 patients were eligible for inclusion, and 2283 (69%) gave consent for data collection. Baseline characteristics were similar, and the median age was 70 years. *S pneumoniae* was detected in 15.9% of patients. About 75% had blood cultures done, and 44% to 47% had sputum cultures; 78% had urinary antigen testing for *S pneumoniae* and 75% for *Legionella*. *H influenzae* was the second most common pathogen at 6.8%, and atypical pathogens were found in 2.1%. On average 83% had no complications and 5% had major complications, which included in-hospital death, respiratory insufficiency, ICU admission, and septic shock. Most had radiographically confirmed pneumonia.[72] In the intention-to-treat analysis, the risk of death was higher by 1.9% points (−0.6 to 4.4) with the β-lactam-macrolide strategy than with the β-lactam strategy and lower by 0.6% points with the fluoroquinolone strategy than with the β-lactam strategy. Thus, there was noninferiority of the β-lactam strategy.[72]

Guideline-concordant antibiotics were associated with decreased mortality among outpatients with pneumonia[73] but not among inpatients.[74] Musher and Thorner[75] indicate that in the United Kingdom and Sweden amoxicillin or penicillin is recommended as empirical therapy for CAP in outpatients.[75] They indicate the following factors are in favor of this approach: most clinicians do not know the level of pneumococcal resistance in their communities; *S pneumoniae* is more susceptible to penicillins than macrolides; if patients do not have a prompt response to a β-lactam, a macrolide or doxycycline can be substituted to treat a possible atypical bacterial infection.[75]

Sligl and colleagues[76] found that macrolide-based therapy was not associated with lower 30-day mortality among adults seriously ill with pneumonia, but receipt of effective antibiotic therapy within 4 hours was strongly predictive of survival. The same investigators did a meta-analysis of the therapy for 9850 seriously ill patients with CAP and found that macrolide use (as part of an antibiotic regimen) was associated with a significantly lower mortality compared with nonmacrolides.[77]

There is support from a randomized trial for the use of a pathway of care in the treatment of pneumonia. Nine hospitals were randomized to a pathway for the treatment of

---

Box 2
Recommendations for empirical ambulatory treatment of community-acquired pneumonia

1. Previously healthy and no use of antimicrobials within the previous 3 months
   a. A macrolide (strong recommendation; level I evidence)
      i. Azithromycin (500 mg day 1 followed by 250 mg once daily days 2–5; or 500 mg once daily for 3 days; or 2-g single dose)
      ii. Clarithromycin XL (two 500-mg tablets once daily for 5 days or until afebrile for 48–72 hours)
   b. Doxycycline (weak recommendation; level III evidence): 100 mg twice daily for 7 to 10 days

2. Presence of comorbidities, such as chronic heart, lung, liver, or renal disease; diabetes mellitus; alcoholism; malignancies; asplenia; immunosuppressing conditions or use of immunosuppressing drugs; or use of antimicrobials within the previous 3 months (in which case an alternative from a different class should be selected)
   a. A respiratory fluoroquinolone (moxifloxacin, gemifloxacin, or levofloxacin [750 mg]) (strong recommendation; level I evidence)
   b. A β-lactam plus a macrolide (strong recommendation; level I evidence) (Recommended β-lactams are high-dose amoxicillin [eg, 1 g 3 times daily] or amoxicillin-clavulanate [2 g 2 times daily]; alternatives include ceftriaxone, cefpodoxime, and cefuroxime [500 mg 2 times daily]; doxycycline [level II evidence] is an alternative to the macrolide.)

3. In regions with a high rate (>25%) of infection with high-level (MIC ≥16 μg/mL) macrolide-resistant *S pneumoniae*, consider use of alternative agents listed earlier in No. 2 for patients without comorbidities (moderate recommendation; level III evidence).

4. Inpatients, non-ICU treatment
   a. A respiratory fluoroquinolone (strong recommendation; level I evidence)
   b. A β-lactam plus a macrolide (strong recommendation; level I evidence)

5. Inpatients, ICU treatment
   a. A β-lactam (cefotaxime, ceftriaxone, or ampicillin-sulbactam) plus either azithromycin (level II evidence)
   b. OR a respiratory fluoroquinolone (level I evidence) (strong recommendation) (for penicillin-allergic patients, a respiratory fluoroquinolone and aztreonam are recommended.)

6. Special concerns
   a. If *Pseudomonas* is a consideration, an antipneumococcal, antipseudomonal β-lactam (piperacillin-tazobactam, cefepime, imipenem, or meropenem) plus either ciprofloxacin or levofloxacin (750 mg)
      OR
   b. The aforementioned β-lactam plus an aminoglycoside and azithromycin
      OR
   c. The aforementioned β-lactam plus an aminoglycoside and an antipneumococcal fluoroquinolone (for penicillin-allergic patients, substitute aztreonam for the aforementioned β-lactam) (moderate recommendation; level III evidence)
   d. If CA-MRSA is a consideration, add vancomycin or linezolid (moderate recommendation; level III evidence)

Abbreviations: CA-MRSA, community-acquired MRSA; MIC, minimal inhibitory concentration.
Adapted from Mandell LA, Wunderink RG, Anzueto A, et al. Infectious Diseases Society of America/American Thoracic Society consensus guidelines on the management of community-acquired pneumonia in adults. Clin Infect Dis 2007;44(Suppl 2):S45; with permission.

---

pneumonia and 10 to usual care. The pathway consisted of an admission guideline, criteria for switch from intravenous to oral levofloxacin, and discharge criteria. There was no difference in quality of life, complications, readmission, or mortality between the two groups. The pathway was associated with a 1.7-day reduction in bed days per patient managed, an 18% decrease in low-risk admissions, 1.7 fewer days of

---

Box 3
Considerations when patients with pneumonia fail to improve or deteriorate during therapy

1. Reconsider the diagnosis. Many conditions can mimic pneumonia, such as pulmonary infarction, malignancy, drug reaction, and eosinophilic pneumonia.

2. Reconsider the etiologic diagnosis: Does your patient have tuberculosis or an infection with a microorganism resistant to the antibiotics you have chosen?

3. Has your patient developed nosocomial pneumonia? In areas where the potable water is contaminated with *Legionella*, consider legionellosis. If your patient has required mechanical ventilation, nosocomial pneumonia is not uncommon.

4. Has metastatic infection occurred? Bacteremic pneumonia can be complicated by endocarditis, meningitis, septic arthritis, or abscess formation in the spleen or liver.

5. Is empyema present?

6. Drug fever should be a consideration in febrile patients who are otherwise well.

---

intravenous antibiotics, and treatment with one class of antibiotics (64% versus 27%).[78]

CMS implemented the hospital inpatient quality reporting program in 2003. For pneumonia this involved 7 processes of care: antibiotic therapy within 4 hours; appropriate antibiotic therapy; blood cultures; blood cultures before antibiotics; smoking cessation counseling; pneumococcal vaccination; and influenza vaccination where appropriate.[38] Lee and colleagues[38] examined these 7 processes of care among 1,819,979 fee-for-service Medicare patients (mean age of 79.7 years and 54% female) who were hospitalized for pneumonia. All measures of care increased over the study period; for example, in 2006, 91.9% of patients received antibiotics within 6 hours and in 2010 this had increased to 96.2%. All pneumonia processes of care were associated with a lower mortality, and 5 of the 7 were associated with lower 30-day readmission rates.[38] The target of 4 hours for antibiotic therapy led to overdiagnosis of pneumonia and inappropriate use of antibiotics. In 2012 the target period was dropped and replaced by the recommendation that treatment be initiated promptly and at the point of care where the diagnosis of pneumonia is made.[74] The only remaining process of care from the original 7 is appropriate empirical antibiotic therapy. Nevertheless, a protocol approach to the treatment of pneumonia is associated with benefits, the so-called halo effect.[79]

An observational study of 1005 patients (mean age 74.7 ±15.1 years) with pneumonia, 390 of whom were receiving 100 mg/d of aspirin, found that the 30-day mortality among the aspirin users was 4.9% compared with 23.4% for the nonusers.[80] There may be some rationale for this as discussed later under long-term outcomes of pneumonia.

In some areas procalcitonin levels are used to determine whether or not to start antibiotics in patients with presumed lower respiratory tract infections. For those with a procalcitonin level of greater than 0.25 mcg/mL, antibiotics are encouraged and strongly encouraged when the level is greater than 0.5 mcg/mL and discouraged when it is less than 0.10 mcg/mL.[35]

Musher and Thorner,[75] in a recent review of CAP, emphasized that clinician judgment should be used in addition to guidelines when considering antibiotic therapy.[75] Thus, if clinical features suggest legionnaires' disease or MRSA, make sure your antibiotic therapy will cover these microorganisms. Clinical features suggestive of MRSA pneumonia include severe pneumonia during the summer months, gross hemoptysis, concurrent influenza, previously healthy young person, skin pustules, erythematous rash, cavitary infiltrate, rapidly increasing pleural effusion, and neutropenia.[37] Legionella infection should be strongly considered in a young, otherwise healthy person with severe pneumonia, usually progression with β-lactam therapy. Other features include recent travel, relative bradycardia, and often confusion.

USE OF GLUCOCORTICOIDS FOR PNEUMONIA

There has been interest in using glucocorticoids as adjunctive therapy to antibiotics in hospitalized patients with CAP in an attempt to reduce the inflammatory response to pneumonia, which is likely to contribute to the morbidity of the disease. Individual randomized trials regarding the efficacy of adjunctive glucocorticoids have shown varying results; but most showing some benefit.[81–88] A recent meta-analysis provides additional evidence of the potential benefit of glucocorticoid use for patients requiring hospitalization for CAP. Siemieniuk and colleagues[87] evaluated 12 randomized clinical trials of the use of glucocorticoids in hospitalized adults with CAP. They evaluated complication rate, mortality, time to clinical stability, and length of hospital stay. Patients who received adjunctive steroids had a reduction in all-cause mortality of borderline significance (RR 0.67, 95% confidence interval 0.45–1.01) as well as a reduction in the use of mechanical ventilation and ARDS. Such patients also had decreased time to clinical stability and decreased duration of hospital stay. They also had an increased frequency of hyperglycemia requiring treatment but no increase in the rate of gastrointestinal bleeding. Subgroup analyses suggested that the relative effect on mortality varied according to severity of CAP, with a mortality benefit observed in those with SCAP but not in those with less severe CAP. Many of the trials in the meta-analysis excluded patients at an increased risk of adverse effects from glucocorticoids, including immunocompromised patients, pregnant women, patients who had gastrointestinal bleeding within the past 3 months, and patients at an increased risk of neuropsychiatric side effects. It should be noted that different glucocorticoid formulations (eg, intravenous methylprednisolone, oral prednisone), doses, and routes of administration were used in different trials; the optimal regimen is unknown. In most trials, patients received glucocorticoids for 5 to 7 days.

Based on the present evidence, it is reasonable to consider adjunctive glucocorticoid therapy for hospitalized patients who are at substantial risk of morbidity and mortality (eg, severe pneumonia requiring ICU admission or those who have elevated C-reactive protein). There remains work to be done in determining the optimal standard of steroid therapy, especially considering the different manifestations of CAP. Currently, the US Department of Veterans Affairs is conducting a trial, the Extended Steroid in CAP (e) (ESCAPe) study, in which hospitalized patients with CAP requiring ICU care are randomly assigned to placebo or methylprednisolone at an initial dosage of either 40 mg or 20 mg/d for 7 days, followed by tapering doses over 13 days.[86] Results will provide further information concerning the utility of steroids.

COMPONENTS OF CARE OTHER THAN ANTIBIOTIC THERAPY

Patients who are ill enough to require admission to the hospital for treatment of pneumonia require careful monitoring with at least a once-daily physician examination. Oxygen should be administered when the oxygen saturation is 92% or less. Treatment of comorbid illnesses should be optimized.[89–92]

In a study of 399 patients with CAP treated on an ambulatory basis, symptoms had resolved within 14 days in 67%. The mean time to return to work in this population was 6 days compared with a median of 22 days for those who required hospitalization.[89] For hospitalized patients, unstable vital signs within 24 hours before discharge (temperature $\geq37.8°C$; heart rate >100/min; respiratory rate >24/min; systolic blood pressure <90 mm Hg; oxygen saturation <90%; inability to maintain oral intake; abnormal mental status) were associated with higher death and readmission rates.[90] Indeed patients with 2 or more instabilities had a 5-fold greater risk-adjusted odds of death or readmission.[90] Thus, patients should not be discharged until vital signs are stable.

About 10% of patients with pneumonia fail to improve or actually get worse over the first few days in the hospital. When this happens, an organized approach is necessary to determine why (see **Box 3**).

LONG-TERM OUTCOMES OF PNEUMONIA

There have been several studies whereby the long-term outcomes of patients with CAP have been studied. In one such study, 3284 patients with pneumonia were followed for a median of 3.8 years.[93] The 30-day, 1-year, and end-of-study mortality rates were 12%, 28%, and 53%, respectively. Of 2950 patients who survived the initial CAP hospitalization, 72% were hospitalized again (median, 2 admissions over follow-up) and 16% were rehospitalized with pneumonia.[93] These data raise the question of whether an episode of pneumonia results in a long-term increase in mortality over what would be expected for an age- and sex-matched population without pneumonia. A total of 6078 patients with pneumonia were age, sex, and site of treatment matched with 5 nonpneumonia controls (n = 29,402).[94] Over a median of 9.8 years, patients with pneumonia experienced 70 deaths per 1000 patient-year's versus 40 per 1000 for the nonpneumonia group (adjusted hazard ratio 1.65 [1.57–1.73] $P<.001$). The highest rate difference was seen among patients less than 25 years of age with 6 versus 2 deaths per 1000 patient-years.[94] These findings are similar to those of Waterer and colleagues.[95] Some investigators have postulated this increased mortality is due to increased procoagulant activity following pneumonia.[96] Brown and colleagues[97] found that patients, monkeys, and mice with S pneumoniae bacteremia developed microscopic lesions within the myocardium. A meta-analysis of the incidence of cardiovascular events within 30 days of hospital admission for CAP found a cumulative rate of heart failure of 14%, arrhythmia of 5%, and acute coronary syndrome of 5%.[98]

REFERENCES

1. Marrie TJ, Campbell GD, Walker DH, et al. Harrisons principles of internal medicine. New York: McGraw- Hill, Medical Publishing Division; 2005.
2. Marston BJ, Plouffe JF, File TM Jr, et al. Incidence of community-acquired pneumonia requiring hospitalization: results of a population-based active surveillance study in Ohio. Arch Intern Med 1997;157:1709–18.
3. Marrie TJ. Epidemiology of community-acquired pneumonia in the elderly. Semin Respir Infect 1990;5:250–8.
4. Marrie TJ, Huang JQ. Epidemiology of community-acquired pneumonia in Edmonton, Alberta: an emergency department based study. Can Respir J 2005; 12:139–42.
5. Jackson ML, Neuzil KM, Thompson WW, et al. The burden of community-acquired pneumonia in seniors: results of a population-based study. Clin Infect Dis 2004;39:1642–50.
6. Wortham JM, Shapiro DJ, Hersh AL, et al. Burden of ambulatory visits and antibiotic prescribing patterns for adults with community-acquired pneumonia in the United States, 1998 through 2009. JAMA Intern Med 2014;174:1520–1.

7. Baik I, Curhan GC, Rimm EB, et al. A prospective study of age and life-style factors in relation to community acquired pneumonia in US men and women. Arch Intern Med 2000;160:3082–8.
8. Koivula I, Stenn M, Makela PH. Risk factors for pneumonia in the elderly. Am J Med 1994;96:313–20.
9. Lipsky BA, Boyko EJ, Inui TS, et al. Risk factors for acquiring pneumococcal infections. Arch Intern Med 1986;146:2179–85.
10. Nuorti JP, Butler JC, Farley MM, et al. Cigarette smoking and invasive pneumococcal disease. N Engl J Med 2000;342:681–9.
11. Plouffe JF, Breiman RE, Facklam RR. Bacteremia with *Streptococcus pneumoniae*. Implications for therapy and prevention. The Franklin County Pneumonia Study Group. JAMA 1996;275:194–8.
12. Marston BJ, Lipman HB, Breiman RF. Surveillance for legionnaires' disease. Risk factors for morbidity and mortality. Arch Intern Med 1994;154:2417–22.
13. Eurich DT, Lee C, Marrie TJ, et al. Inhaled corticosteroids and risk of recurrent pneumonia: a population based, nested case-control study. Clin Infect Dis 2013;57:1138–44.
14. Gambassi G, Sultana J, Trifiro G. Antipsychotic use elderly patients and risk of pneumonia. Expert Opin Drug Saf 2015;14:1–6.
15. Paul KJ, Walker RL, Dublin S. Anticholinergic medications and risk of community-acquired pneumonia in elderly adults: a population based case-control study. J Am Geriatr Soc 2015;63:476–85.
16. Linuma T, Arai Y, Abe Y, et al. Denture wearing during sleep doubles the risk of pneumonia in the very elderly. J Dent Res 2015;94(3 Suppl):28S–36S.
17. Morens DM, Taubenberger JK, Fauci AS. Predominant role of bacterial pneumonia as a cause of death in pandemic influenza: implications for pandemic influenza preparedness. J Infect Dis 2008;198:962–70.
18. Campigotto A, Mubareka S. Influenza-associated bacterial pneumonia; managing and controlling infection on two fronts. Expert Rev Anti Infect Ther 2015;13:55–68.
19. Weinberger DM, Klugman KP, Steiner CA, et al. Association between respiratory syncytial virus activity and pneumococcal disease in infants: a time series analysis of United States hospitalization data. PLoS Med 2015;12(1):e1001776.
20. Shah S, McArthur E, Farag A, et al. Risk of hospitalization for community-acquired pneumonia with renin-angiotensin blockade in elderly patients: a population based study. PLoS One 2014;9(10):e110165.
21. Quinton LJ, Mizgerd JP. Dynamics of lung defense in pneumonia: resistance, resilience and remodeling. Annu Rev Physiol 2015;77:407–30.
22. Johanson WG, Pierce AK, Sanford JP. Changing pharyngeal bacterial colonization during viral illness. N Engl J Med 1969;281:1137–40.
23. Fuxench-Lopea Z, Ramirez-Ronda C. Pharyngeal flora in ambulatory alcoholic patients: prevalence of gram negative bacilli. Arch Intern Med 1978;138:1815–6.
24. Valenti WM, Trudell RG, Bentley DW. Factors predisposing to oropharyngeal colonization with gram negative bacteria in the aged. N Engl J Med 1978;298:1108–11.
25. Woods DE, Strauss DC, Johanson WG Jr, et al. Role of salivary protease activity in adherence of gram-negative bacilli to mammalian buccal epithelial cells in vivo. J Clin Invest 1981;68:1435–40.
26. Woods DE, Strauss DC, Johanson WG Jr, et al. Role of fibronectin in the prevention of adherence of *Pseudomonas aeruginosa* to buccal cells. J Infect Dis 1981;143:784–90.

27. Kikuchi R, Watabe N, Konno T, et al. High incidence of silent aspiration in elderly patients with community-acquired pneumonia. Am J Respir Crit Care Med 1994; 150:251–3.

28. Horner J, Alberts MJ, Davison DV, et al. Swallowing in Alzheimer's disease. Alzheimer Dis Assoc Disord 1994;8:177–89.

29. Horner J, Massey EW, Riski JE, et al. Aspiration following stroke: clinical correlates and outcome. Neurology 1988;38:1359–62.

30. Croghan JE, Burke EM, Caplan S, et al. Pilot study of 12-month outcomes of nursing home patients with aspiration on videofluoroscopy. Dysphagia 1994;9: 141–6.

31. Weir DL, Majumdar SR, McAlister FA, et al. The impact of multimorbidity on short-term events in patients with community-acquired pneumonia – a prospective cohort study. Clin Microbiol Infect 2015;21(3):264.e7–13.

32. Fine MJ, Stone RA, Singer DE, et al. Processes and outcomes of care for patients with community-acquired pneumonia. Results from the Pneumonia Patient Outcomes Research Team (PORT) study. Arch Intern Med 1999;159:970–80.

33. Clegg A, Young J, Lliffe S, et al. Frailty in elderly people. Lancet 2013;381: 752–62.

34. Torres A, Blasi F, Peetermans WE, et al. The aetiology and antibiotic management of community-acquired pneumonia in adults in Europe: a literature review. Eur J Clin Microbiol Infect Dis 2014;33:1065–79.

35. Prina E, Ranzani OT, Torres A. Community-acquired pneumonia. Lancet 2015; 386(9998):1097–108.

36. Jeong BH, Koh WJ, Yoo H, et al. Risk factors for acquiring potentially drug resistant pathogens in immunocompetent patients with pneumonia developed out of hospital. Respiration 2014;88:190–8.

37. Wunderink RG, Waterer GW. Community-acquired pneumonia. N Engl J Med 2014;370:543–50.

38. Lee JS, Nsa W, Hausmann LRM, et al. Quality of care for elderly patients hospitalized for pneumonia in the United States, 2006 to 2010. JAMA Intern Med 2014; 174:1806–14.

39. Templeton KE, Scheltinga SA, van den Eden WC, et al. Improved diagnosis of the etiology of community-acquired pneumonia with real time polymerase chain reaction. Clin Infect Dis 2005;41:345–51.

40. Musher DM, Roig IL, Cazares G, et al. Can an etiologic agent be identified in adults who are hospitalized for community-acquired pneumonia: results of a one-year study. J Infect 2013;67:11–8.

41. Jain S, Self WH, Wunderink S, et al. Community-acquired pneumonia requiring hospitalization among United States adults. N Engl J Med 2015;373:415–27.

42. Falsey AR, Becker KL, Swinburne AJ, et al. Bacterial complications of respiratory tract viral illness: a comprehensive evaluation. J Infect Dis 2013;208:432–41.

43. Marrie TJ, Haldane EV, Faulkner RS, et al. Community-acquired pneumonia is it different in the elderly. J Am Geriatr Soc 1985;33:671–80.

44. StrauB R, Ewig S, Richler K, et al. The prognostic significance of respiratory rate in patients with pneumonia. Dtsch Arztebl Int 2014;111:503–8.

45. Warnier MJ, Rutten FH, de Boer A, et al. Resting heart rate is a risk factor for mortality in chronic obstructive pulmonary disease, but not for exacerbations or pneumonia. PLoS One 2014;9(8):e105152.

46. Majumdar SR, Eurich DT, Gamble JM, et al. Oxygen saturations less than 92% are associated with major adverse events in outpatients with pneumonia: a population-based cohort study. Clin Infect Dis 2011;521:325–31.

47. Metlay JP, Schulz R, Yi-Hwei L, et al. Influence of age on symptoms at presentation in patients with community-acquired pneumonia. Arch Intern Med 1997;157: 1453–9.

48. El-Solh AA, Niederman MS, Drinka P. Nursing home acquired pneumonia: a review of risk factors and therapeutic approaches. Curr Med Res Opin 2010;26: 2707–14.

49. Hagaman JT, Rouan GW, Shipley RT, et al. Admission chest radiograph lacks sensitivity in the diagnosis of community-acquired pneumonia. Am J Med Sci 2009;337:236–40.

50. Hayden GE, Wrenn KW. Chest radiography vs computed tomography scan in the evaluation of pneumonia. J Emerg Med 2009;36:266–70.

51. Basi SJ, Marrie TJ, Huang JQ, et al. Patients admitted to hospital with suspected pneumonia and normal chest radiographs: epidemiology, microbiology and outcomes. Am J Med 2004;117:305–11.

52. Hopstaken RM, Witbraad T, van Engelshoven JMA, et al. Inter-observer variation in the interpretation of chest radiographs for pneumonia in community-acquired lower respiratory tract infections. Clin Radiol 2004;59:743–52.

53. Loeb MB, Carusone SBC, Marrie TJ, et al. Inter observer reliability of radiologists' interpretation of mobile chest radiographs for nursing home-acquired pneumonia. J Am Med Dir Assoc 2006;7:416–9.

54. Chavez MA, Shams N, Ellington LE, et al. Lung ultrasound for the diagnosis of pneumonia in adults: a systematic review and meta-analysis. Respir Res 2014; 15:50.

55. Lisboa T, Blot S, Waterer GW, et al. Radiologic progression of pulmonary infiltrates predicts a worse prognosis in severe community-acquired pneumonia than bacteremia. Chest 2009;135:165–72.

56. Ahmed RA, Marrie TJ, Huang JQ. Thoracic empyema in patients with community-acquired pneumonia. Am J Med 2006;119:877–83.

57. El Sohl A, Aquilna A, Gunen H, et al. Radiographic resolution of community-acquired pneumonia in the elderly. J Am Geriatr Soc 2004;52:224–9.

58. Tang KL, Eurich DT, Minhas-Sandhu JK, et al. Incidence, correlates, and chest radiographic yield of new lung cancer in 3398 patients with pneumonia. Arch Intern Med 2011;171:1193–8.

59. Yin J, Marrie TJ, Carriere KC, et al. Variation in management of community-acquired pneumonia requiring admission to Alberta, Canada hospitals. Epidemiol Infect 2003;130:41–51.

60. Fine MJ, Auble TE, Yealy DM, et al. A prediction rule to identify low-risk patients with community-acquired pneumonia. N Engl J Med 1997;336:243–50.

61. Niederman MS, Feldman C, Richards GA. Combining information from prognostic scoring tools for CAP: an American view on how to get the best of all worlds. Eur Respir J 2006;27:9–11.

62. Lim WS, van der Eerden MM, Laing R, et al. Defining community acquired pneumonia severity on presentation to hospital: an international derivation and validation study. Thorax 2003;58:377–82.

63. Mandell LA, Wunderink RG, Anzueto A, et al. Infectious Diseases Society of America/American Thoracic Society consensus guidelines on the management of community-acquired pneumonia in adults. Clin Infect Dis 2007;44(Suppl 2): S27–72.

64. Phua J, See KC, Chan YH, et al. Validation and clinical implications of the IDSA/ATS minor criteria for severe community-acquired pneumonia. Thorax 2009;64: 598–603.

65. Chalmers JD, Taylor JK, Mandal P, et al. Validation of the Infectious Diseases Society of America/American Thoracic Society minor criteria for intensive care unit admission in community-acquired pneumonia patients without major criteria or contraindications to intensive care unit care. Clin Infect Dis 2011;53:503–11.

66. Liapikou A, Ferrer M, Polverino E, et al. Severe community-acquired pneumonia: validation of the Infectious Diseases Society of America/American Thoracic Society guidelines to predict an intensive care unit admission. Clin Infect Dis 2009;48: 377–85.

67. Charles PG, Wolfe R, Whitby M, et al. SMART-COP: a tool for predicting the need for intensive respiratory or vasopressor support in community-acquired pneumonia. Clin Infect Dis 2008;47:375–84.

68. Espana PP, Capelastegui A, Mar C, et al. Performance of proadrenomedullin for identifying adverse outcomes in community-acquired pneumonia. J Infect 2015; 70:457–66.

69. Valley TS, Sjoding MW, Ryan AM, et al. Association of intensive care unit admission with mortality among older patients with pneumonia. JAMA 2015;314:1272–9.

70. Rautanen A, Mills TC, Gordon AC, et al. Genome-wide association study of survival from sepsis due to pneumonia: an observational cohort study. Lancet Respir Med 2015;3:53–60.

71. Misch EA, Verban A, Prins JM, et al. A TLR6 polymorphism is associated with an increased risk of legionnaires' disease. Genes Immun 2013;14:420–6.

72. Postma DF, van Werkhoven CH, van Elden LJR, et al. Antibiotic treatment strategies for community-acquired pneumonia in adults. N Engl J Med 2015;372: 1312–23.

73. Asadi L, Eurich DT, Gamble JM, et al. Guideline adherence and macrolides reduced mortality in outpatients with pneumonia. Respir Med 2012;106:451–8.

74. Asadi L, Eurich DT, Gamble M, et al. Impact of guideline concurrent antibiotics and macrolide beta lactam combinations in 3202 patients hospitalized with community-acquired pneumonia: prospective cohort study. Clin Microbiol Infect 2013;19:257–64.

75. Musher DM, Thorner AR. Community-acquired pneumonia. N Engl J Med 2014; 371:1619–28.

76. Sligl WI, Hoang H, Eurich DT, et al. Macrolide use in treatment of critically ill patients with pneumonia: incidence, correlates, timing and outcomes. Can J Infect Dis Med Microbiol 2013;24:e107–12.

77. Sligl WI, Asadi L, Eurich DT, et al. Macrolides and mortality in critically ill patients with community-acquired pneumonia: a systematic review and meta-analysis. Crit Care Med 2014;42:420–32.

78. Marrie TJ, Lau CY, Wheeler SL, et al. A controlled trial of a critical pathway for treatment of community-acquired pneumonia. CAPITAL Study Investigators. Community-Acquired Pneumonia Intervention Trial Assessing Levofloxacin. JAMA 2000;283:749–55.

79. Marrie TJ. The halo effect of adherence to guidelines extends to patients with severe pneumonia admitted to an intensive care unit. Clin Infect Dis 2005;41: 1717–9.

80. Falcone M, Russo A, Congemi RE, et al. Lower mortality with community-acquired pneumonia on treatment with aspirin. J Am Heart Assoc 2015;4:e001595.

81. Confalonieri M, Urbino R, Potena A, et al. Hydrocortisone infusion for severe community-acquired pneumonia: a preliminary randomized study. Am J Respir Crit Care Med 2005;171:242.

82. Garcia-Vidal C, Calbo E, Pascual V, et al. Effects of systemic steroids in patients with severe community-acquired pneumonia. Eur Respir J 2007;30:951.

83. Snijders D, Daniels JM, de Graaff CS, et al. Efficacy of corticosteroids in community-acquired pneumonia: a randomized double-blinded clinical trial. Am J Respir Crit Care Med 2010;181:975.

84. Meijvis SC, Hardeman H, Remmelts HH, et al. Dexamethasone and length of hospital stay in patients with community-acquired pneumonia: a randomised, double-blind, placebo-controlled trial. Lancet 2011;377:2023.

85. Blum CA, Nigro N, Briel M, et al. Adjunct prednisone therapy for patients with community-acquired pneumonia: a multicentre, double-blind, randomised, placebo-controlled trial. Lancet 2015;385:1511.

86. Torres A, Sibila O, Ferrer M, et al. Effect of corticosteroids on treatment failure among hospitalized patients with severe community-acquired pneumonia and high inflammatory response: a randomized clinical trial. JAMA 2015;313:677.

87. Siemieniuk RA, Meade MO, Alonso-Coello P, et al. Corticosteroid therapy for patients hospitalized with community-acquired pneumonia: a systematic review and meta-analysis. Ann Intern Med 2015;163(7):519–28.

88. Clinicaltrials.gov. Extended Steroid in CAP(e) (ESCAPe). Available at: https://clinicaltrials.gov/ct2/show/NCT01283009?term=Extended+Steroid+in+CAP%28e%29+%28ESCAPe%29&rank=1. Accessed August 24, 2015.

89. Sin DD, Man SF, Marrie TJ. Arterial carbon dioxide tension on admission as a marker of in-hospital mortality in community-acquired pneumonia. Am J Med 2005;118(2):145–50.

90. McAlister FA, Rowe BH, Majumdar SR, et al. The relation between hyperglycemia and outcomes in 2,471 patients admitted to the hospital with community-acquired pneumonia. Diabetes Care 2005;28:810–5.

91. Marrie TJ, Beecroft MD, Herman-Gnjidic Z. Resolution of symptoms in patients with community-acquired pneumonia treated on an ambulatory basis. J Infect 2004;49(4):302–9.

92. Halm EA, Fine MJ, Kapoor WN, et al. Instability on hospital discharge and the risk of adverse outcomes in patients with pneumonia. Arch Intern Med 2002;162:1278–84.

93. Johnstone J, Eurich DT, Majumdar SR, et al. Long term morbidity and mortality after hospitalization with community acquired pneumonia. A population based cohort study. Medicine (Baltimore) 2008;87:329–34.

94. Eurich DT, Marrie TJ, Minhas-Sandhu JK, et al. Ten year mortality following community-acquired pneumonia. Am J Respir Crit Care Med 2015;192:597–604.

95. Waterer GW, Kessler LA, Wunderink RG. Medium-term survival after hospitalization with community-acquired pneumonia. Am J Respir Crit Care Med 2004;169:910–4.

96. Corrales-Medina VF, Alvarez KN, Weissfeld LA, et al. Association between hospitalization for pneumonia and subsequent risk of cardiovascular disease. JAMA 2015;313:264–74.

97. Brown AO, Mann B, Gao G. *Streptococcus pneumoniae* translocates into the myocardium and forms unique microlesions that disrupt cardiac function. PLoS Pathog 2014;10(9):e1004383.

98. Corrales-Medina VF, Suh KN, Rose G, et al. Cardiac complications in patients with community-acquired pneumonia: a systematic review and meta-analysis of observational studies. PLoS Med 2011;8:e1001048.

Tuberculosis in Older Adults

Shobita Rajagopalan, MD, MSCR, MPH[a,b,]*

KEYWORDS

- Tuberculosis • Infection • Aging • Long-term care

KEY POINTS

- Tuberculosis (TB) remains one of the world's most lethal infectious diseases.
- Preventive and control strategies among other high-risk groups such as the elderly population continues to be a challenge.
- Clinical features of TB in older adults may be atypical and confused with age-related diseases.
- Underlying diseases, malnutrition, and biological changes with aging can contribute to age-associated decline in cellular immune responses to infecting agents such as *Mycobacterium tuberculosis*.
- Diagnosis and management of TB in the elderly person may be difficult; treatment can be associated with adverse drug reactions; the institutionalized elderly adult is at high risk both for reactivation of latent TB and to new TB infection.

INTRODUCTION

Tuberculosis (TB) continues to be a significant global health concern and ranks alongside the human immunodeficiency virus (HIV) as the leading cause of death from infectious diseases worldwide. Although since 1990, there has been a steady decline in TB cases each year, the current mortality rates for this treatable illness remain relatively high.

In the United States, during the past 3 decades, the excess in morbidity reflected a changing epidemiologic pattern. Human immunodeficiency virus (HIV) infection, poverty, homelessness, substance abuse, and immigration from countries with a high prevalence of TB have all contributed to this TB morbidity. Since the mid-1990s, aggressive TB control measures, and implementation and enhanced resource frameworks have resulted in a substantial decline in the overall incidence of TB.

[a] Los Angeles County Department of Public Health, 123 West Manchester Boulevard, Inglewood, CA 90301, USA; [b] Charles R. Drew University of Medicine and Science, Los Angeles, CA, USA
* 123 West Manchester Boulevard, Inglewood, CA 90301.
E-mail address: srajagopalan@ph.lacounty.gov

Clin Geriatr Med 32 (2016) 479–491
http://dx.doi.org/10.1016/j.cger.2016.02.006   **geriatric.theclinics.com**
0749-0690/16/$ – see front matter © 2016 Elsevier Inc. All rights reserved.

The geriatric population across all racial and ethnic groups and both genders is at substantial risk for *Mycobacterium tuberculosis* infection, perhaps because of both biological (compromised nutrition and immune status, underlying disease, medications, and possible racial predisposition) and socioeconomic factors (poverty, living conditions, and access to health care). Frail elderly residents of nursing homes and other long-term care settings are the most vulnerable group. Because of the highly communicable potential of *M tuberculosis,* the inevitable endemic transmission between residents and from residents to staff remains a concern in such facilities. (For clarity, TB infection, or latent TB, refers to contained and asymptomatic primary infection with a positive TB screening test [tuberculin skin test reaction or interferon-gamma release assay (IGRA) test], whereas TB disease indicates overt clinical manifestations of TB.)

This article reviews the current global epidemiology, pathogenesis, clinical characteristics, diagnosis, management, and prevention of *M tuberculosis* infection in community-dwelling and institutionalized aging adults.

EPIDEMIOLOGY

More than 2 billion people (approximately one-third of the world's population) are reported to be infected with TB.[1] Recent reports on the TB burden of disease from the World Health Organization (WHO) estimate 9.9 million incident cases (of whom 13% were HIV-positive in 2013), 9.6 to 13.3 million prevalent cases, 1.5 million deaths, 1.1 million of whom were among HIV-negative persons, and 0.4 million among HIV-positive people.[1] Among these deaths 210,000 were attributed to multiple drug–resistant (MDR)-TB, a relatively high total compared with 480,000 incident cases of MDR-TB.

In the United States since 1992, there has been an overall decline in the absolute number of TB cases and the TB case rates by greater than 45%.[2,3] The total case count of 9421 and case rate of 3.0 per 100,000 persons represent steady progress toward the goal of TB elimination in the United States (<1 case per 1,000,000 population). This downward trend in TB cases has been largely because of improved funding resources channeled into TB control programs, which allowed for the implementation of directly observed therapy (DOT). However, despite consistent declines in TB cases and case rates over the past 60 years, this year's decline in the rate of TB (−2.2%) was the smallest decrease in more than a decade. In addition, the percentage of cases among foreign-born persons has continued to rise disproportionately. In 2014, a total of 66% of reported TB cases in the United States occurred among foreign-born persons. The case rate among foreign-born persons (15.4 cases per 100,000 persons) was approximately 13 times higher than among US-born persons (1.2 cases per 100,000 persons).

US national data indicate that the rate of TB is 30% higher in older adults than their younger counterparts; US-born and non-Hispanic whites are more commonly affected and Asians have the highest TB incidence rates per 100,000.[4] Elders living in communal settings, such as nursing homes or other long-term care facilities (LTCFs), have a TB incidence rate approximately 4 times greater than the general population.[5] The aggregate TB incidence rate for nursing home residents is 1.8 times higher than the rate seen in community-dwelling elderly adults.[6] The enhanced efficiency of TB transmissibility within congregate settings, such as prisons, nursing facilities (nursing homes), chronic disease facilities, and homeless shelters, has raised concerns about TB infection and disease in the institutionalized elderly group.[7,8] Positive tuberculin reactivity associated with

prolonged stay among residents of long-term care facilities for the elderly population has been demonstrated, implying an increasing risk of TB infection. A recent
prospective surveillance study of nursing home and community-dwelling older
adults in California from 2000 to 2009 demonstrated that although there was a
lower incidence of TB infection in nursing home residents compared with
community elders, the mortality in nursing home–residing elderly adults was significantly higher; this difference was attributed to increased comorbid illnesses, debil-
ity, and frailty in nursing home residents, which enhances the risk of TB
reactivation.[9]

Thus, TB control measures must focus on highest-risk populations for TB, such as
persons born in high-burden countries and residents of congregate settings, such as
elderly residents of LTCFs. Strong emphasis must be placed on refined surveillance
strategies, contact investigations, and screening and treating of contacts with latent
TB infection (LTBI).

PATHOGENESIS

The pathogenesis of TB infection and disease begins in most cases with the inhalation
of the tubercle bacilli.[9] The usual inoculum is no more than 1 to 3 organisms, which are
taken up by alveolar macrophages and carried to regional lymph nodes. Spread may
occur via the lymphohematogenous route with dissemination to multiple organs. From
2 to 8 weeks after infection, cell-mediated immunity (CMI) and delayed-type hypersensitivity (DTH) responses develop, leading to the characteristic reactive tuberculin test
and to the containment of infection. Chemoattractants cause monocytes to enter the
area and become transformed into histiocytes forming granulomas. Although the
bacilli may persist within macrophages, additional multiplication and spread is cur-
tailed. Healing usually follows with calcification of the infected focus. Caseous necrosis may result secondary to the immune response. Erosion into a bronchiole causes
cavity formation where bacilli can multiply and spread. Solid necrosis can result
from production of hydrolases from inflammatory cells causing tissue liquefaction
and creating a prime medium for microbial replication, generating up to 10 billion
bacilli per milliliter. Individuals who develop active disease either fail to contain the primary infection or develop reactivation as a result of relative or absolute immune suppression at a point remote from primary infection. This is most likely to occur in
immunocompetent adults within the first 3 years after exposure. Factors related to
progression of disease reflect a weakened immune status and include physiologic
states, for example, normal aging; associated intercurrent disease, particularly diabetes mellitus, malignancies causing primary immunosuppression, or requiring toxic
chemotherapy, or corticosteroid-dependent diseases, such as asthma or collagen
vascular disease; poor nutritional status particularly related to alcohol and drug abuse;
smoking; and HIV infection. Although it is likely that the increased frequency of TB in
the elderly person could partly be due to CMI that is impaired by senescence (shown in
murine models), other concomitant age-related diseases (diabetes mellitus, malignancy), chronic kidney disease, and renal insufficiency, poor nutrition, and immunosuppressive drugs may also contribute to this increase.[10] In the elderly population,
approximately 90% of TB disease cases are due to reactivation of primary infection.
Persistent infection without disease may occur in 30% to 50% of individuals. Some
elderly persons previously infected with *M tuberculosis* may eventually eliminate the
viable tubercle bacilli and revert to a negative tuberculin reactor state. These individuals are therefore at risk for new infection (reinfection) with *M tuberculosis*. There are
therefore 3 subgroups of older persons potentially at risk for TB: one subgroup never

exposed to TB that may develop primary TB disease, a second subgroup with persistent and latent primary infection that may reactivate, and a third subgroup that is no longer infected and consequently at risk for reinfection.

CLINICAL CHARACTERISTICS

Clinicians must be aware that frail older persons with TB disease may not demonstrate the overt and characteristic clinical features of TB, such as fever, night sweats, or hemoptysis. They may exhibit atypical and subtle clinical manifestations of "failure to thrive" with loss of appetite, functional decline, and low-grade fever or weight loss.[8] Although several published works have attempted to delineate clear differences between younger and older TB patients, such studies have provided variable findings. In a meta-analysis of published studies, comparing pulmonary TB in older and younger patients, evaluating the differences in the clinical, radiologic, and laboratory features of pulmonary TB, no differences were found in the prevalence of cough, sputum production, weight loss, fatigue/malaise, radiographic upper lobe lesions, positive acid-fast bacilli (AFB) in sputum, anemia or hemoglobin level, and serum aminotransferases.[11] A lower prevalence of fever, sweating, hemoptysis, cavitary disease, and positive purified protein derivative (PPD), and also lower levels of serum albumin and blood leukocytes, were noticed among older patients. In addition, the older population had a greater prevalence of dyspnea and some underlying comorbid conditions, such as cardiovascular disorders, chronic obstructive pulmonary disease, diabetes mellitus, gastrectomy history, and malignancies. This meta-analytical review identified some subtle differences in clinical presentations of older TB patients compared with their younger TB counterparts. However, most of these differences can be explained by the already known physiologic changes that occur during aging. Most older patients with TB (75%) with *M tuberculosis* disease manifest active disease in their lungs.[11] Extrapulmonary TB in elderly adults is similar to that in younger persons and may involve the meninges, bone and joint, and genitourinary systems or disseminate in a military pattern.[12–17] Infection of lymph nodes, pleura, pericardium, peritoneum, gall bladder, small and large bowel, the middle ear, and carpal tunnel have been described in the literature. Because TB can involve virtually any organ in the body, this infection must be kept in the differential diagnosis of unusual presentations of diseases, especially in the elderly. Thus, TB has been aptly described as "the great masquerader" of many diseases.

DIAGNOSIS

Clinicians caring for the elderly must maintain a high index of suspicion for TB when possible, so as to recognize and treat infected individuals promptly.

Tuberculin Skin Testing

The Mantoux method of tuberculin skin testing (TST) using the Tween-stabilized PPD antigen is one of the diagnostic modalities readily available to screen for TB infection, despite its potential for false-negative results.[18] In the elderly person, because of the increase in anergy to cutaneous antigens, the 2-step TST is suggested as part of the initial geriatric assessment to avoid overlooking potentially false-negative reaction.[19] The American Geriatrics Society routinely recommends 2-step TST as part of the baseline information for all institutionalized elderly.[20] The 2-step TST involves initial intradermal placement of 5 tuberculin units of PPD and the results are read at 48 to 72 hours. Patients are retested within 2 weeks after a negative response (induration of <10 mm). A positive "booster effect," and therefore a positive TST reaction, is a skin test of 10 mm or more and an increase of 6 mm or more over the first skin test reaction. It is important to distinguish the booster phenomenon from a true tuberculin conversion. The booster effect occurs in a person previously infected with *M tuberculosis* but who has a false-negative skin test; repeat skin test elicits a truly positive test. Conversion (not to be confused with the booster phenomenon) occurs in persons previously uninfected with *M tuberculosis* and who have had a true negative tuberculin skin test, but who become infected within 2 years as demonstrated by a repeat skin test induration that is a positive 10 mm or more during this period. Several factors influence the results and interpretation of the TST. Decreased skin test reactivity is associated with waning DTH with time, disseminated TB, corticosteroids and other drugs, and other diseases in addition to the elimination of TB infection. False-positive TST results occur with cross-reactions with nontuberculous mycobacteria and in persons receiving the Bacillus Calmette-Guerin (BCG) vaccine, the latter having been administered to some foreign-born elderly persons, which has an unpredictable effect on the TST reactivity and is presumed to wane after 10 years. The use of anergy testing has been debated because of lack of a standardized protocol for selection of the number and type of antigens to be used, the criteria for defining positive and negative reactions, and administration and interpretation techniques.[21]

Interferon-Gamma Release Assays

In 2005, the Centers for Disease Control and Prevention (CDC) published guidelines for using an interferon-gamma release assay (IGRA) known as the QuantiFERON-TB Gold test (QFT-G) (Cellestis, Carnegie, Victoria, Australia).[22] Subsequently, 2 new IGRAs were approved by the US Food and Drug Administration (FDA) as aids in diagnosing both TB infection and disease. These tests are the QuantiFERON-TB Gold In-Tube test (QFT- GIT) (Cellestis) and the T-SPOT TB test (T-Spot) (Oxford Immunotec, Abingdon, UK). The antigens, methods, and interpretation criteria for these assays differ from those for IGRAs approved previously by the FDA. This in vitro test measures by an enzyme-linked immunosorbent assay (ELISA) the concentration of interferon-gamma (IFN-gamma) released from tuberculin. PPD sensitized lymphocytes in heparinized whole blood incubated for 16 to 24 hours. Interpretation of QFT results is stratified by estimated risk for *M tuberculosis* infection in a manner similar to the tuberculin skin test using different induration cutoff values.

Currently, IGRAs are the preferred method of testing for persons who have poor rates of return for TST reading and interpretation (eg, homeless persons), previous BCG vaccination, and for immunocompromised patients with high likelihood of TST anergy. TST is the preferred method for testing of immunocompetent US-born adults and for children younger than 5 years. Either TST or IGRA may be used without preference for other groups that are tested for LTBI.

Chest Radiography and Computer-Aided Diagnosis

Chest radiography is indicated in all individuals with suspected TB infection, regardless of the primary site of infection. In the elderly population, 75% of all TB disease occurs in the respiratory tract and largely represents reactivation disease; 10% to 20% of cases may be as a result of primary infection.[23] Although reactivation TB disease characteristically involves the apical and posterior segments of the upper lobes of the lungs, several studies have shown that many elderly patients manifest their pulmonary infection in either the middle or lower lobes or the pleura, and also present with interstitial, patchy, or cavitary infiltrates that may be bilateral. Primary TB can involve any lung segment, but more often tends to involve the middle or lower lobes in addition to mediastinal or hilar lymph nodes. Therefore, caution must be exercised in dismissing the radiographic diagnosis of pulmonary TB in the elderly adult because of the atypical location of the infection in the lung fields. Computer-aided diagnosis (CAD) with digital chest radiograph (CXR) programs for scoring CXRs of patients with presumptive TB is being considered in resource-poor settings. A recent study showed that the CAD program had high sensitivity but low specificity and positive predictive value.[24]

Laboratory Diagnosis

Laboratory tests currently include microscopy, culture (liquid and sold media), and traditional drug susceptibility testing, nucleic acid amplification technologies (NAATs), and sequencing methods for drug resistance (GeneXpert [Cepheid, Inc, Sunnyvale, CA, USA] and pyrosequencing [PSQ]), biomarkers to detect active or latent TB, serodiagnostic assays, and volatile organic compounds (VOC).[25–27]

Sputum samples must be collected from all patients, regardless of age, with pulmonary symptoms or CXR changes compatible with TB disease and who have not been previously treated with antituberculous agents. In elderly patients unable to expectorate sputum, other diagnostic techniques such as sputum induction or bronchoscopy should be considered. Flexible bronchoscopy to obtain bronchial washings and to perform bronchial biopsies has been shown to be of diagnostic value for TB disease in the elderly adult; however, in frail and very old patients, the risk of such a procedure must be carefully balanced against the benefits of potentially making a definite diagnosis of TB.[28] In the case of pulmonary and genitourinary TB, 3 consecutive early-morning sputum or urine specimens, respectively, are recommended for routine mycobacteriologic studies. Sputum samples are examined initially by smear before and after concentration and then cultured for *M tuberculosis*. Because routine mycobacterial culture methods may require up to 6 weeks for growth of *M tuberculosis*, many laboratories now use radiometric procedures for the isolation and susceptibility testing of this organism; this method may identify the organisms as early as after 8 days. Sterile body fluids and tissues can be inoculated into liquid media, which also allow the growth and detection of *M tuberculosis* 7 to 10 days earlier than in the solid media techniques. Histologic examination of tissue from various sites, such as the liver, lymph nodes, bone marrow, pleura, or synovium, may show the characteristic tissue reaction (caseous necrosis with granuloma formation) with or without AFB, which would also strongly support the diagnosis of TB disease.

Other Tuberculosis Diagnostics

In 2015, the TB diagnostics landscape included a robust pipeline of novel molecular assays for rapid detection and drug resistance testing; this should improve time to treatment, enable point-of-care (POC) testing programs, and support greater access to drug susceptibility (DST) testing.[25,26] Improved alignment between diagnostics and novel TB drug regimens are needed in addition to biomarker-based tests for cure, triage, and predicting progression of LTBI progression of latent *M tuberculosis* infection.

Molecular diagnostics

The molecular diagnostic methods for TB that have been clinically evaluated include serology and NAATs, such as polymerase chain reaction and other methods for amplifying DNA and RNA.[29] The latter may facilitate rapid detection of *M tuberculosis* from respiratory specimens; the interpretation and use of the NAAT results has been updated by the CDC. Similar techniques using DNA probes for genotyping of TB strains can be used to track the spread of the organism in epidemiologic studies and may be used to predict drug resistance before the availability of standard results; such methods are currently being used in some laboratories. The rapid diagnosis of TB is especially important in elderly patients, in addition to HIV-infected persons and patients with multidrug-resistant (MDR) TB. The availability of the GeneXpert MTB/rifampin (RIF) assay has been an important breakthrough in the TB diagnostics market. GeneXpert is a cartridge-based, automatic NAAT, for TB case detection and rifampin resistance testing. It purifies, amplifies, and identifies targeted nucleic acid sequences in the TB genome, and provides results from unprocessed sputum samples in less than 2 hours.[30] This assay showed a high sensitivity in both pulmonary and extrapulmonary TB.[30,31] It was endorsed by the WHO for use in TB-endemic countries; data suggest that this test is most applicable in selected patients at risk of resistance or co-infection with HIV, and not for early case detection in all patients with presumed TB. The newly established PSQ assay is a rapid method for the detection of resistance to RIF, isoniazid (INH), streptomycin (SM), ethambutol (EMB), levofloxacin, and amikacin in *M tuberculosis*.[26] PSQ can be used as a practical molecular diagnostic tool for screening and predicting the resistance of retreatment in patients with pulmonary TB.

Biomarkers

Among the TB biomarkers, one of the most promising antigens that are being evaluated is lipoarabinomannan (LAM). LAM is a structurally important component of the outer cell wall of all bacteria of the genus *Mycobacterium* that is shed from metabolically active or degrading cells, is cleared by the kidney, and detectable in urine.[32,33] Antigen detection assays were described for LAM, most of which are based on a sandwich capture ELISA format to detect LAM in sputum[34] or urine.[35] In the TB diagnostic field, antigen detection technologies and biomarker discovery strategies are rapidly evolving.

Serologic tests

Evaluation of the clinical use of serology for the rapid detection of HIV-associated smear-negative pulmonary and extrapulmonary cases warrants large cohort studies. The observation of higher rates of antibody (Ab) responses in certain TB suspects, especially those who are HIV-infected and from TB-endemic regions suggests that Ab reactivity may represent a true serologic response to *M tuberculosis*.

Volatile organic compounds

The strategy of developing tests based on TB-associated VOC biomarkers offers substantial advantages over other approaches in that such tests are simple, noninvasive, and suitable for POC testing. The widespread use of VOC remains to be evaluated and holds promise as a novel diagnostic adjunct for TB diagnosis in aging individuals.

TREATMENT OF TUBERCULOSIS DISEASE

The recommended treatment regimens are for the most part based on evidence from clinical trials and are rated on the basis of a system developed by the US Public Health Service (USPHS) and the Infectious Diseases Society of America (IDSA)[36] The recommended regimens for treating patients with TB caused by drug-susceptible organisms consist of an initial phase of 2 months followed by a choice of several options for the continuation phase of either 4 or 7 months. The recommended treatment algorithm and regimens are shown in **Fig. 1** and **Table 1**, respectively.[36] Because of the relatively high proportion of adult patients with TB caused by organisms that are resistant to INH, 4 drugs are necessary in the initial phase for the 6-month regimen to be maximally

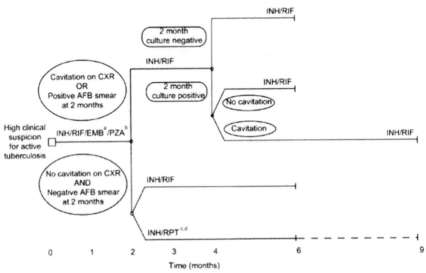

Fig. 1. Treatment algorithm for tuberculosis. Patients in whom tuberculosis is proved or strongly suspected should have treatment initiated with INH, RIF, PZA, and EMB for the initial 2 months. A repeat smear and culture should be performed when 2 months of treatment has been completed. If cavities were seen on the initial chest radiograph or the acid-fast smear is positive at completion of 2 months of treatment, the continuation phase of treatment should consist of INH and RIF daily or twice weekly for 4 months to complete a total of 6 months of treatment. If cavitation was present on the initial CXR and the culture at the time of completion of 2 months of therapy is positive, the continuation phase should be lengthened to 7 months (total of 9 months of treatment). If the patient has HIV infection and the CD4+ cell count is <100/μL, the continuation phase should consist of daily or 3 times weekly INH and RIF. In HIV-uninfected patients having no cavitation on CXR and negative acid-fast smears at completion of 2 months of treatment, the continuation phase may consist of either once weekly INH and RIF, or daily or twice weekly INH and RIF, to complete a total of 6 months (*bottom*). Patients receiving INH and RIF and whose 2-month cultures are positive should have treatment extended by an additional 3 months (total of 9 months). [a] EMB may be discontinued when results of drug susceptibility testing indicate no drug resistance. [b] PZA may be discontinued after it has been taken for 2 months (56 doses). [c] RPT should not be used in HIV-infected patients with TB or in patients with extrapulmonary TB. [d] Therapy should be extended to 9 months if 2-month culture is positive. (*From* Centers for Disease Control and Prevention, American Thoracic Society, Infectious Disease Society of America. Treatment of tuberculosis. MMWR Recomm Rep 2003;52(RR–11):1–77.)

effective. Thus, in most circumstances, the treatment regimen for all adults including the elderly with previously untreated TB should consist of a 2-month initial phase of INH, RIF, pyrazinamide (PZA), and EMB. If (when) drug susceptibility test results are known and the organisms are fully susceptible, EMB need not be included. If PZA cannot be included in the initial phase of treatment, or if the isolate is resistant to PZA alone (an unusual circumstance), the initial phase should consist of INH, RIF, and EMB given daily for 2 months. However, because most TB in the elderly adult is due to reactivation (from infection acquired before 1950), the organism will generally be sensitive to INH and other antituberculous drugs. The first-line injectable agent SM is reserved for patients with drug-sensitive TB who cannot tolerate one or more of the other first-line agents.

Table 1 Basic tuberculosis disease treatment regimens		
Preferred Regimen	**Alternative Regimen**	**Alternative Regimen**

Initial phase
  Daily INH, RIF, PZA, and
    EMB[a] for 56 doses (8 wk)
	Initial phase
	  Daily INH, RIF, PZA, and
	    EMB[a] for 14 doses (2 wk),
	    then twice weekly for 12
	    doses (6 wk)
		Initial phase
		  Thrice-weekly INH, RIF,
		    PZA, and EMB[a] for 24
		    doses (8 wk)

Continuation phase
  Daily INH and RIF for 126
    doses (18 wk)
  Or
  Twice-weekly INH and RIF
    for 36 doses (18 wk)
	Continuation phase
	  Twice-weekly INH and RIF
	    for 36 doses (18 wk)
		Continuation phase
		  Thrice-weekly INH and RIF
		    for 54 doses (18 wk)

A continuation phase of once-weekly INH/rifapentine can be used for human immunodeficiency virus–negative patients who do not have cavities on the chest film *and* who have negative acid-fast bacilli smears at the completion of the initial phase of treatment.

Abbreviations: EMB, ethambutol; INH, isoniazid; PZA, pyrazinamide; RIF, rifampin; RPT, rifapentine.

[a] EMB can be discontinued if drug-susceptibility studies demonstrate susceptibility to first-line drugs.

Data from Centers for Disease Control and Prevention, American Thoracic Society, Infectious Disease Society of America. Treatment of tuberculosis. MMWR Recomm Rep 2003;52(RR–11):1–77.

Treatment of MDR-TB is complex and often needs to be individualized, requiring the addition of a minimum of 2 additional antituberculous agents to which the organism is presumably susceptible, preferably in consultation with a TB expert who is familiar with *M tuberculosis* drug resistance. Alternative drugs, such as capreomycin, kanamycin, amikacin, ethionamide, and cycloserine, and more recently levofloxacin, moxifloxacin, linezolid, delamanid, and bedaquiline may have to be used for treatment in such cases.[37]

Monitoring of Response to Drug Therapy

Patients with active pulmonary TB should be monitored on a monthly basis with sputum examination until conversion to negative by culture is achieved; this usually occurs within 3 months in 90% of cases. Continued positive sputum cultures for *M tuberculosis* beyond 3 months of initiation therapy should raise the suspicion for drug resistance or noncompliance (if not on DOT); such patients should have sputum culture and susceptibility repeated and started on DOT pending results of these data. Follow-up CXR is indicated 2 to 3 months after initiation of drug therapy. Older patients are at greater risk for hepatic toxicity from INH. Although INH therapy poses a small but significant risk for hepatitis, the hepatitis is relatively low in frequency and mild in severity. Therefore, presumably with careful monitoring of the older patient, antituberculous chemotherapy is a relatively safe intervention in this population. It is recommended that clinical assessments and also baseline liver function tests be performed before the administration of INH and RIF (and PZA) in older patients.

Monthly clinical evaluations and periodic measurements of the serum aminotransferase (SGOT) level should be performed in the elderly person. If the SGOT rises to 5 times above normal or if the patient exhibits symptoms or signs of hepatitis, INH and other hepatotoxic agents must be discontinued. After clinical symptoms improve or the SGOT level normalizes, or both, INH may be resumed at a lower dose and gradually increased to a full dose if symptoms and the SGOT level remain stable. In case of relapse of the hepatitis with the INH challenge, the drug should be replaced with an alternative regimen. There is some disagreement among clinicians regarding the monitoring of liver function tests in older patients on INH. Because frail, elderly patients may often be asymptomatic in the presence of worsening hepatitis and may not be able to communicate symptoms, laboratory monitoring seems prudent. The frequency of such monitoring (eg, monthly or every 2–3 months) remains less clear. RIF, in addition to hepatitis, is also associated with orange discoloration of body fluids. EMB may cause loss of color discrimination, diminished visual acuity, and central scotomata; older patients receiving this drug should have frequent evaluation of visual acuity and color discrimination. SM is associated with irreversible auditory and vestibular damage and generally should not be prescribed in the elderly patient. Adverse effects of PZA include hyperuricemia, hepatitis, and flushing. Dose adjustment of antituberculous drugs is necessary with streptomycin, when used in the presence of renal impairment; however, no adjustment is needed for INH, RIF, or PZA in most elderly patients.

TREATMENT OF LATENT TUBERCULOSIS INFECTION

Table 2 shows the interpretation of TST results is based on the measurement of the reaction in millimeters, the person's risk of acquiring TB infection, or the risk of progression to disease if infected.[38] Drug treatment for LTBI based on this risk stratification by skin test induration criteria considerably decreases the risk of progression of TB infection to TB disease. Because the LTBI treatment recommendations address

Table 2 Classification of tuberculin skin test reaction	
TST Induration Size	
≥5 mm	• HIV-infected persons • Recent contacts of a person with infectious TB disease • Persons with fibrotic changes on chest radiograph consistent with prior TB • Patients with organ transplants and other immunosuppressed patients (including patients taking the equivalent of ≥15 mg/d of prednisone for 1 mo or more or those taking TNF-α antagonists)
≥10 mm	• Recent arrivals to the United States (within last 5 y) from high-prevalence areas • Injection drug users • Residents or employees of high-risk congregate settings (eg, correctional facilities, long-term care facilities, hospitals and other health care facilities, residential facilities for patients with HIV infection/AIDS, and homeless shelters) • Mycobacteriology laboratory personnel • Persons with clinical conditions that increase the risk for progression to TB disease • Children younger than 5 y • Infants, children, and adolescents exposed to adults in high-risk categories
≥15 mm	Persons with no known risk factors for TB

Abbreviations: HIV, human immunodeficiency virus; TB, tuberculosis; TNF, tumor necrosis factor.
Adapted from Centers for Disease Control and Prevention. Screening for tuberculosis and tuberculosis infection in high-risk populations: recommendations of the Advisory Council for the Elimination of Tuberculosis. MMWR 1995;44(No. RR-11):19–34.

adults in general, targeted skin testing and treatment of high-risk populations can be applied to the elderly adult.

Table 3 outlines the current CDC-recommended LTBI treatment regimens.[39] The INH daily regimen for 9 months has recently replaced the previously recommended 6-month schedule for treatment of LTBI. In a community-based study conducted in Bethel, Alaska, persons who took less than 25% of the prescribed annual dose had a threefold higher risk for TB than those who took more than 50% of the annual dose. In addition, the efficacy decreased significantly if INH was taken for less than 9 months. Randomized, prospective trials in HIV-negative persons have indicated that a 12-month regimen is more effective than 6 months of treatment; subgroup analyses of several trials indicate that the maximum beneficial effect of INH is likely.

More recently, shorter-course regimens of rifampin for 4 months and higher-dose daily INH and rifapentine (3HP regimen) via DOT have been added to the recommended LTBI treatment options.[38,39] In instances of known exposure to drug-resistant organisms, alternative preventive therapy regimens may be recommended.

Although these recommendations do not specifically address aging adults, the concept of targeted skin testing and revised LTBI treatment guidelines for high-risk populations to include the elderly adult can be applied. Elderly persons receiving INH should continue to be monitored for hepatitis and peripheral neuropathy induced by the drug.

INFECTION CONTROL ISSUES

The primary goal of an infection control program is to detect TB disease early and to isolate and treat persons with infectious TB promptly. Prevention of transmission of TB in any health care environment is of the utmost importance, for both patients and health care workers. Enhanced awareness of drug-resistant TB has prompted public health agencies to institute strict TB identification, isolation, treatment, and prevention guidelines. The TB infection control program in most acute care and LTCFs should consist of 3 types of control measures: administrative actions (ie, prompt detection of suspected cases, isolation of infectious patients and rapid institution of appropriate treatment), engineering control (negative-pressure ventilation rooms, high-efficiency particulate air filtration and ultraviolet germicidal irradiation) and personal respiratory protection requirements (masks). The Advisory Committee for the Elimination of Tuberculosis of the CDC has established recommendations for surveillance, containment, assessment, and reporting of TB infection and disease in LTCFs; health care professionals, administrators, and staff of such extended care programs should be made aware of these recommendations.[40]

Table 3
Latent tuberculosis infection treatment regimens

Drugs	Duration, mo	Interval	Minimum Doses
Isoniazid	9	Daily	270
		Twice weekly[a]	76
Isoniazid	6	Daily	180
		Twice weekly[a]	52
Isoniazid and Rifapentine	3	Once weekly[a]	12
Rifampin	4	Daily	120

[a] Use directly observed therapy.

Data from Centers for Disease Control and Prevention. Treatment for latent TB infection. Available at: http://www.cdc.gov/tb/topic/treatment/ltbi.htm. Accessed October 1, 2015.

REFERENCES

1. World Health Organization. Global tuberculosis report 2015. Geneva (Switzerland): WHO; 2015. p. 1–204.
2. Centers for Disease Control and Prevention. Reported tuberculosis - United States, 2014. p. 1–204. Available at: http://www.cdc.gov/tb/statistics/reports/2014/pdfs/tb-surveillance-2014-report.pdf. Accessed September 25, 2015.
3. Centers for Disease Control and Prevention. Decrease in reported tuberculosis cases - United States, 2009. MMWR Morb Mortal Wkly Rep 2010;59:289–94.
4. Pratt RH, Winston CA, Kammerer SF, et al. Tuberculosis in older adults in the United States, 1993-2008. J Am Geriatr Soc 2011;59:851–7.
5. Narain J, Lofgren J, Warren E, et al. Epidemic tuberculosis in a nursing home: a retrospective cohort study. J Am Geriatr Soc 1985;33:258–63.
6. Schultz M, Hernandez JM, Hernandez NE, et al. Onset to tuberculosis disease: new converters in long-term care settings. Am J Alzheimers Dis Other Demen 2001;16:313–8.
7. Hutton MD, Cauthen GM, Bloch AB. Results of a 29-state survey of tuberculosis in nursing homes and correctional facilities. Public Health Rep 1993; 108:305–14.
8. Ijaz K, Dillara JA, Yang Z, et al. Unrecognized tuberculosis in a nursing home causing death with spread of tuberculosis to the community. J Am Geriatr Soc 2002;50:1213–7.
9. Chitnis AS, Robsky K, Schecter GF, et al. Trends in tuberculosis cases among nursing home residents, California, 2000 to 2009. J Am Geriatr Soc 2015;63: 1098–104.
10. Donald PR, Marais BJ, Barry CR. Age and the epidemiology and pathogenesis of tuberculosis. Lancet 2010;375:1852–4.
11. Perez-Guzman C, Vargas MH, Torres-Cruz A, et al. Does aging modify pulmonary tuberculosis? A meta-analytical review. Chest 1999;116:961–7.
12. Yoshikawa TT. Tuberculosis in aging adults. J Am Geriatr Soc 1992;40:178.
13. Mert A, Bilir M, Tabak F. Miliary tuberculosis: clinical manifestations, diagnosis and outcome in 38 adults. Respirology 2001;6:217–624.
14. Kalita J, Misra UK. Tuberculous meningitis with pulmonary miliary tuberculosis: a clinicoradiological study. Neurol India 2004;52:194–6.
15. Shah AH, Joshi SV, Dhar HL. Tuberculosis of bones and joints. Antiseptic 2001; 98:385–7.
16. Malaviya A. Arthritis associated with tuberculosis. Best Pract Res Clin Rheumatol 2003;17:319–43.
17. Lenk S, Schroeder J. Genitourinary tuberculosis. Curr Opin Urol 2001;11:93–8.
18. Markowitz N, Hansen NI, Wilcosky TC, et al. Tuberculin and anergy testing in HIV-seropositive and HIV-seronegative persons. Ann Intern Med 1993;119:185–93.
19. Tort J, Pina JM, Martin-Ramos A, et al. Booster effect in elderly patients living in geriatric institutions. Med Clin (Barcelona) 1995;105:41–4.
20. American Geriatrics Society. Two-step PPD testing for nursing home patients on admission, 1993. Available at: www.info.amger@americangeriatrics.org. Accessed September 26, 2015.
21. Slovis BS, Plitman JD, Haas DW. The case against anergy testing as a routine adjunct to tuberculin skin testing. JAMA 2000;283:2003–7.
22. Mazurek GH, Jereb J, Vernon A, et al, IGRA Expert Committee, Centers for Disease Control and Prevention. Updated guidelines for using interferon gamma

release assays to detect *Mycobacterium tuberculosis* infection - United States, 2010. MMWR Recomm Rep 2010;54(RR-15):49–55.

23. Woodring JH, Vandiviere HJV, Fried AM, et al. Update: the radiographic features of pulmonary tuberculosis. AJR Am J Roentgenol 1986;146:497–506.

24. Muyoyeta M, Maduskar P, Moyo M, et al. The sensitivity and specificity of using a computer aided diagnosis program for automatically scoring chest x-rays of presumptive TB patients compared with Xpert MTB/RIF in Lusaka Zambia. PLoS One 2014;9:1–9.

25. UNITAID. Tuberculosis: diagnostics technology and market landscape. 3rd edition. Geneva (Switzerland): WHO; 2014. p. 1–42.

26. Pai M, Shito M. Tuberculosis diagnostics: landscape, needs and prospects. J Infect Dis 2015;211(Suppl 2):S21–8.

27. Zheng R, Zhu C, Guo Q, et al. Pyrosequencing for rapid detection of tuberculosis resistance in clinical isolates and sputum samples from re-treatment pulmonary tuberculosis patients. BMC Infect Dis 2014;14:200–8.

28. Patel YR, Mehta JB, Harvill L, et al. Flexible bronchoscopy as a diagnostic tool in the evaluation of pulmonary tuberculosis in an elderly population. J Am Geriatr Soc 1993;41:629–32.

29. Centers for Disease Control and Prevention. Nucleic acid amplification tests for tuberculosis. Morb Mortal Wkly Rep 2000;49:593–4.

30. Boehme CC, Nabeta P, Hillemann D, et al. Rapid molecular detection of tuberculosis and rifampin resistance. N Engl J Med 2010;363:1005–15.

31. Hillemann D, Rüsch-Gerdes S, Boehme C, et al. Rapid molecular detection of extrapulmonary tuberculosis by the automated GeneXpert MTB/RIF System. Clin Microbiol 2011;49:1202–5.

32. Hunter SW, Gaylord H, Brennan PJ. Structure and antigenicity of the phosphorylated lipopolysaccharide antigens from the leprosy and tubercle bacilli. Biol Chem 1986;261:12345–51.

33. Chan J, Fan XD, Hunter SW, et al. Lipoarabinomannan, a possible virulence factor involved in persistence of *Mycobacterium tuberculosis* within macrophages. Infect Immun 1991;59:1755–61.

34. Pereira Arias-Bouda LM, Nguyen LN, Ho LM, et al. Development of antigen detection assay for diagnosis of tuberculosis using sputum samples. Clin Microbiol 2000;38:2278–83.

35. Hamasur B, Bruchfeld J, Haile M, et al. Rapid diagnosis of tuberculosis by detection of mycobacterial lipoarabinomannan in urine. J Microbiol Methods 2001;45:41–52.

36. Centers for Disease Control and Prevention, American Thoracic Society and Infectious Disease Society of America. Treatment of tuberculosis. MMWR Recomm Rep 2003;52(RR-11):1–77.

37. Zumla AI, Gillespie SH, Hoelscher M, et al. New antituberculosis drugs, regimens, and adjunct therapies: needs, advances, and future prospects. Lancet Infect Dis 2014;14:327–40.

38. American Thoracic Society. Targeted skin testing and treatment of latent tuberculosis infection. Am J Respir Crit Care Med 2000;161:5221–47.

39. Centers for Disease Control and Prevention. Treatment for latent TB infection. Available at: http://www.cdc.gov/tb/topic/treatment/ltbi.htm. Accessed September 27, 2015.

40. Centers for Disease Control and Prevention. Control of tuberculosis in facilities providing long-term care to the elderly: recommendations of the Advisory Committee for the Elimination of Tuberculosis. Morb Mortal Wkly Rep 1990; 39(RR-10):7–20.

Intraabdominal Infections in Older Adults

Ana Berlin, MD, MPH[a], Jason Michael Johanning, MD, MS[b],*

KEYWORDS

- Acute abdomen • Atypical presentation • Intraabdominal infection
- Geriatric surgery • Frailty • Surgical outcomes

KEY POINTS

- Intraabdominal infections may be confined, localized, or diffuse.
- Compared with younger patients, elderly patients with intraabdominal infection tend to present in delayed or atypical fashion and have a narrow therapeutic window, both of which are associated with significantly increased morbidity and mortality.
- Treatment of intraabdominal infections is based on source control and judicious use of antibiotics. In elderly patients, this requires a balanced approach, taking into consideration the invasiveness and inherent risk of a procedure as well as its efficacy for producing the desired outcomes.
- Multimodal and aggressive preventative management of geriatric syndromes and collateral damage of diagnostic and therapeutic interventions decreases the risk of adverse outcomes in geriatric acute-surgery patients.

GENERAL PRINCIPLES

Intraabdominal infections are a leading cause of illness in the elderly population.[1] The pillars of treatment of any intraabdominal infection are antibiotics and source control (drainage or removal of the infecting agent when possible). To appropriately choose and direct therapy, it is helpful to classify intraabdominal infections according to their anatomic extent and recognize the patterns of presentation typical for each category. Perhaps most important, it is important to recognize the unique presentation of intraabdominal infections in the elderly patient and understand the outcomes of available management options in the geriatric population.

Anatomic Classification

Intraabdominal infections can be broadly classified as localized or diffuse. Localized infections may be solely confined to an organ or hollow viscus (eg, uncomplicated

[a] Department of Surgery, Rutgers New Jersey Medical School, 185 South Orange Avenue, Newark, NJ 07103, USA; [b] Department of Surgery, University of Nebraska Medical Center, 4101 Woolworth Avenue, Omaha, NE 68105, USA
* Corresponding author.
E-mail address: Jason.johanning@va.gov

Clin Geriatr Med 32 (2016) 493–507
http://dx.doi.org/10.1016/j.cger.2016.02.002
0749-0690/16/$ – see front matter Published by Elsevier Inc.
geriatric.theclinics.com

cholecystitis or *Clostridium difficile* colitis), producing localized symptoms. Additionally, these localized infections may create systemic effects (eg, severe cholangitis or fulminant *C difficile* colitis) or, with rupture or progression of local infection, may create a colocalized abscess. Diffuse intraabdominal infections, on the other hand, extend throughout the peritoneal cavity. Peritonitis may be primary, as in the case of spontaneous bacterial peritonitis; secondary, as in the case of perforated appendicitis or diverticulitis with diffuse peritoneal purulence or spillage of enteric contents; or tertiary, which represents incompletely eradicated or recurrent secondary peritonitis. Elderly patients are especially susceptible to tertiary peritonitis due to their decreased physiologic reserve and prevalence of malnutrition. Whereas primary and secondary peritonitis are predominantly associated with normal enteric flora (*Escherichia coli*, *Bacteroides fragilis*, and *Streptococcus* species), the pathogens responsible for tertiary peritonitis include frequently resistant nosocomial and opportunistic organisms such as *Pseudomonas aeruginosa*, multidrug-resistant *Klebsiella* and *Enterobacter*, and *Candida* species.[2]

Clinical Evaluation

The constellation of symptoms and signs that herald an intraabdominal infection in a young, healthy patient (ie, abdominal pain, guarding, rebound, fever, and leukocytosis, with or without hemodynamic changes such as tachycardia) are often absent or atypical in elderly patients. In patients with a decreased range of verbal expression due to dementia, aphasia, or other cognitive impairments, history may be difficult to obtain. Delirium and worsening cognitive function may be related to systemic effects of infection and/or decreased end-organ perfusion. Due to physiologic alterations associated with aging, abdominal pain may be vague and elusive, manifesting as social withdrawal, irritability, and disinterest in food or activity. The tachycardia common in children and young adults with intraabdominal infections may be absent in older patients, especially those on beta blockers. Because of changes in the immune system associated with advanced age and frailty, fever and leukocytosis may not develop. In fact, hypothermia and leukopenia are equally if not more ominous signs of intraabdominal infection in older patients (See Norman DC: Clinical Features of Infection in Older Adults, in this issue.) Given the altered presentation, sepsis diagnosis can be late and the resultant hypotension can be sudden and profound. In addition to abdominal infections, due to the multiple chronic conditions encountered in this population, acute abdominal infections in the elderly person may be overshadowed or coexist with significant distracting diagnoses, including urinary tract infection and acute coronary syndrome.[3] In summary, an inability to rely on obvious physiologic derangements is a hallmark in the geriatric population and is often associated with delays in diagnosis and treatment. Although this phenomenon is widely reported and well known to the geriatrician, the atypical presentation cannot be overemphasized and should be promulgated to surgeons, both established and in training, to reinforce this well-established fact.

The abdominal examination in the elderly patient with a suspected intraabdominal infection deserves particular mention. Because of connective tissue and immune changes associated with age, peritonitis in older patients who have insufficient skeletal muscle mass and inability to mount an appropriate inflammatory response does not produce the classic physical signs of involuntary guarding, rebound tenderness, and abdominal rigidity in response to peritoneal irritation characteristic of younger patients. Pain out of proportion to physical examination findings (ie, severe abdominal pain in the absence of objective physical examination signs of peritonitis) usually indicates intestinal ischemia associated with vascular inflow or outflow occlusion due to arterial thromboembolic events, mesenteric venous thrombosis, or mechanical factors such as volvulus and closed-loop obstruction. These alterations in elderly patients create a tenderness that may be subtle and diffuse, rather than focal and specific, even if a process is confined to a specific organ. Pain may also be referred, such as the right shoulder and scapular pain classically associated with acute biliary processes. Abdominal distension should be further classified according to the presence of tympani or dullness to percussion, indicating the presence of intraluminal or free air, or ascites or free fluid, respectively. Finally, the rectal examination is an essential component of the abdominal examination in any patient but especially so in the elderly person. The presence or absence of gross blood, indicating intestinal hemorrhage or mucosal ischemia; tenderness or fluctuance of the anal canal, indicating a perianal or perirectal abscess; an obstructing mass in the anal lumen or peritoneal reflection, indicating possible malignancy; or mere fecal impaction, a common and treatable finding among elderly patients, are all important observations.

Management Options

Intraabdominal infections frequently require multimodal therapy, as indicated previously. With the exception of contained intraabdominal abscesses limited to less than 3 to 4 cm in diameter, antibiotics alone are unlikely to be sufficient without source control.[4,5] Conversely, source control alone cannot address the systemic response to infection or bacteremia that may ensue. The choice of initial antibiotics should be based on guidelines for empirical therapy coupled with local antibiotic susceptibility profiles. Piperacillin-tazobactam, or a fluoroquinolone plus metronidazole, are recommended choices in advanced age and high-risk infections.[2] Carbapenems and third-generation cephalosporins, the latter in combination with metronidazole, are also acceptable choices but may be less cost-effective. Empirical therapy against methicillin-resistant *Staphylococcus aureus* (MRSA) with vancomycin is recommended in patients known or suspected to be colonized with MRSA who acquire an intra-abdominal infection in the nosocomial setting.[2] The duration of antibiotic therapy for established infection in which source control has been achieved should be limited to 7 days, given that longer durations of therapy have not been shown to demonstrate improved outcomes. In fact, emerging evidence suggests that courses as short as 4 days may be equivalent.[6] In many instances, including organ-confined disease (eg, acute appendicitis without evidence of generalized peritonitis or perforation, or acute cholecystitis) and intraoperative spillage of enteric contents, antibiotic therapy should be limited to less than or equal to 24 hours.[2]

Options for source control vary in invasiveness and may be definitively therapeutic or temporizing. Surgical approaches offer the option of definitive management and include laparotomy and laparoscopy. Laparoscopy has a proven record of safety in elderly patients and, in many circumstances, produces outcomes favorable to open surgery.[7–9] However, it requires general anesthesia and has some relative contraindications, including hypertension and pulmonary compromise, that may limit its applicability in select cases. Abdominal surgery under local, epidural, or spinal anesthesia is another a potential option for the treatment of localized disease in high–operative risk patients. Although not standard therapy, these anesthetic modalities can and have been used to perform appendectomy, sigmoid colon resection, and ileostomy or colostomy procedures.[10–13]

In addition to surgery, percutaneous interventions guided by ultrasound, fluoroscopy, or computed tomography may be suitable for controlling the source of infection while avoiding the morbidity and mortality associated with more invasive surgical approaches. Percutaneous drainage may be considered a temporizing measure, as in the case of a cholecystostomy tube used to manage a patient with acute calculous cholecystitis who may or may not be a future candidate for cholecystectomy. Post-cholecystostomy patients with gallstones should be managed according to a patient-centered approach, taking into account their specific operative risks, goals of care, and clinical variables such as the presence or absence of continued cystic duct obstruction on repeat cholangiography. In certain instances, a cholecystostomy tube for life may be considered the best available option. In contrast, patients with acalculous cholecystitis who are not operative candidates are well served by chole-cystostomy tube decompression followed by simple removal of the tube after recovery. Additional therapeutic interventions include percutaneous abscess drainage, for example for perforated appendicitis or complicated diverticulitis, which carries a success rate as high as 90% in combination with antibiotics.[4]

In choosing the right intervention, one should adhere to the principles of shared decision-making and patient-centered care. Whenever possible, knowledge of patient's preferences, goals, and values should inform therapeutic choices so that these are concordant with patient wishes. Patients who prioritize comfort-directed measures above those with curative intent may nonetheless benefit from multimodal therapy, including minimally invasive interventional techniques, to palliate the significant pain and discomfort associated with intraabdominal infections.

Important Considerations

Interventions for intraabdominal infections for elderly patients need to be taken in the context of 3 specific issues: the age of the patient, frailty, and the increasing invasiveness of intervention. Age alone is not a simple predictor of whether or not someone will tolerate and intraabdominal infection and its treatment. However, in multiple studies, age has been shown to increase risk of complications and mortality in surgical patients, with nonagenarians especially at risk. Thus, when treating patients of advanced age, one must be cognizant of the impact age has on both in 30-day and 1-year mortality in the oldest of the old.

In contrast to age, frailty seems to be the most prominent risk factor for morbidity and mortality related to infections and subsequent interventional and surgical treatment of those infections. Multiple studies have now documented that frailty confers a marked risk of complications related to intraabdominal surgical intervention.[14–16] One would ideally perform a detailed individualized risk assessment of the patient to guide the decision-making and discussion about alternatives of treatment based on a physical phenotype (weakness, exhaustion, somatic shrinking, slow walking speed, and low physical activity) and deficit accumulation index approach based on the research, which clearly demonstrates that frailty confers a marked increase in surgical risk of mortality and morbidity.[16–18] Unfortunately, intraabdominal infections do not often present with the luxury of time to perform classic frailty assessments. Decisions regarding intervention are time-sensitive in the setting of rapid and progressive decline. However, there are multiple tools, such as the Edmonton Frail Scale, Risk Analysis Index, and Rockwood Clinical Frailty Scale, that can be rapidly performed and provide a guide for risk compared with a nonfrail individual and inform the shared decision-making process.[19,20] At a minimum, surgical intervention in the setting of a major intraabdominal infection should prompt a preintervention discussion to include a complication rate of approximately 40% to 50%. Although this figure may seem high, multiple investigators across multiple settings have documented significant morbidity associated with major elective operations on abdominal organs of the intraperitoneal cavity.

Regarding the invasiveness of intervention, a systematic thought process of advancing invasiveness of intervention should be entertained with each patient that is based on increasing levels of intervention to achieve the optimal outcome. The first and obvious step is to start with antibiotics because this should be the cornerstone of treatment. Antibiotics can be used as treatment in and of itself or in conjunction with invasive intervention. Consideration for antibiotic treatment alone in particular conditions that were once considered obvious surgical conditions should be considered, especially in the elderly frail patient (see later discussion on appendicitis). Source control of the infection to eradicate the infection and prevent progression is well recognized to accompany antibiotic treatment. Because source control is the primary goal of any invasive treatment of intraabdominal infection, percutaneous drainage remains an attractive option for treating the elderly frail patient because it removes the infectious source without major physiologic insult. In patients with a localized process and coexistent abscess (appendicitis or diverticulitis with abscess), the ability to treat the abscess and convert definitive treatment to an elective setting is attractive. Should surgical intervention be needed, one must give thought immediately to laparoscopic intervention, which has been shown to have markedly reduced physiologic insult compared with standard laparotomy.[15,21–23] Although one should lean toward the least invasive intervention for source control, in certain situations, maximal intervention in the form of open laparotomy is often necessary to rapidly obtain source control and eradicate the infectious process.

Structured communication techniques and time-limited trials are strategies for improving the patient-centeredness and goal-concordance of treatment of acute intraabdominal processes in the elderly, frail, or chronically ill.[24,25] Structured communication involves (1) clarifying the patient's decisional capacity, expectations, and understanding regarding the situation, treatment options, and overall prognosis; (2) identifying the patient's priorities and goals; (3) determining the fears, worries, and health states that the patient would find unacceptable; (4) recommending a course of action that is best aligned with patient goals and wishes; (5) identifying objective markers and time points to evaluate for improvement or deterioration (time-limited trial); and (6) affirming one's commitment to the patient's well-being.[24] In a time-limited trial of therapy, patients who fail to improve according to the selected parameters within the predetermined time period for evaluation should be managed according to the paradigm of "changing hopes," whereby a transition is made from resuscitative and life-saving treatment toward comfort-directed measures.[25]

SPECIFIC CONDITIONS

Intraabdominal infections may be associated with both hollow and solid organs. This section reviews the presentation, management options, and potential complications associated with infection arising from the various anatomic locations and organ systems within the abdomen.

Biliary Tract

Cholecystitis and cholangitis are common problems in the elderly person, with acute cholecystitis representing the leading cause (32%) of acute abdomen among the elderly population in a recent analysis from Finland, where the incidence of biliary tract disease may well be lower than that in the United States.[26] Acute cholecystitis often occurs in isolation but may also occur in the setting of hospitalization or decompensation due to other causes. Acute cholecystitis after a period of decreased oral intake or physiologic stress is well-described and illustrated by the recent finding of a higher than expected rate of acute cholecystitis among hip fracture patients, with a 2-month incidence of approximately 0.75%.[27] Clinical history and examination revealing right-upper quadrant tenderness, fever or hypothermia, leukocytosis or leukopenia, and gallstones on ultrasound are sufficient to establish the diagnosis of acute cholecystitis, regardless of the presence of gallbladder wall thickening and pericholecystic fluid, which are less specific. Liver enzymes and bilirubin are normal in uncomplicated cholecystitis and, if elevated, may represent biliary obstruction or hepatocellular injury associated with severe inflammation extending to the livery parenchyma surrounding the gallbladder. Patients should be treated with intravenous fluids, nothing by mouth, and early antibiotics. For lower risk patients with uncomplicated disease and early presentation, cefazolin and metronidazole or ampicillin-sulbactam provide adequate coverage. Higher risk patients with more severe presentations warrant piperacillin-tazobactam or a quinolone plus metronidazole.[2] Multiple studies, albeit many with a high risk of bias, document the risks associated with delayed definitive treatment of acute cholecystitis in elderly patients. In fact, a recent study of more than 4000 subjects using the National Surgical Quality Improvement Program database found that early laparoscopic cholecystectomy, within 24 hours of admission, was associated with shorter postoperative stay and no increase in postoperative complications or conversion to open cholecystectomy compared with delayed cholecystectomy in elderly patients with significant comorbidities.[28] This suggests that delays in definitive management, whether due to delays in diagnosis or systematic delays introduced by the perceived need for preoperative risk stratification and optimization, or other factors, may be detrimental to older patients.

Cholangitis, which may be due to obstructing biliary stone disease, malignancy, or benign strictures, has a presentation similar to that of acute cholecystitis, with the addition of increased markers of biliary obstruction (ie, jaundice or hyperbilirubinemia, elevated alkaline phosphatase, and elevated gamma-glutamyl transferase). Severe cholangitis, indicating systemic involvement, includes the triad of cholangitis, as well as hypotension and mental status change. Early antibiotics, urgent biliary decompression via endoscopic retrograde pancreatography (ERCP), and monitoring in a high-acuity level of care are indicated for severe cholangitis. If ERCP is unsuccessful, percutaneous transhepatic cholangiography with external decompression of the biliary tract is an alternative. Because elderly patients with biliary stone disease have a high risk of recurrent complications (more than 40% in patients treated noninvasively), and because these recurrent complications are often accompanied by high morbidity and mortality, cholecystectomy should be recommended to elderly patients during the index presentation. Patients who are not operative candidates should undergo ERCP with sphincterotomy as an alternative.[29]

Stomach and Duodenum

Although perforated peptic ulcer has decreased in incidence since the advent of therapy suppressing gastric acid production and targeted against *Helicobacter pylori,* it is still an important cause of acute abdomen. This is especially so among older patients, who have increased risk factors, including pharmacologic interruption of mucosal barrier protection associated with nonsteroidal anti-inflammatory drugs, corticosteroids, and other treatments. Elderly patients may lack the precise history of sudden onset intense upper abdominal pain, are more likely to have a delayed presentation, and have high mortality (34%–44%) associated with perforated peptic ulcer, especially when presenting with shock.[30,31]

Up to half of perforated gastric and duodenal ulcers self-seal with omentum or surrounding viscera.[32] This provides a justification for the observed success of nonoperative management in up to 73% of patients.[33] Patients without shock and with evidence of sealed perforation on a water-soluble contrast study can be treated supportively with a low (<5%) risk of intraabdominal abscess and reperforation.[34] Supportive treatment includes rapid resuscitation, prompt surgical evaluation, and early antibiotics. The choice of antibiotics is dictated by knowledge of the microbiology of the condition rather than high-level empirical evidence. Gastric juice, in normal circumstances, consists primarily of gram-positive cocci and fungi, whereas under conditions of acid suppression or malignancy is enriched for total organisms, including enteric. Empirical antifungal therapy is not indicated except in nosocomial settings or when documented infection is established. When source control is achieved expeditiously, either surgically or by self-sealing, and diffuse peritonitis does not exist, therapy need not extend beyond 24 hours.[2] In addition, all patients should be tested for *H pylori* infection and treatment should be directed accordingly. Patients who do not meet criteria for nonoperative intervention should undergo prompt operation. Gastric ulcers should be biopsied or excised to rule out malignancy. Ulcers less than 10 mm in diameter can be safely managed laparoscopically with omental patch repair.[35] Definitive acid-reducing procedures should be performed only in highly select patients.[36]

An important percentage of intraabdominal infections associated with proximal gastrointestinal tract perforation in the elderly population are iatrogenic. Due to the prevalence of dysphagia in the setting of acute and chronic neurologic deterioration caused by cerebrovascular accident and neurodegenerative disorders, and acute and chronic serious illness accompanied by the inability to meet nutritional needs through oral intake, the elderly patient is frequently subjected to placement of gastrostomy tubes for enteral nutrition. Although the evidence-based indications for feeding gastrostomy tube placement are actually quite restrictive, health care system realities drive local practice patterns in complex ways. For instance, up to one-third of long-term care residents with advanced cognitive impairment have feeding tubes, despite any demonstrated benefit in preventing aspiration pneumonia or prolonging life.[37]

Unfortunately, the burdens associated with feeding gastrostomy tubes are significant, including diarrhea, increased rate of pressure ulcer formation, and multiple complications culminating in intraabdominal infection. Chief among these is leakage of gastric contents, sometimes admixed with tube feeds, into the abdominal cavity, producing peritonitis. Early mild leakage associated with the procedure and an insufficiently tightened retention ring or external bolster may be managed by placing the gastrostomy tube to gravity, and initiating bowel rest and antibiotic therapy with consideration of antifungal coverage, until symptoms resolve (**Fig. 1**). Severe leakage, often associated with complete traumatic dislodgment of the tube by the patient or staff during the course of moving or transferring the patient, can only be successfully addressed by prompt laparotomy, lavage of the peritoneal cavity, appropriate antibiotic therapy (gram-positive or mixed flora coverage if the patient had acid suppressive therapy, with or without antifungal coverage), gastrorrhaphy, and resiting of the gastrostomy tube in a new location.[38,39]

Other gastrostomy tube complications, namely acute tube migration and the more chronic buried bumper syndrome, result when outward traction along the tube produces displacement of the internal balloon or deformable dome (bumper) of the gastrostomy tube into the abdominal wall (**Fig. 1**). This can occur if the external bolster is excessively tightened against the skin, causing the internal balloon or bolster to exert pressure necrosis on the gastric mucosa, eventually pulling the internal bolster into the gastrocutaneous tract. Instillation of feeds directly into the abdominal wall may produce a collection initially mistaken for, and subsequently developing into, an abscess. These abscesses are notoriously difficult to manage but should be done so aggressively, with early antibiotics, incision and drainage, interruption of feeds, placement of the gastrostomy tube to gravity drainage, and potentially resiting of the tube to a remote location to allow for local healing to take place. Finally, abdominal wall

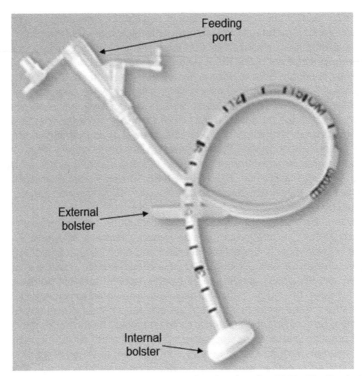

Feeding port

External bolster

Internal bolster

Fig. 1. Percutaneous endoscopic gastrostomy (PEG) tube. (© 2015 C.R. Bard, Inc; used with permission. Bard and Ponksy PEG are trademarks and/or registered trademarks of C. R. Bard, Inc.)

hematomas occurring on tube placement can become secondarily infected and produce an abscess. This is managed in the same way as those associated with buried bumper syndrome.[40–42]

Small Bowel

Small bowel obstruction and ischemia can produce intraabdominal infection when treatment delays or failures result in intestinal necrosis and perforation, or as complications of initial surgical treatment. Secondary and tertiary peritonitis, in these circumstances, should be managed according the general principles outlined above. Goal-directed resuscitation and early antibiotics (piperacillin-tazobactam or a carbapenem, or metronidazole plus a third-generation cephalosporin or a quinolone) should be initiated; source control should be achieved percutaneously, if possible. Diffuse peritonitis mandates emergency surgical intervention if the probable outcomes are consistent with the patient's previously expressed goals and wishes.[2,43,44]

Appendix

Acute appendicitis is an important cause of intraabdominal infection in the elderly person, accounting for up to 28% of cases and constituting the diagnosis in 10% to 15% of emergency operations in this age group.[45–48] A true intestinal diverticulum, the appendix is subject to luminal obstruction from fecalith (20%–40%), lymphoid hyperplasia, or malignancy, all of which contribute to bacterial overproliferation, overdistension, venous congestion, mucosal ischemia, and, eventually, necrosis and perforation. Elderly patients are at especially high risk of perforation, with rates of this complication as high as 50% in several recent studies.[49,50] The morbidity and mortality of appendicitis in the elderly patient are as high as 15% and 40%, respectively, likely reflective of a combination of delayed diagnosis and underlying pathophysiologic factors.[51]

The gold standard for treatment of acute appendicitis in the elderly patient is appendectomy, open or laparoscopically, to the extent the patient can tolerate the required pneumoperitoneum.[52] Management decisions should be made on an individualized basis taking into account each patient's operative risk, the risks of nonoperative treatment, and overall goals. Although recent interest has grown in the nonoperative management of acute appendicitis, randomized controlled trials comparing antibiotics alone to antibiotics with surgery have failed to demonstrate noninferiority of antibiotics alone in the elderly population.[53–55] Importantly, none of these studies have targeted enrollment of elderly subjects who may have a different risk profile for nonresolution or recurrence based on underlying causal factors such as malignancy. Indeed, elderly patients with perforated appendicitis who are treated nonoperatively should be referred for colonoscopy 4 to 6 weeks after the index event, due to the relatively high incidence of cecal or appendiceal cancer in this age group. A high index of suspicion for malignancy should be also maintained in elderly patients with uncomplicated appendicitis who undergo appendectomy. Postoperative surveillance is recommended if screening is not up-to-date or if any risk factors for malignancy exist, such as unexplained anemia or weight loss.

Colon

More than one-third of elderly patients with intraabdominal sepsis will be found to have a colonic source.[45] The most important causes are diverticulitis, infectious colitis, and ischemia and subsequent perforation in the setting of obstruction due to malignancy or volvulus. Diverticulitis may be uncomplicated or complicated. Uncomplicated diverticulitis represents local inflammation associated with bacterial overproliferation in a diverticulum and can be treated with oral antibiotics, although the exact role of antibiotics in uncomplicated diverticulitis is not well-defined.[56] Complicated diverticulitis, on the other hand, results from diverticular perforations that may result in contained abscesses or diffuse peritonitis. Because of the increased prevalence of diverticulosis, as well as age-related connective tissue changes in the bowel wall that predispose to perforation, older patients are more likely than younger patients to have complicated diverticulitis with diffuse peritonitis. Unfortunately, the mortality rate is also excessive compared with younger patients (17% vs 6%).[45,57,58]

Treatment of complicated diverticulitis depends on the overall condition of the patient and the extent of disease. Stable patients with focal abdominal examination findings, and pericolic or mesenteric abscesses on cross-sectional imaging (Hinchey stage I disease), should be treated with intravenous fluids, bowel rest, and early broad-spectrum antibiotics (piperacillin-tazobactam or metronidazole plus a quinolone). For patients with walled-off pelvic or retroperitoneal abscesses (Hinchey stage II disease), image-guided percutaneous abscess drainage should be added to the treatment armamentarium. After recovery, decisions about elective surgery should be made on a case-by-case basis, taking into account the risk of recurrence, the risks of surgery, and the patient's goals and preferences.[59]

For patients with diffuse peritonitis, shock, or evidence of free air and fluid on radiographic imaging, emergent surgical intervention is required for source control. The goals of the operation are not only to drain and lavage the peritoneal cavity of purulent

(Hinchey stage III) or feculent (Hinchey stage IV) spillage but also to remove the focus of infection and prevent recurrent attacks. The question of whether to undertake a definitive resection in the acutely ill patient with Hinchey stage III disease, with either a primary anastomosis or an end colostomy (Hartmann procedure), is the subject of ongoing controversy in the surgical literature. Although the appeal of minimally invasive laparoscopic lavage and drainage is clear and small studies in the elderly population have been promising,[60] current evidence does not convincingly support its superiority compared with sigmoidectomy, and it may even contribute to worse outcomes.[61,62] These patients are at high risk of ongoing secondary and tertiary peritonitis and undiagnosed malignancy, and should be managed according to the general principles previously outlined.

Sigmoid volvulus, obstructing masses, and mesenteric ischemia can lead to intra-abdominal infection through the final common pathway of necrosis and perforation, or through direct extension of a tumor into the peritoneal cavity in the case of malignancy. In the elderly patient with obstructing carcinomas of the cancer and rectum, proximal perforation is more likely.[63,64] Given the poor long-term survival associated with perforated colon cancer in the elderly patient, early palliative care and excellent communication with patients and families about expected outcomes, goals, and priorities are of paramount importance in formulating treatment plans that are concordant with patient's values and preferences.[24,65]

Clostridium difficile Infection

Despite being preventable, *C difficile*–associated diarrhea or infection (CDI) is an increasingly prevalent problem that disproportionately affects the elderly population (See White MB, Rajagopalan S, Yoshikawa T: Infectious Diarrhea: Norovirus and Clostridium Difficile in Older Adults, in this issue.) It is the most common infectious cause of acute diarrhea in both inpatient and outpatient health care settings, carries a high morbidity and mortality, and its economic costs are estimated at $500 million annually in the United States. The spore-forming anaerobic gram-positive bacillus produces a toxin that causes pseudomembranous colitis. Although asymptomatic carriage and mild infection can occur, the most dreaded consequence is the toxic megacolon seen in severe disease, which can lead to full-thickness colonic ischemia and perforation along with septic shock due to the systemic inflammatory response.[66]

CDI should be suspected in any elderly patient presenting with diarrhea, though it is important to note that CDI may present with obstipation as well, particularly in severe disease with toxic megacolon. Abdominal cramping or pain and leukocytosis should raise the index of suspicion, although any 1 or more of these features may be absent in the elderly population. Mild and moderate disease is defined as diarrhea and cramping without criteria of severe illness, which include abdominal distension and tenderness, leukocytosis (white blood cell [WBC] count>15,000 cells/mm^3), and hypoalbuminemia (albumin<3 g/dL). Complicated CDI is defined by any of the following criteria: WBC greater than 35,000 cells/mm^3 or less than 2000 cells/mm^3, lactate greater than 2.2 mmol/L, admission to the intensive care unit, hypotension with or without vasopressor support, fever greater than 38.5°C (to which hypothermia should be added for the elderly), ileus or abdominal distension, mental status changes, and end-organ failure.[67] The cornerstones of medical management of CDI include discontinuation of initial antibiotics if possible, and early therapy with appropriate antibiotics according to the severity of illness. Metronidazole for mild-moderate disease should be given intravenously if patient has vomiting, ileus, or other reason to suspect that absorption of the drug and delivery to the colonic lumen via the enterohepatic circulation will not be optimal; with the addition of vancomycin 500 mg orally every 6 hours for severe disease; as well as vancomycin enemas in patients with ileus.[66]

Surgical consultation should be requested early in the course of illness (ie, for mild-moderate disease) so that decisions regarding operative management can be made proactively. Diffuse peritonitis, metabolic acidosis, and signs of septic shock, including refractory hypotension, altered mental status, and end-organ dysfunction, unfortunately portend a mortality rate in excess of 50%, even with emergency surgical intervention. Although subtotal colectomy has been the standard treatment, recent success with loop ileostomy and antegrade colonic lavage, which can be performed laparoscopically, has resulted in success with substantially less morbidity and mortality.[68] Nevertheless, this approach remains untested in prospective randomized fashion.

Solid Organs: Pancreas, Spleen, and Liver

Most infectious complications of the abdomen in the elderly population occur in the hollow viscus organs described previously. However, the solid organs of the abdomen are also susceptible to infection. Specific and notable patterns of infection are seen, although at a rate far less than for other intraabdominal structures. For the pancreas, infection occurs secondarily in the setting of necrotizing pancreatitis. Infection is more common in younger patients than the elderly adult but when present in the elderly patient the mortality rate approaches 30%. Because the primary cause of death in these patients is systemic sepsis, adjunctive invasive treatment is directed at establishing source control. Dogmatic surgical approaches for infected necrotizing pancreatitis, including early debridement and wide drainage, have generally evolved into a step-up approach using percutaneous and minimally invasive techniques in a progressively more invasive algorithmic fashion until source control is established.[69,70] Early and aggressive nutritional support has been associated with improved outcomes and is likely to be especially beneficial in elderly patients who may already be nutritionally depleted.[71,72] Although controversial, prophylactic antibiotic administration with beta-lactams in the setting of necrotizing pancreatitis in the elderly patient seems reasonable based on current data.[73,74]

Liver infections in the elderly patient in the form of pyogenic liver abscess are rare but a well-described entity. These infections previously carrying a high mortality have now become treatable based on the advent of high-quality computed tomographic imaging and accurate percutaneous aspiration and drainage, allowing for minimally invasive treatment. Most liver infections were from a biliary source.[75] Splenic bacterial infections are rare. It should be recognized that either congenital or acquired asplenia (previous surgery or infiltrative diseases), leading to splenic nonfunction that predisposes the patient to infection of encapsulated bacteria.[76]

REFERENCES

1. Esposito AL, Gleckman RA. Fever of unknown origin in the elderly. J Am Geriatr Soc 1978;26(11):498–505.

2. Solomkin JS, Mazuski JE, Bradley JS, et al. Diagnosis and management of complicated intra-abdominal infection in adults and children: guidelines by the Surgical Infection Society and the Infectious Diseases Society of America. Clin Infect Dis 2010;50(2):133–64.

3. Agaba EA, Goon P, Pushdary K, et al. Perforated appendicitis in the elderly masquerading as acute coronary syndrome. Surg Infect (Larchmt) 2004;5(2): 195–9.
4. Golfieri R, Cappelli A. Computed tomography-guided percutaneous abscess drainage in coloproctology: review of the literature. Tech Coloproctol 2007; 11(3):197–208.
5. American College of Radiology. ACR practice guideline for specifications and performance of image-guided percutaneous drainage/aspiration of abscesses and fluid collections (PDAFC) in adults. In: Practice guidelines and technical standards, 2003. Reston (VA): American College of Radiology; 2003. p. 319–26.
6. Sawyer RG, Claridge JA, Nathens AB, et al. Trial of short-course antimicrobial therapy for intraabdominal infection. N Engl J Med 2015;372(21):1996–2005.
7. Lu J, Huang CM, Zheng CH, et al. Short- and long-term outcomes after laparoscopic versus open total gastrectomy for elderly gastric cancer patients: a propensity score-matched analysis. J Gastrointest Surg 2015;19(11):1949–57.
8. Wang XT, Wang HG, Duan WD, et al. Pure laparoscopic versus open liver resection for primary liver carcinoma in elderly patients: a single-center, case-matched study. Medicine (Baltimore) 2015;94(43):e1854.
9. Xie M, Qin H, Luo Q, et al. Laparoscopic colorectal resection in octogenarian patients: is it safe? A systematic review and meta-analysis. Medicine (Baltimore) 2015;94(42):e1765.
10. Abreu RA, Vaz FA, Laurino R, et al. Randomized clinical trial comparing spinal anesthesia with local anesthesia with sedation for loop colostomy closure. Arq Gastroenterol 2010;47(3):270–4.
11. Haagmans MJ, Brinkert W, Bleichrodt RP, et al. Short-term outcome of loop ileostomy closure under local anesthesia: results of a feasibility study. Dis Colon Rectum 2004;47(11):1930–3.
12. Kapala M, Meterissian S, Schricker T. Neuraxial anesthesia and intraoperative bilevel positive airway pressure in a patient with severe chronic obstructive pulmonary disease and obstructive sleep apnea undergoing elective sigmoid resection. Reg Anesth Pain Med 2009;34(1):69–71.
13. Sharma LB, Agarwal M, Chaudhary L, et al. Appendicectomy under local anaesthesia. Eur J Surg 1999;165(11):1091–2.
14. Watt DG, Wilson MS, Shapter OC, et al. 30-day and 1-year Mortality in emergency general surgery laparotomies: an area of concern and need for improvement? Eur J Trauma Emerg Surg 2015;41(4):369–74.
15. Soreide K, Desserud KF. Emergency surgery in the elderly: the balance between function, frailty, fatality and futility. Scand J Trauma Resusc Emerg Med 2015;23:10.
16. Farhat JS, Velanovich V, Falvo AJ, et al. Are the frail destined to fail? Frailty index as predictor of surgical morbidity and mortality in the elderly. J Trauma Acute Care Surg 2012;72(6):1526–30.
17. Joseph B, Pandit V, Zangbar B, et al. Superiority of frailty over age in predicting outcomes among geriatric trauma patients: a prospective analysis. JAMA Surg 2014;149(8):766–72.
18. Oresanya LB, Lyons WL, Finlayson E. Preoperative assessment of the older patient: a narrative review. JAMA 2014;311(20):2110–20.
19. Kenig J, Zychiewicz B, Olszewska U, et al. Six screening instruments for frailty in older patients qualified for emergency abdominal surgery. Arch Gerontol Geriatr 2015;61(3):437–42.

20. Ernst KF, Hall DE, Schmid KK, et al. Surgical palliative care consultations over time in relationship to systemwide frailty screening. JAMA Surg 2014; 149(11):1121–6.
21. Frasson M, Braga M, Vignali A, et al. Benefits of laparoscopic colorectal resection are more pronounced in elderly patients. Dis Colon Rectum 2008;51(3):296–300.
22. Person B, Cera SM, Sands DR, et al. Do elderly patients benefit from laparoscopic colorectal surgery? Surg Endosc 2008;22(2):401–5.
23. Popa D, Soltes M, Uranues S, et al. Are there specific indications for laparoscopic appendectomy? A review and critical appraisal of the literature. J Laparoendosc Adv Surg Tech A 2015;25(11):897–902.
24. Cooper Z, Courtwright A, Karlage A, et al. Pitfalls in communication that lead to nonbeneficial emergency surgery in elderly patients with serious illness: description of the problem and elements of a solution. Ann Surg 2014;260(6):949–57.
25. Neuman MD, Allen S, Schwarze ML, et al. Using time-limited trials to improve surgical care for frail older adults. Ann Surg 2015;261(4):639–41.
26. Ukkonen M, Kivivuori A, Rantanen T, et al. Emergency abdominal operations in the elderly: a multivariate regression analysis of 430 consecutive patients with acute abdomen. World J Surg 2015;39(12):2854–61.
27. Choo SK, Park HJ, Oh HK, et al. Acute cholecystitis in elderly patients after hip fracture: incidence and epidemiology. Geriatr Gerontol Int 2015;16(3):380–3.
28. Haltmeier T, Benjamin E, Inaba K, et al. Early versus delayed same-admission laparoscopic cholecystectomy for acute cholecystitis in elderly patients with comorbidities. J Trauma Acute Care Surg 2015;78(4):801–7.
29. Garcia-Alonso FJ, de Lucas Gallego M, Bonillo Cambrodon D, et al. Gallstone-related disease in the elderly: is there room for improvement? Dig Dis Sci 2015;60(6):1770–7.
30. Irvin TT. Mortality and perforated peptic ulcer: a case for risk stratification in elderly patients. Br J Surg 1989;76(3):215–8.
31. Christensen S, Riis A, Norgaard M, et al. Short-term mortality after perforated or bleeding peptic ulcer among elderly patients: a population-based cohort study. BMC Geriatr 2007;7:8.
32. Donovan AJ, Vinson TL, Maulsby GO, et al. Selective treatment of duodenal ulcer with perforation. Ann Surg 1979;189(5):627–36.
33. Crofts TJ, Park KG, Steele RJ, et al. A randomized trial of nonoperative treatment for perforated peptic ulcer. N Engl J Med 1989;320(15):970–3.
34. Donovan AJ, Berne TV, Donovan JA. Perforated duodenal ulcer: an alternative therapeutic plan. Arch Surg 1998;133(11):1166–71.
35. Siu WT, Leong HT, Law BK, et al. Laparoscopic repair for perforated peptic ulcer: a randomized controlled trial. Ann Surg 2002;235(3):313–9.
36. Kauffman GL Jr. Duodenal ulcer disease: treatment by surgery, antibiotics, or both. Adv Surg 2000;34:121–35.
37. Mitchell SL, Teno JM, Roy J, et al. Clinical and organizational factors associated with feeding tube use among nursing home residents with advanced cognitive impairment. JAMA 2003;290(1):73–80.
38. Schulenberg E, Schule S, Lehnert T. Emergency surgery for complications related to percutaneous endoscopic gastrostomy. Endoscopy 2010;42(10): 872–4.
39. Singh A, Gelrud A. Adverse events associated with percutaneous enteral access. Gastrointest Endosc Clin N Am 2015;25(1):71–82.
40. Oh DJ, Kim B, Lee JK, et al. Can percutaneous endoscopic gastrostomy be carried out safely in the elderly? Geriatr Gerontol Int 2015. [Epub ahead of print].

41. Udd M, Lindstrom O, Mustonen H, et al. Assessment of indications for percutaneous endoscopic gastrostomy–development of a predictive model. Scand J Gastroenterol 2015;50(2):245–52.

42. Rahnemai-Azar AA, Rahnemaiazar AA, Naghshizadian R, et al. Percutaneous endoscopic gastrostomy: indications, technique, complications and management. World J Gastroenterol 2014;20(24):7739–51.

43. Ballus J, Lopez-Delgado JC, Sabater-Riera J, et al. Surgical site infection in critically ill patients with secondary and tertiary peritonitis: epidemiology, microbiology and influence in outcomes. BMC Infect Dis 2015;15:304.

44. Barie PS, Hydo LJ, Eachempati SR. Longitudinal outcomes of intra-abdominal infection complicated by critical illness. Surg Infect (Larchmt) 2004;5(4):365–73.

45. Podnos YD, Jimenez JC, Wilson SE. Intra-abdominal sepsis in elderly persons. Clin Infect Dis 2002;35(1):62–8.

46. Cooper GS, Shlaes DM, Salata RA. Intraabdominal infection: differences in presentation and outcome between younger patients and the elderly. Clin Infect Dis 1994;19(1):146–8.

47. Kaiser M, Wilson S. Intra-abdominal infections. In: Norman D, Yoshikawa T, editors. Infectious disease in the aging. New York: Humana Press; 2009. p. 125–41.

48. Addiss DG, Shaffer N, Fowler BS, et al. The epidemiology of appendicitis and appendectomy in the United States. Am J Epidemiol 1990;132(5):910–25.

49. Omari AH, Khammash MR, Qasaimeh GR, et al. Acute appendicitis in the elderly: risk factors for perforation. World J Emerg Surg 2014;9(1):6.

50. Sirikurnpiboon S, Amornpornchareon S. Factors associated with perforated appendicitis in elderly patients in a tertiary care hospital. Surg Res Pract 2015; 2015:847681.

51. Kraemer M, Franke C, Ohmann C, et al. Acute appendicitis in late adulthood: incidence, presentation, and outcome. Results of a prospective multicenter acute abdominal pain study and a review of the literature. Langenbecks Arch Surg 2000;385(7):470–81.

52. Moazzez A, Mason RJ, Katkhouda N. Thirty-day outcomes of laparoscopic versus open appendectomy in elderly using ACS/NSQIP database. Surg Endosc 2013;27(4):1061–71.

53. Vons C, Barry C, Maitre S, et al. Amoxicillin plus clavulanic acid versus appendicectomy for treatment of acute uncomplicated appendicitis: an open-label, noninferiority, randomised controlled trial. Lancet 2011;377(9777):1573–9.

54. Mason RJ, Moazzez A, Sohn H, et al. Meta-analysis of randomized trials comparing antibiotic therapy with appendectomy for acute uncomplicated (no abscess or phlegmon) appendicitis. Surg Infect (Larchmt) 2012;13(2):74–84.

55. Salminen P, Paajanen H, Rautio T, et al. Antibiotic therapy vs appendectomy for treatment of uncomplicated acute appendicitis: the APPAC randomized clinical trial. JAMA 2015;313(23):2340–8.

56. Shabanzadeh DM, Wille-Jorgensen P. Antibiotics for uncomplicated diverticulitis. Cochrane Database Syst Rev 2012;(11):CD009092.

57. Watters JM, Blakslee JM, March RJ, et al. The influence of age on the severity of peritonitis. Can J Surg 1996;39(2):142–6.

58. Arenal JJ, Bengoechea-Beeby M. Mortality associated with emergency abdominal surgery in the elderly. Can J Surg 2003;46(2):111–6.

59. Ambrosetti P, Chautems R, Soravia C, et al. Long-term outcome of mesocolic and pelvic diverticular abscesses of the left colon: a prospective study of 73 cases. Dis Colon Rectum 2005;48(4):787–91.

60. Gentile V, Ferrarese A, Marola S, et al. Perioperative and postoperative outcomes of perforated diverticulitis Hinchey II and III: open Hartmann's procedure vs. laparoscopic lavage and drainage in the elderly. Int J Surg 2014;12(Suppl 2):S86–9.

61. Schultz JK, Yaqub S, Wallon C, et al. Laparoscopic lavage vs primary resection for acute perforated diverticulitis: the SCANDIV randomized clinical trial. JAMA 2015;314(13):1364–75.

62. Vennix S, Musters GD, Mulder IM, et al. Laparoscopic peritoneal lavage or sigmoidectomy for perforated diverticulitis with purulent peritonitis: a multicentre, parallel-group, randomised, open-label trial. Lancet 2015;386(10000):1269–77.

63. Chen HS, Sheen-Chen SM. Obstruction and perforation in colorectal adenocarcinoma: an analysis of prognosis and current trends. Surgery 2000;127(4):370–6.

64. Kelley WE Jr, Brown PW, Lawrence W Jr, et al. Penetrating, obstructing, and perforating carcinomas of the colon and rectum. Arch Surg 1981;116(4):381–4.

65. Zielinski MD, Merchea A, Heller SF, et al. Emergency management of perforated colon cancers: how aggressive should we be? J Gastrointest Surg 2011;15(12): 2232–8.

66. Keller JM, Surawicz CM. *Clostridium difficile* infection in the elderly. Clin Geriatr Med 2014;30(1):79–93.

67. Surawicz CM, Brandt LJ, Binion DG, et al. Guidelines for diagnosis, treatment, and prevention of *Clostridium difficile* infections. Am J Gastroenterol 2013; 108(4):478–98.

68. Neal MD, Alverdy JC, Hall DE, et al. Diverting loop ileostomy and colonic lavage: an alternative to total abdominal colectomy for the treatment of severe, complicated *Clostridium difficile* associated disease. Ann Surg 2011;254(3):423–7.

69. van Santvoort HC, Besselink MG, Bakker OJ, et al. A step-up approach or open necrosectomy for necrotizing pancreatitis. N Engl J Med 2010;362(16):1491–502.

70. Logue JA, Carter CR. Minimally Invasive necrosectomy techniques in severe acute pancreatitis: role of percutaneous necrosectomy and video-assisted retroperitoneal debridement. Gastroenterol Res Pract 2015;2015:693040.

71. Zou L, Ke L, Li W, et al. Enteral nutrition within 72 h after onset of acute pancreatitis vs delayed initiation. Eur J Clin Nutr 2014;68(12):1288–93.

72. Sanford DE, Sanford AM, Fields RC, et al. Severe nutritional risk predicts decreased long-term survival in geriatric patients undergoing pancreaticoduodenectomy for benign disease. J Am Coll Surg 2014;219(6):1149–56.

73. Ukai T, Shikata S, Inoue M, et al. Early prophylactic antibiotics administration for acute necrotizing pancreatitis: a meta-analysis of randomized controlled trials. J Hepatobiliary Pancreat Sci 2015;22(4):316–21.

74. Villatoro E, Mulla M, Larvin M. Antibiotic therapy for prophylaxis against infection of pancreatic necrosis in acute pancreatitis. Cochrane Database Syst Rev 2010;(5):CD002941.

75. Chen CH, Wu SS, Chang HC, et al. Initial presentations and final outcomes of primary pyogenic liver abscess: a cross-sectional study. BMC Gastroenterol 2014; 14:133.

76. Chattopadhyay B. Splenectomy, pneumococcal vaccination and antibiotic prophylaxis. Br J Hosp Med 1989;41(2):172–4.

Infectious Diarrhea

Norovirus and *Clostridium difficile* in Older Adults

Mary B. White, MD[a], Shobita Rajagopalan, MD, MSCR, MPH[b],*,
Thomas T. Yoshikawa, MD[a]

KEYWORDS

- Norovirus • Gastroenteritis • Long-term care • Elderly • *Clostridium difficile* infection
- Infectious diarrhea • Long-term care facilities • Aging

KEY POINTS

- Norovirus infection is a highly contagious illness which usually results in an acute gastroenteritis, often with incapacitating nausea, vomiting, and diarrhea.
- Community dwelling older adults as well as residents of long-term care facilities are disproportionately affected by complications that may result in hospitalization and/or death.
- *Clostridium difficile* infection is the leading cause of health care-associated diarrhea in the United States; antibiotic use is the most common risk factor for *C difficile* colonization and infection.
- Frail older adults are commonly affected by complications from *C difficile* infection, hospitalization, or death.
- Appropriate preventative and infection control measures can mitigate the morbidity and mortality associated with both these infections.

NOROVIRUS

Introduction

Noroviruses are a group of nonenveloped single-stranded RNA viruses in the Caliciviridae family, and are the leading cause of acute gastroenteritis, with 21 million cases, greater than 70,000 hospitalizations, and 800 deaths in the United States annually **(Fig. 1)**.[1]

The norovirus **(Fig. 2)** was originally called the Norwalk virus, because the first confirmed outbreak occurred in the town of Norwalk, Ohio, in 1968. There are 6 known

[a] Department of Veterans Affairs, VA Greater Los Angeles Healthcare System, 11300 Wilshire Boulevard, Los Angeles, CA 90073, USA; [b] County of Los Angeles Department of Public Health, Curtis Tucker Health Center, 123 West Manchester Boulevard, Inglewood CA 90301, USA
* Corresponding author. 123 West Manchester Boulevard, Suite 220C, Inglewood, CA 90301.
E-mail address: srajagopalan@ph.lacounty.gov

Clin Geriatr Med 32 (2016) 509–522
http://dx.doi.org/10.1016/j.cger.2016.02.008   geriatric.theclinics.com

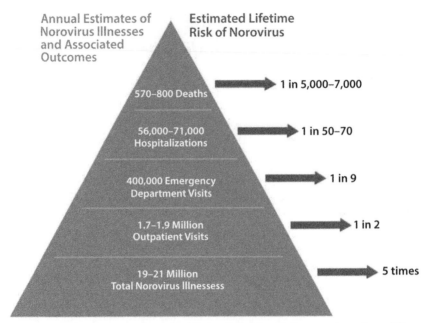

Fig. 1. Burden of norovirus in the United States. Estimates of the annual number of illnesses and associated outcomes for norovirus disease in the United States, across all age groups. Lifetime risks of disease are based on a life expectancy of 79 years of age. Ranges represent point estimates from different studies, not uncertainty bounds. (*From* Centers for Disease Control. Burden of norovirus illness and outbreaks. Available at: http://www.cdc.gov/norovirus/php/illness-outbreaks.html. Accessed April 8, 2016.)

genogroups of the virus, and more than 25 genotypes, but only genogroups I, II, and IV are known to cause disease in people.[2] Most outbreaks since 2002 have been caused by variations of the genotype GII.4.[3] It is not yet possible to grow the human norovirus in a cell culture, and this has hampered the development of a vaccine.[4]

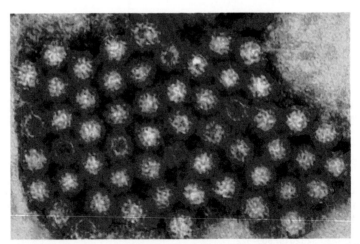

Fig. 2. Transmission electron micrograph of norovirus virions. (*Courtesy of* Public Health Image Library, no. 10708, CDC, Atlanta, GA. CDC/ Charles D. Humphrey.)

Norovirus is highly contagious. Once infected, the onset of illness is rapid, usually 12 to 48 hours. Symptoms usually include nausea, vomiting, and/or diarrhea. Because of the close quarters and communal living areas, nursing homes provide an ideal breeding ground for norovirus. Elderly persons, particularly those residing in nursing homes, are more susceptible to, and more likely to develop severe complications of norovirus infection due to altered immunity, comorbid medical conditions, compromised nutritional status, and use of medications such as statins,[5] proton pump inhibitors (PPIs), and antibiotics.[6]

Hospitalization may be required for treatment of volume depletion, renal failure, hypokalemia, arrhythmias, and delirium. Patients age 65 and older are at the highest risk of death from norovirus infection. Eighty-three percent of the deaths from acute diarrhea occur in patients 65 and older, with the leading cause being hospital-associated *Clostridium difficile-* associated diarrhea, followed by norovirus infection.[7]

Elderly patients typically do not recover as rapidly as the young. Residual thirst, anorexia, lethargy, vertigo, and malaise may last up to 4 weeks and may prevent patients from returning to their premorbid functional status. There is also an increased risk of falls during this more prolonged recovery period.[8] Because of the severe implications of norovirus infection in the elderly population, it is important to identify and control an outbreak at the earliest possible stage.

Transmission

Transmission occurs via the fecal–oral route and is very efficient. While affected patients can shed billions of virus particles daily, exposure to as few as 18 particles may cause a new infection.[9] It can be transmitted via person-to-person contact, contact with contaminated surfaces, inadvertent swallowing of aerosolized vomitus, and consumption of contaminated water and food. In fact, it is the most common cause of food-borne illness and is usually transmitted via contaminated produce, followed by seafood. Oysters are frequently implicated, but outbreaks have also been associated with consumption of mussels, cockles, and clams. Contamination of fishing waters by human sewage has played a major role in seafood-associated outbreaks.[10]

Long-term care facilities (LTCFs) seem particularly vulnerable to norovirus outbreaks, with nearly two-thirds of all norovirus outbreaks reported in the United States occurring in nursing homes, and most of these outbreaks reportedly caused by person-to-person transmission.[7,11] Food and drink contamination, often caused by infected food service workers, accounts for some of the outbreaks observed at long-term care facilities. Infected visitors may also introduce the virus to the facility.

Long-term care residents frequently suffer from incontinence, dementia, and musculoskeletal problems, often resulting in compromised hygiene. Shared bathroom facilities and inadequate hand washing only add to the ease with which norovirus is spread in residential facilities.[12] It is understandable why norovirus infection, once established in a residential care facility, is rapidly transmitted and difficult to eradicate.

In 1 study of an outbreak in an aged-care hostel in Melbourne, Australia, in 2003, an asymptomatic staff member had a stool specimen that was positive for norovirus 1 day prior to developing symptoms of acute illness. In the same study, while the vomiting and diarrhea usually resolved after 3 days, the median norovirus excretion time was 8.6 days, with a range of 2 to 15 days.[13] Other studies have shown norovirus excretion for up to 22 days post onset of acute illness.[14] For this reason, it is recommended that infection control measures remain active for at least 2 weeks following resolution of the last known case. The prolonged postacute shedding state, combined with the prodromal shedding, may also contribute to the difficulty eradicating the organism once it has a foothold in a long-term care facility.

Both the emesis and stools of norovirus patients are infectious. Attack rates in long-term care facilities vary depending on degree of exposure and host factors, but residents are more likely to become infected than staff. For example, 1 meta-analysis of observational studies indicated an overall attack rate (AR) of 32.9%, with a resident AR of 43.5% and a staff AR of 23.9%. Risk factors for patients included a high degree of dependence, and for staff, a high degree of contact with residents. Exposure to vomit without the use of facemasks was also a risk factor for infection.[8,15]

Clinical Manifestations

Norovirus is also known as winter vomiting bug, with nausea, vomiting, and diarrhea being the most common symptoms. Elderly patients are at greater risk of developing complications of norovirus, such as: volume depletion, electrolyte disturbances, acute kidney injury, arrhythmia, and death. They may also suffer from nonspecific symptoms such as headache, vertigo, thirst, and weakness to a greater degree than the general population, and these symptoms can persist for days or weeks after recovery from the acute phase.[16] Elderly patients afflicted with diarrhea tend to have longer hospital stays (7.4 days in patients older than 75 years vs 4.1 days in those patients 20–49 years old) and a higher mortality rate.[2,7,14,17] These factors should prompt the clinician to take a more aggressive approach in treating this more vulnerable group.

Complete recovery from norovirus gastroenteritis does not confer lasting immunity. It is unknown how long immunity from a particular strain of norovirus lasts, but because of the many variants of each genotype, it is possible for an individual to have multiple episodes of norovirus gastroenteritis over a lifetime.[18]

Diagnosis

Reverse transcriptase polymerase chain reaction (RT-PCR) is the diagnostic method of choice and can be used to detect norovirus from stool, vomit, and on surfaces or objects. RT-PCR is sensitive, detecting as few as 10 to 100 viral particles per reaction. It can quantify the viral load and identify the specific strain of virus by analysis of the genetic sequence. An enzyme immunoassay may also be used to identify norovirus, but because of low sensitivity of less than 50%, this type of test is not recommended to detect the infection in individual cases. However, it may be useful for preliminary screening early in a suspected outbreak. Stool specimens should be collected within 48 to 72 hours of the onset of acute symptoms and should be refrigerated at 39° F [40° C].[19]

If RT-PCR testing is not available or if results are delayed, the Kaplan criteria can be used to identify a norovirus outbreak. To satisfy the Kaplan criteria, more than half of symptomatic cases should experience vomiting; the mean or median incubation period should be 24 to 48 hours. The mean or median duration of illness should be 12 to 60 hours, and no bacterial pathogen should be isolated from stool cultures of affected individuals.[6]

Treatment

Treatment is mainly supportive, as there are no available antiviral treatment options. Because of the severe and often disabling symptoms, particularly in elderly persons, fluid resuscitation should be instituted without delay. If patients are unable to tolerate oral hydration, antiemetics and/or intravenous fluids should be administered.[20] Hypokalemia caused by excessive vomiting and diarrhea is common. Other metabolic disturbances may be present, such as hypochloremic metabolic alkalosis from vomiting and loss of gastric acid.[21] Hyperchloremic metabolic acidosis from excessive diarrhea may also be present. This occurs when the kidney is no longer able to compensate for the loss of bicarbonate and is often accompanied by volume depletion and hypotension. Hypovolemic shock, lactic acidosis caused by hypoperfusion, arrhythmia, and death may occur in extreme cases without appropriate supportive therapy.[22]

Because of the high frequency of renal impairment and cardiovascular comorbidities in the elderly population, severe acid–base derangements should be treated in a monitored setting, with careful attention to volume status, electrolytes, and blood gas measurements.[21] Antidiarrheals such as loperamide can be used when fluid loss from vomiting and diarrhea exceeds the ability to replenish it orally, but only at the lowest effective dose, as overuse may result in constipation following resolution of the diarrhea.[20]

Prevention/Intervention

The Centers for Disease Control and Prevention (CDC) recommend isolating suspected or confirmed norovirus cases. Such patients may be given private rooms or placed with similar patients. Patient transfers in and out of affected wards should be minimized, although patients can be discharged home with proper precautions. Visitors should be kept to a minimum. Infected staff should not return to work until at least 48 to 72 hours after complete resolution of symptoms.[23] However, studies have shown that asymptomatic (recovered) health care workers rarely contribute to the nosocomial transmission of norovirus despite continued viral shedding.[1,24,25] Disposal of contaminated waste should be done in accordance with Occupational Safety and Health Administration guidelines. Local health authorities should be notified in all cases of norovirus outbreaks to assist with proper management and containment.[22, 23]

Hand hygiene is of paramount importance, as the most frequent mode of transmission is fecal–oral. Hand washing involving rubbing the fingers together using soap and water is more effective than using an alcohol-based hand sanitizer.[26] However, hand washing alone cannot be relied upon to completely eliminate the virus, which can be present in concentrations of up to 10^{12} copies per gram of stool. Therefore, the use of disposable gloves is recommended when providing care to infected patients.[1]

Norovirus is stable on dry surfaces and can survive for several weeks in this state.[22] Contaminated and/or frequently touched surfaces should be cleaned regularly with a disinfectant approved by the Environmental Protection Agency (EPA) for activity against norovirus, and this heightened disinfection protocol should be maintained for at least 2 weeks after the resolution of the last known case. In caring for norovirus patients, personal protective equipment including masks with eye shields is recommended, because the virus can be readily transmitted through aerosolization of vomitus. Affected patients should be on contact precautions for the duration of symptoms plus an additional 48 hours.[22,23]

Vaccines and Antivirals

Norovirus vaccine development is ongoing. A bivalent GI.1/GII.4 virus-like particle injectable vaccine has been shown to reduce vomiting and/or diarrhea, as well as duration and quantity of viral shedding in infected volunteers.[27] The vaccine seems to be protective against different strains of GI.1 and GII.4 strains. However, volunteer studies have shown a lack of long-term immunity against reinfection.[28] Even if an effective bivalent (vs GI.1 and GII.4) vaccine were available, it would not be useful in the immunocompromised patient, or in rapidly evolving outbreaks. In such cases, an antiviral approach may be more effective. The most promising target for inhibition is viral RNA polymerase using nucleoside and non-nucleoside inhibitors.[29]

To summarize, norovirus is the most common cause of acute gastroenteritis and tends to cause more severe symptoms in the elderly population. It is highly transmissible and difficult to eradicate. Outbreaks frequently occur in long-term care facilities.

Due to their higher rate of complications and death, elderly patients should be treated with supportive therapy without delay. As no vaccine or antiviral is yet commercially available, aggressive measures must be taken to contain the spread of virus. These measures should include hand and environmental hygiene, the use of personal protective equipment, the isolation of suspected cases, the testing of patients and staff, and cooperation with local health authorities to control the outbreak.

CLOSTRIDIUM DIFFICILE

Clostridium difficile infection is the leading cause of health care-associated diarrhea in the United States. Antibiotic use is by far the most common risk factor for *C difficile* colonization and infection. Frail older adults are disproportionally affected by complications from *C difficile* infection, hospitalization, or death. Ongoing outbreaks of *C difficile* infection continue to be reported from long-term care facilities affecting a large proportion of elderly residents. Appropriate preventive measures and judicious use of antibiotics can help mitigate the morbidity and mortality associated with *C difficile* infection.

Introduction

Clostridium difficile (C difficile) causes a wide spectrum of human infection ranging from asymptomatic intestinal colonization to severe diarrhea, pseudomembranous colitis, toxic megacolon, perforation of the colon, sepsis syndrome, and death.[30] It is the leading cause of gastrointestinal illness and epidemics of diarrhea in hospitals and long-term care facilities (LTCFs).[31] Recent epidemiologic data suggest that *C difficile* is also becoming an important pathogen in the community, with a significant proportion of symptomatic *C difficile* infection (CDI) developing outside the health care setting.[32] Antibiotic-resistant CDI has also recently been reported.[33] Older adults with antibiotic exposure, prolonged antacid use, gastrointestinal surgery, long institutional stays, or serious underlying illness are at increased risk of acquiring CDI and its complications.[34] CDI is primarily precipitated by antimicrobial therapy, which disrupts the normal colonic microbiota, predisposing to *C difficile* intestinal colonization. The pathogenicity of *C difficile* is mediated by 2 potent cytotoxic enzyme exotoxins; other virulence factors such as proteolytic enzymes and adhesins may play a role in adherence and intestinal colonization. Age-related changes in fecal flora, immunosenescence, decreased antibody production to *C difficile* toxins, and impaired phagocytosis all contribute to an increased risk of complications, relapse, and reinfection.[34] The clinical diagnosis is best confirmed by PCR testing of the stools. Treatment modalities include antibiotics, alternative therapies such as probiotics and immune therapy, fecal microbiota transplantation (FMT), and surgery. Antibiotic stewardship is an important preventive strategy CDI. Strict infection control practices can help curb the spread of this infection. This section provides an update on the current epidemiology, risk factors, pathogenesis, clinical manifestations, laboratory diagnosis, treatment, recurrence, and prevention of CDI in older adults, both in the community and long-term care settings.

Epidemiology

C.difficile is the most common cause of health care-associated infectious diarrhea and accounts for 15% to 30% of all episodes of antibiotic-associated diarrhea; 11% of cases are attributed to elderly residents living in nursing homes.[35,36] A 2008 national point prevalence survey for CDI in 648 US hospitals (12.5% of all acute care hospitals) showed a prevalence of 13.1 cases per 1000 inpatients; 69% of affected patients were 60 years and older; 75% of cases were health care associated.[35,37] An upward trend in

CDI from health care settings has been reported in the United States from 2001 through 2010, with a 47% increase in cases of C difficile colitis in the second half of the decade compared with the first half.[36] Sporadic cases, as well as outbreaks of CDI, frequently occur in LTCF residents. The prevalence of C difficile colonization in LTCF residents ranges between 4% and 30%.[38–40] A significant proportion of residents may already be colonized with C difficile on admission to the LTCF, and an additional 10% to 20% of patients may acquire the organism during their stay in an LTCF.

The incidence rate (2.3 cases/10,000 resident–days) and recurrence rate (1.0 case/ 10,000 resident–days) of CDI in LTCFs is comparable to that of acute-care hospitals.[1] The highest incidence and greatest morbidity occurs in elderly persons. The mortality from CDI in the United States quadrupled from 1999 (5.7 cases per 1,000,000 persons) to 2005 (32.7 cases per 1,000,000 persons), with the highest rate in the elderly greater than 75 years (104 cases per 1.000,000 persons).[36]

A recent report from the CDC highlighted the emergence of a highly quinolone-resistant C difficile BI/NAP1/027 strain associated with severe disease secondary to enhanced toxin A and B production and hypersporulation, calling for high priority and aggressive measures to prevent and control this infection.[41]

Pathogenesis

C.difficile is a noninvasive gram-positive, spore-forming bacterium usually spread by the fecal–oral route. CDI is typically precipitated by antimicrobial therapy, which alters the normal protective colonic microbiota. Endogenous or exogenous contamination by C difficile spores result in germination of the spores and multiplication of the vegetative forms. C difficile can then adhere to and penetrate the mucus layer at the base of the enterocytes via flagella and proteases; adherence to enterocytes by multiple adhesins results in colonization. The primary virulence factors are the 2 large potent clostridial cytotoxic enzymes toxins A and B (TcdA and TcdB), which damage the human colonic mucosa.[42] A combination of asymptomatic colonization or carriage with a toxigenic strain of C difficile, antibiotic use, and low antibody production by the host is associated with a high risk for symptomatic CDI.

Risk Factors

Four major risk factors identified for CDI include advancing age, antibiotic exposure, admission to a hospital or nursing home, and low antibody response to the C difficile toxin. Advanced age-related factors (impaired immunity, reduced gastric acid, greater exposure to the organism due to institutionalization and antibiotic use) lead to a several-fold higher age-adjusted rate of CDI among persons more than 64 years of age.[34,43] Admission to a hospital or nursing home is associated with a daily increase in the risk of C difficile acquisition due to longer exposure to the organism from other patients with CDI, providers, and/or contaminated objects in the environment and invasive procedures and/or devices.[44,45] The key modifiable risk factor for the development of C difficile colonization and/or symptomatic disease is exposure to antimicrobial agents regardless of the number of antimicrobials or the duration of use. Although many antibiotics have been implicated, the highest risk for CDI has been linked to clindamycin, cephalosporins, penicillins, and β lactam/β lactamase inhibitor drugs because of their suppression of anaerobes and aerobes.[46] The relative risk of therapy with a given antimicrobial agent and its association with CDI depends on the local prevalence of strains that are highly resistant to that particular antimicrobial agent. Low antibody production (immunoglobulin M [IgM] and IgG) to C difficile toxin is associated with the highest risk for CDI and its recurrence. Contributing factors include immunosenesence, immunosuppression from cancer chemotherapy, human immunodeficiency virus infection, gastrointestinal surgery, or manipulation of the gastrointestinal tract, including tube feeding and use of acid-suppressing medications such as histamine-2 blockers and PPIs.[47]

Clinical Manifestations

The clinical presentation of infection with toxin-producing strains of C difficile in older adults, similar to their younger counterparts, can range from asymptomatic carriage; mild or moderate diarrhea; severe diarrhea with systemic manifestations (fever, leukocytosis, dehydration); to fulminant and sometimes fatal pseudomembranous colitis, toxic megacolon, sepsis, and death.[46] Several studies have shown that 50% or more of hospital patients colonized by C difficile are asymptomatic carriers, possibly reflecting natural immunity. Olson and colleagues[48] reported that 96% of patients with symptomatic C difficile infection had received antimicrobials within the 14 days before the onset of diarrhea and that all had received an antimicrobial within the previous 3 months. Symptoms of CDI usually begin soon after colonization, with a median time to onset of 2 to 3 days.

Mild disease is associated with watery malodorous stool. Fever, cramping, abdominal discomfort, and leukocytosis are common but found in fewer than half of patients and are suggestive of moderate disease. Severe disease is associated with colitis with pseudomembranes, presence of fecal leukocytes, and hypoalbuminemia, while fulminant disease can present with toxic megacolon, paralytic ileus, and sepsis.[49] Extraintestinal manifestations, such as arthritis or bacteremia, are rare. Complications of severe C difficile colitis are common in elderly persons and include dehydration, electrolyte disturbances, bowel perforation, hypotension, renal failure, systemic inflammatory response syndrome, septic shock, and death. Recurrences are also more common in older persons. Clinical diagnosis of mild, moderate, severe, or fulminant CDI can be confirmed by laboratory testing of stool.

Laboratory Diagnosis

Diagnostic testing for C difficile has rapidly evolved in the past decade. Laboratory diagnosis of C difficile infection requires demonstration of C difficile toxin(s) or detection of toxigenic C difficile organism(s) from stool samples.[50]

Nucleic acid amplification tests such as polymerase chain reaction tests

Real-time PCR tests that detect toxin A and B genes are highly sensitive and specific. The sensitivity of PCR is greater than enzyme immunoassay (EIA) and comparable to cytotoxicity assay. In addition, PCR results can be available within as little as 1 hour. Given its high sensitivity and the potential, therefore, for false-positive results, some favor use of PCR in an algorithm together with other assays such as EIA for glutamate dehydrogenase (GDH) and toxins A and B.

Enzyme immunoassay for Clostridium difficile glutamate dehydrogenase

GDH antigen is an essential enzyme produced constitutively by all C difficile isolates; its detection cannot distinguish between toxigenic and nontoxigenic strain. Therefore, testing for GDH antigen is useful as an initial screening step in a multistep approach, which also consists of subsequent testing with more specific assays such as PCR on specimens that are GDH antigen positive. GDH antigen testing is highly sensitive, and results are available in less than 1 hour.

Enzyme immunoassay for Clostridium difficile toxins A and B

Most C difficile strains produce both toxins A and B, although some strains produce toxin A or B only. The sensitivity of EIA for toxins A and B is about 75%; the specificity is high (up to 99%). There is a relatively high false-negative rate, since 100 to 1000 pg of toxin must be present for the test to be positive. Several inexpensive assays are commercially available, and test results are available within hours. If the initial EIA test is negative, the value of repeating the test is limited, and repeat testing is generally discouraged. Three studies found fewer than 10% more cases by repeated testing, while 2 others found 19% and 20% more cases with 1 or 2 further tests.

Cell culture cytotoxicity assay
The cell culture cytotoxicity assay is the gold standard test for diagnosis of *C difficile* and is the standard against which other tests should be compared. It is performed by adding a prepared stool sample (diluted, buffered, and filtered) to a monolayer of cultured cells. If *C difficile* toxin is present, it exerts a cytopathic effect characterized by rounding of fibroblasts in tissue culture. This assay is more sensitive than EIA but is slow and labor intensive.

Selective anaerobic culture
Culture on selective medium with toxin testing of isolated *C difficile* is the most sensitive diagnostic method, although culture alone cannot distinguish toxin-producing strains from nontoxin–producing strains. Prior treatment with heat or alcohol to select spores is sometimes used to improve yield. Culture is useful for epidemiologic studies, but is generally too slow and labor-intensive for clinical use. Several multistep algorithms have been developed in an attempt to improve the accuracy of diagnostic testing for CDI.

Treatment

Patients diagnosed with CDI must be placed in contact isolation, and any inciting antimicrobial agent (s) must be discontinued. Strong pretest probability for CDI should prompt the initialization of empiric therapy for CDI regardless of the laboratory testing results.

Treatment modalities include antimicrobial treatment; alternative therapies such as cholestyramine, probiotics, immunotherapy (intravenous immune globulin [IVIG]) and monoclonal antibodies to toxins; fecal microbiota transplant (FMT); and surgery.[51–56]

Antibiotics
Table 1 summarizes the current recommended antimicrobial treatment for mild, moderate, severe, fulminant, and recurrent CDI.

Alternative therapies
Cholestyramine Resin binding of toxin has shown limited benefit.

Probiotics (*Saccharomyces boulardi*; lactobacillus; bifidobacterium) Recent evidence suggests beneficial effects of probiotics in the prevention and treatment of recurrent CDI; they may cause bacteremia in immunosuppressed individuals. Further validation of these studies is needed for routine recommendations.[53]

Immunotherapy IVIG may be helpful in patients with hypogammaglobulinemia. Randomized trials are needed to determine the dose and duration of use in CDI. Monoclonal antibodies against toxins A and B may lower the recurrence rate (7% vs 25%).

Fecal microbiota transplant FMT is increasingly accepted as an effective and safe intervention in patients with recurrent disease, likely because of the restoration of a disrupted microbiome. A recent review in 115 patients age 60 to 101 years over a 2-month to 5-year follow-up period demonstrated cure rates of greater than 90%,

Table 1
Clostridium difficile severity and summary of recommended treatment regimens

Severity	Clinical Presentation	Treatment	Comment
Mild-to-moderate disease	Soft stool with greater frequency or watery with foul odor plus any additional signs or symptoms not meeting severe or complicated criteria Recurrent CDI within 8 wk of completion of therapy	Metronidazole 500 mg orally 3 times a day for 10 d; if unable to take metronidazole, vancomycin 125 mg orally 4 times a day for 10 d (standard dose) First recurrence: repeat course of standard dose metronidazole or change to vancomycin	If no improvement in 5–7 d, consider change to vancomycin at standard dose (vancomycin 125 mg 4 times per day for 10 d); a more costly alternative antibiotic is fidaxomicin (200 mg orally 2 times per day for 10 d); more data are needed to routinely recommend its use
Severe disease	Mild disease with fever, serum albumin <3 g/dL plus 1 of the following: White blood cell (WBC) count ≥15,000 cells/mm³ or abdominal tenderness Recurrent CDI within 8 wk of completion of therapy	Vancomycin 125 mg orally 4 times a day for 10 d First recurrence: higher dose vancomycin (500 mg every 6 h) and/or longer duration (3–4 weeks)	—
Severe complicated (fulminant) disease	Fever ≥38.5°C, sepsis, shock with multiorgan failure, ileus or abdominal distention, mental status changes, colitis, with pseudomembranes, presence of fecal WBCs, hypoalbuminemia, WBC ≥35,000 cells/mm³ or <2000 cells/mm³, serum lactate levels >2.2 mmol/L	Vancomycin 500 mg orally 4 times a day (high dose) and metronidazole 500 mg intravenously every 8 h, and vancomycin per rectum (vancomycin 500 mg in 500 mL saline as enema) 4 times a day	Surgical consultation is recommended
Multiple recurrent CDI	Recurrent CDI within 8 wk of completion of therapy	1. Vancomycin: standard or high dose followed by tapered dose for 21 d 2. Vancomycin standard dose followed by pulse dose (every 6 h): day 1: 125 mg; day 2: 250 mg; Day 3: 500 mg; repeat every 3 d for 27 d 3. Fidoxamycin: 200 mg orally twice a day for 10 d (fewer recurrences than vancomycin)	Consider FMT after 3 recurrences

Drugs with limited success include rifampin, ritazoxanide, rifaximin, bacitracin and tigecycline.[59]

also consistently reported from multiple centers.[55] Transplantation can be provided through a variety of methodologies, either to the lower proximal, lower distal, or upper gastrointestinal tract.

Surgery

Surgery is recommended for severe fulminant complicated cases associated with toxic megacolon or colonic perforation.

Infection Control and Prevention

Besides the affected patients, other important reservoirs for *C difficile* include spore-contaminated environments and equipment such as rectal thermometers, bedside commodes, and telephones. Hands of health care workers who directly care for patients with CDI are transiently contaminated with *C difficile* and may also contribute to spread.

Infection control and prevention strategies can help to reduce the incidence of CDI and must include several steps:

- Institution of a strong antibiotic stewardship program in health care facilities to guide the judicious use of antibiotics[55]
- Observation of contact precautions for patients with CDI at least until the resolution of diarrhea
- Patients with known or suspected CDI should be placed in a private room or in a room with another patient with documented CDI when feasible
- Hand hygiene and barrier precautions, including gloves and gowns, should be strongly reinforced and consistently used by all health care workers and visitors entering the room of any patient with known or suspected CDI
- Single-use disposable equipment should be used for prevention of CDI transmission. Nondisposable medical equipment must be dedicated to the patient's room; other equipment should be thoroughly cleaned after use in a patient with CDI
- Disinfection of environmental surfaces is recommended using an EPA-registered disinfectant with *C difficile*-sporicidal label claim or 5000 parts per million; chlorine-containing cleaning agents in areas of potential contamination by *C difficile*

The American College of Gastroenterology has published clinical practice guidelines that supplement the Infectious Disease Society of America/Society of Hospital Epidemiologists of America, and European Society of Clinical Microbiology and Infectious Diseases guidelines for prevention and control of *C difficile* infection.[57–59]

REFERENCES

1. Lopman B, Gastanaduy P, Park GW, et al. Environmental transmission of norovirus gastroenteritis. Curr Opin Virol 2012;2(1):96–102.
2. Glass RI, Parashar UD, Estes MK. Current concepts: norovirus gastroenteritis. N Engl J Med 2009;361:1776–85.
3. Bull RA, Tu ETV, McIver CJ, et al. Emergence of a new norovirus genotype II.4 variant associated with global outbreaks of gastroenteritis. J Clin Microbiol 2006;44:327–33.
4. Duizer E, Schwab KJ, Neill FH, et al. Laboratory efforts to cultivate noroviruses. J Gen Virol 2004;85(Pt 1):79–87.
5. Rondy M, Koopans M, Rotsaert C, et al. Norovirus disease associated with excess mortality and use of statins: a retrospective cohort study of an outbreak following a pilgrimage to Lourdes. Epidemiol Infect 2011;139:453–63.

6. Dupont HL. Acute infectious diarrhea in immunocompetent adults. N Engl J Med 2014;370:1532–40.

7. Trivedi TK, DeSalvo T, Lee L, et al. Hospitalizations and mortality associated with norovirus outbreaks in nursing homes, 2009-2010. JAMA 2012;308:1668–75.

8. Goller JL, Dimitriadis A, Tan A, et al. Long-term features of norovirus gastroenteritis in the elderly. J Hosp Infect 2004;58:286–91.

9. Teunis PF, Moe CL, Liu P, et al. Norwalk virus: how infectious is it? J Med Virol 2008;80:1468–76.

10. Weissfeld AS. Infections from eating raw or undercooked seafood. Clin Microbiol Newsl 2014;36(3):18.

11. Mody L. Establishing an infection control program. In: Yoshikawa TT, Ouslander JG, editors. Infection management for geriatrics in long-term care facilities. 2nd edition. New York: Informa Healthcare; 2007. p. 115–30.

12. Said MA, Perl TB, Sears CL. Gastrointestinal flu: norovirus in health care and long-term care facilities. Clin Infect Dis 2008;47:1202–8.

13. Rockx B, de Wit M, Vennema H, et al. Natural history of human calcivirus infection: a prospective cohort study. Clin Infect Dis 2002;35:246–53.

14. Petrignani M, van Beek J, Borsboom G, et al. Norovirus introduction routes into nursing homes and risk factors for spread: a systematic review and meta-analysis of observational studies. J Hosp Infect 2015;89:163–78.

15. Hall AJ, Vinjé J, Lopman B, et al. Updated norovirus outbreak management and disease prevention guidelines. MMWR Recomm Rep 2011;60(RR03):1–15.

16. Mounts AW, Holman RC, Clarke MJ, et al. Trends in hospitalizations associated with gastroenteritis among adults in the United States, 1979–1995. Epidemiol Infect 1999;123:1–8.

17. Harris JP, Lopman BA, O'Brien SJ. Infection control measures for norovirus: a systematic review of outbreaks in semi-enclosed settings. J Hosp Infect 2010;74:1–9.

18. CDC Norovirus Specimen Collection. Available at: http://www.cdc.gov/norovirus/lab-testing/collection.html. Accessed September 3, 2015.

19. Kaplan JE, Feldman R, Campbell DS, et al. The frequency of a Norwalk-like pattern of illness in outbreaks of acute gastroenteritis. Am J Public Health 1982;72(12):1329–32.

20. Seifter JL. Integration of acid–base and electrolyte disorders. N Engl J Med 2014;371:1821–31.

21. Kraut JA, Kurtz I. Treatment of acute non-anion gap metabolic acidosis. Clin Kidney J 2014;8(1):93–9.

22. MacCannell T, Umscheid CA, Agarwal RK, et al. Guideline for the prevention and control of norovirus gastroenteritis outbreaks in healthcare settings. Infect Control Hosp Epidemiol 2011;32:939–69.

23. Huttenen R, Syrjanen J. Health care workers as vectors of infectious diseases. Eur J Clin Microbiol Infect Dis 2014;33:1477–88.

24. Sukhrie FH, Teunis P, Vennema H, et al. Nosocomial transmission of norovirus is mainly caused by symptomatic cases. Clin Infect Dis 2012;54:931–7.

25. Atmar RL, Opekun AR, Gilger MA, et al. Norwalk virus shedding after experimental human infection. Emerg Infect Dis 2008;14:1553–7.

26. Blany DD, Daly ER, Kirkland KB, et al. Use of alcohol-based hand sanitizers as a risk factor for norovirus outbreaks in long-term care facilities in northern New England: December 2006 to March. Am J Infect Control 2011;39:296–301.

27. Bernstein DI, Atmar RL, Lyon GM, et al. Norovirus vaccine against experimental human GII.4 virus illness: a challenge study in healthy adults. J Infect Dis 2015; 211:875–7.

28. Simmons K, Gambhir M, Leon J, et al. Duration of immunity to norovirus gastro-enteritis. Emerg Infect Dis 2013;19:1260–7.

29. Arias A, Emmott E, Vashist S, et al. Progress towards the prevention and treat-ment of norovirus infections. Future Microbiol 2013;8(11):1475–87.

30. Gerding DN, Johnson S, Peterson LR, et al. *Clostridium difficile*-associated diar-rhea and colitis. Infect Control Hosp Epidemiol 1995;16:459–77.

31. Hall AJ, Cums AT, McDonald MD, et al. The roles of *Clostridium difficile* and nor-ovirus among gastroenteritis-associated deaths in the United States 1999-2007. Clin Infect Dis 2012;55:216–23.

32. Centers for Disease Control and Prevention (CDC). Surveillance for community-associated Clostridium difficile-Connecticut, 2006. Morb Mortal Wkly Rep 2008; 54:1201–5.

33. CDC Antibiotic resistance threats in the United States 2013. US Department of Health and Human Services 2013. Available at: http://www.cdc.gov/drug resistance/threat-report-2013/. Accessed October 1, 2015.

34. Morrison RH, Hall NS, Said M, et al. Risk factors associated with complications and mortality in patients with *Clostridium difficile* infection. Clin Infect Dis 2011; 53:860–9.

35. Simor AE, Yake SL, Tsimidis K. Infection due to *Clostridium difficile* among elderly residents of a long-term care facility. Clin Infect Dis 1993;17:672–8.

36. Halabi W, Carmichael J, Pigazzi A, et al. *Clostridium difficile* colitis in the United States: a decade of trends, outcomes, risk factors for colectomy, and mortality af-ter colectomy. J Am Coll Surg 2013;217:802–12.

37. Simor AE, Bradley SF, Strausbaugh LJ, et al. Clostridium difficile in long-term care facilities for the elderly. Infect Control Hosp Epidemiol 2002;23:696–703.

38. Walker KJ, Gilliland SS, Vance-Bryan L, et al. *Clostridium difficile* colonization in residents of long-term care facilities: prevalence and risk factors. J Am Geriatr Soc 1993;41:940–6.

39. Loo VG, Bourgault A-M, Poirier L, et al. Host and pathogen factors for *Clostridium difficile* infection and colonization. N Engl J Med 2011;365:693–703.

40. Pawar D, Tsay R, Nelson DS, et al. Burden of *Clostridium difficile* infection in long-term care facilities in Monroe County, New York. Infect Control Hosp Epidemiol 2012;33:1107–12.

41. See I, Mu Y, Cohen J, et al. NAP1 strain type predicts outcomes from *Clostridium difficile* infection. Clin Infect Dis 2014;58:1394–400.

42. Denève C, Janoir C, Poilane I. New trends in *Clostridium difficile* virulence and pathogenesis. Int J Antimicrob Agents 2009;33(S1):S24–8.

43. Zilberberg MD, Shorr AF, Micek ST, et al. *Clostridium-difficile*-associated disease and mortality among the elderly critically ill. Crit Care Med 2009;37:2583–9.

44. Kim KH, Fekety R, Batts DH, et al. Isolation of *Clostridium difficile* from the envi-ronment and contacts of patients with antibiotic-associated colitis. J Infect Dis 1981;143:42–50.

45. Brooks SR, Vail RO, Kramer M, et al. Reduction in the incidence of *Clostridium difficile* associated diarrhea in an acute care hospital and a skilled nursing facility following replacement of electronic thermometers with single-use disposables. Infect Control Hosp Epidemiol 1992;12:98–103.

46. Bartlett JG, Gerding DN. Clinical recognition and diagnosis of *Clostridium difficile* infection. Clin Infect Dis 2008;46(Suppl 1):12–8.

47. Leekha S, Aronhalt KC, Sloan LM, et al. Clostridium difficile colonoziation in a tertiary care hospital: admission, prevalence and risk factors. Am J Infect Control 2013;41:390–3.
48. Olson M, Yan Y, Reske KA, et al. Impact of *Clostridium difficile* recurrence on hospital readmissions. Am J Infect Control 2015;43:318–22.
49. Jump RLP. *Clostridium difficile* infection in older adults. Aging Health 2013;4: 403–14.
50. Tenover FC, Barren EJ, Peterson LR. Laboratory diagnosis of *Clostridium difficile* infection: can molecular amplification methods move us out of uncertainty. J Mol Diagn 2011;13:573–82.
51. Zar FA, Bakkanagari SR, Moorthi KM, et al. A comparison of vancomycin and metronidazole for the treatment of *Clostridium difficile*-associated diarrhea, stratified by disease severity. Clin Infect Dis 2007;45:302–7.
52. Connely OA, Miller MA, Louie TJ, et al. Treatment of first recurrence of *Clostridium difficile* Infection: fidaxomicin versus vancomycin. Clin Infect Dis 2012;55(Suppl 2): S154–61.
53. Evans CT, Johnson S. Prevention of *Clostridium difficile* infection with probiotics. Clin Infect Dis 2015;60(Suppl 2):122–8.
54. Adalja AA, Kellum JA. Clostridium difficile: moving beyond antimicrobial therapy. Crit Care 2010;14:320.
55. Nood E, Speelman P, Nieuwdorp M, et al. Fecal microbiota transplantation: facts and controversies. Curr Opin Gastroenterol 2014;30:34–9.
56. Chopra T, Goldstein EJ. *Clostridium difficile* infection in Long-term care facilities: a call to action for antimicrobials stewardship. Clin Infect Dis 2015;60(Suppl 2): S72–6.
57. Cohen SH, Gerding DN, Johnson S, et al. Clinical practice guidelines for *Clostridium difficile* infection in adults: 2010 update by the Society for healthcare epidemiology of America (SHEA) and the infectious diseases Society of America (IDSA). Infect Control Hosp Epidemiol 2010;31:431–55.
58. Bauer MP, Kuijper EJ, van Dissel T. European Society of clinical Microbiology and infectious diseases (ESCMID): treatment guidance for *Clostridium difficile* infection. Clin Microbiol Infect 2009;15:1067–79.
59. Surawicz CM, Brandt LJ, Binion DG, et al. Guidelines for diagnosis, treatment, and prevention of *Clostridium difficile* infections. Am J Gastroenterol 2013;108: 478–98.

Urinary Tract Infections in the Older Adult

Lindsay E. Nicolle, MD, FRCPC[a,b,*]

KEYWORDS

- Urinary infection • Cystitis • Pyelonephritis • Asymptomatic bacteriuria • Elderly
- Long-term care facility • Urinary catheter

KEY POINTS

- Symptomatic urinary tract infection and asymptomatic bacteriuria are very common in elderly populations.
- Major risk factors for infection are female sex, functional impairment, and use of indwelling urethral catheters.
- Clinical diagnosis of symptomatic urinary tract infection in long-term care facility residents is compromised by impaired communication and chronic genitourinary symptoms. Non-localizing symptoms, together with the high prevalence of asymptomatic bacteriuria, promote overdiagnosis and overtreatment of urinary infection.
- Residents of long-term care facilities with chronic indwelling catheters are always bacteriuric. The most common presentation of symptomatic infection in these patients is fever without localizing genitourinary symptoms or signs.
- Antimicrobial treatment is selected based on clinical presentation, presumed or known infecting organism, and patient tolerance.

INTRODUCTION

Urinary infection is an important clinical problem affecting older populations across the clinical spectrum of well, elderly men and women living independently in the community to the highly functionally impaired nursing home resident with multiple comorbidities. The site of infection may be the bladder (cystitis or acute lower tract infection) or kidney (pyelonephritis or acute upper tract infection). Acute or chronic bacterial prostatitis are additional presentations for men but will not be discussed further. Urinary infection in women with a normal genitourinary tract is referred to as acute uncomplicated urinary tract infection. Complicated urinary tract infection occurs in

[a] Department of Internal Medicine, Health Sciences Centre, University of Manitoba, Room GG443, 820 Sherbrook Street, Winnipeg, Manitoba R3A 1R9, Canada; [b] Department of Medical Microbiology, Health Sciences Centre, University of Manitoba, Room GG443, 820 Sherbrook Street, Winnipeg, Manitoba R3A 1R9, Canada
* Department of Medical Microbiology, Health Sciences Centre, University of Manitoba, Room GG443, 820 Sherbrook Street, Winnipeg, Manitoba R3A 1R9, Canada.
E-mail address: lnicolle@hsc.mb.ca

Clin Geriatr Med 32 (2016) 523–538
http://dx.doi.org/10.1016/j.cger.2016.03.002
0749-0690/16/$ – see front matter © 2016 Elsevier Inc. All rights reserved.
geriatric.theclinics.com

patients with functional or structural abnormalities of the genitourinary tract.[1] Asymptomatic bacteriuria is identified when the urine culture is positive without accompanying symptoms or signs attributable to genitourinary infection.[2] Individuals managed with a chronic indwelling urethral catheter have unique considerations with respect to diagnosis, complications, and management.[3]

EPIDEMIOLOGY
Community Populations

Asymptomatic bacteriuria increases with increasing age in elderly women living in the community, reaching a prevalence of 20% or more in those older than 80 years.[4] For healthy men, asymptomatic bacteriuria is unusual before 60 years of age; however, 5% to 10% of men older than 80 years have bacteriuria.[2,4] Individuals with bacteriuria also experience an increased frequency of symptomatic infection but symptomatic episodes are not directly attributable to the bacteriuria. Survival, and long-term negative outcomes such as renal failure or hypertension are not associated with bacteriuria.[2]

Older women in the community experience a higher frequency of symptomatic infection than men but the magnitude of the gender difference is less than in younger populations[4–12] (Table 1). There is limited morbidity associated with symptomatic urinary infection in healthy older individuals. Hospitalization rates for acute pyelonephritis increase with age and are highest for the oldest age groups.[10,11] Frequent recurrent infections may occur in some individuals, especially those with complicated infection.

Mortality directly attributable to urinary infection is uncommon.[7] For 270 Spanish subjects of mean age 83.7 years (14% from nursing homes) admitted with severe

Table 1
Occurrence of asymptomatic bacteriuria and symptomatic urinary infection in older populations

	Asymptomatic Prevalence (%)	Symptomatic Incidence
Community		
Women		
>80 y	20[4]	—
55–75 y		7/100 patient years[5]
86–90 y		12.8/100 patient years[6]
Hospitalization, pyelonephritis >60 y		1.4–2.3/10,000 population[7]
Men		
>80 y	8.0–9.5[4]	0–17/1000 d[8]
75–84 y	—	2.8–6.7/1000 population[9]
>85 y	—	4.3–7.8/1000 population[9]
86–90 y		7.8/100 patient years[6]
Hospitalization, pyelonephritis >60 y		6–1.3/10,000 population[7]
Women and men		
Hospitalization, pyelonephritis >70 y	—	1.0–1.5/10,000[10]
Long-term care	15–50[1]	—
United States	—	0.57/1000 d[11]
Germany	—	0.49/1000 d[12]
Chronic indwelling catheter	100[3]	3.2/1000 catheter days[11]
		3.5/1000 catheter days[12]

Data from Refs.[3–12]

urinary tract infection to a nonintensive care ward, the in-hospital mortality was 8.9%.[13] Independent risk factors for mortality were inappropriate empiric antimicrobial treatment, Acute Physiologic Assessment and Chronic Health Evaluation (APACHE) II greater than or equal to 15 on admission, dementia, and presence of a solid neoplasm. An Israeli review of 191 subjects ages 75 to 105 years admitted to a community-based geriatric hospital (35% from a nursing home)with bacteremic urinary infection reported the in-hospital mortality was 33%.[14] Hospital stay more than 20 days, dementia, and number of diagnoses were significantly associated with mortality but not more advanced age or gender.

Institutionalized Populations

A remarkable aspect of the long-term care facility population is the very high prevalence of asymptomatic bacteriuria, which is present in 25% to 50% of women and 15% to 40% of men.[1,2] Bacteriuria is dynamic. About one-third of bacteriuric individuals will have negative urine cultures by 3 to 6 months, and a further one-third of individuals without bacteriuria become bacteriuric in the same time period. Bacteriuria persists for years in many residents. Asymptomatic bacteriuria is not associated with negative clinical outcomes but promotes unnecessary antimicrobial use, leading to emergence of antimicrobial-resistant organisms, increased risk of *Clostridium difficile* infection, and adverse drug effects.[2,15]

Symptomatic urinary tract infection is the second most frequent infection in residents of long-term care facilities. The reported incidence for noncatheterized residents is 0.5 per 1000 resident days[11,12] (see **Table 1**). Although 45% to 56% of episodes of bacteremia in long-term care facilities are attributable to a urinary source, bacteremic infection occurs predominantly in residents with chronic indwelling catheters.[1,16] Urinary tract infection is a common reason for transfer of long-term care facility residents to an acute care facility but an infrequent cause of mortality.

PATHOGENESIS
Host Factors

Community population

Host determinants are similar for asymptomatic and symptomatic urinary infection. For well postmenopausal women, recurrent urinary infection is most strongly associated with a history of urinary tract infection at a younger age,[5,17] suggesting genetic determinants remain important in the postmenopausal period. One well-established association is being a nonsecretor of the blood group substances.[17] Sexual intercourse is not an important contributor to urinary infection in postmenopausal women.[5,18,19] In diabetic women aged 55 to 75 years, the incidence of symptomatic urinary infection was 12.2 per 100 person-years, compared with 6.7 per 100 for nondiabetic women.[20] The increased risk was observed primarily in women on insulin treatment or with diabetes for 10 or more years.

Lactobacilli spp are major components of the vaginal flora and maintain the acid pH of the vagina. Colonization by these strains is decreased in postmenopausal women, presumably because of a loss of estrogen.[21,22] The higher pH allows colonization with uropathogens such as *Escherichia coli* and *Enterococcus* spp. This change in flora may contribute to the increased frequency of urinary infection in elderly women. Estrogen replacement therapy can restore vaginal colonization with *Lactobacilli* spp and re-establish the acid pH.[21,23,24] However, women receiving systemic or topical estrogen therapy do not have a decreased incidence of symptomatic urinary tract infection compared with those without replacement therapy,[5,17,25–27] so the association of infection and estrogen is not straightforward (**Table 2**).

Prostate hypertrophy is the most important contributor to urinary infection in older men. It causes urethral obstruction and turbulent urine flow, which facilitates ascension of organisms into the bladder. Bacteria established in the prostate may persist indefinitely because of restricted diffusion of antimicrobials into the gland and the persistence of bacteria in some prostate stones. This is a source for recurring cystitis or febrile urinary infection for some men. Elderly women and men with genitourinary abnormalities that impair voiding, such as obstruction of the urethra or ureters, cystoceles in women, or bladder diverticulae, have an increased frequency of urinary tract infection. Urinary incontinence is a consistent association of infection in older women and men.[17,27,28] Incontinence is a marker for genitourinary voiding abnormalities, which also promote bacteriuria, rather than a cause of infection.

Ambulatory women aged 62 to 94 years with a prior history of urinary infection had a significantly higher mean postvoid residual volume, 70 mL versus 33 mL, compared with women without prior infection.[29] In ambulatory men of median age 62 years, the mean postvoid residual volume was 257 mL (range 150–560 mL) with bacteriuria and 133 mL (10–340 mL) in nonbacteriuric individuals.[30] However, another study in postmenopausal women reported no independent association of recurrent urinary infection with increased postvoid residual volume.[17] A prospective study in women ages 55 to 75 years reported symptomatic urinary infection was not correlated with postvoid residual volume stratified as less than 50, 50 to 100, or greater than 100 mL.[5] Thus, the association of residual urine volume and infection is inconsistent among different groups.

A Swedish study reported independent risk factors for bacteriuria in women older than 80 years in the community were reduced mobility, urinary incontinence, and receiving estrogen treatment and, in men, prostatic disease, history of stroke, and living in supervised housing.[27] The Netherlands study in the very elderly (86–90 years)[6] identified severe cognitive impairment, disability in daily living, urinary infection between the ages of 85 and 86 years, and self-reported urinary incontinence but not gender or residence as variables associated with urinary infection.

Table 2
Association of systemic and topical estrogen therapy with urinary infection or bacteriuria in postmenopausal women

Population (Reference)	Study Design	Estrogen Delivery	Outcomes[a] OR (95% CI)[b]
66 ± 6.9 y[17]	Matched, case control	Systemic or topical	2.14 (0.89–5.68)
55–75 y[5]	Prospective, cohort	Oral <1 mo	1.0 (0.5–1.2)
55–75 y[25]	Population-based, case control	Oral <0.625 mg/d	0.94 (0.69–1.27)
		0.625 mg/d	0.81 (0.62–1.06)
		>0.625 mg/d	1.61 (0.99–2.63)
50–69 y[26]	Case control, administrative data	Cream, patch, or oral ≥1 y	1.1 (0.8–1.5)
>80 y[27]	Case control	systemic or topical	2.01 (1.24–3.24)

[a] Symptomatic urinary infection, unless noted otherwise.
[b] Odds ratio for infection or bacteriuria in population receiving estrogen therapy (95% confidence intervals).
Data from Refs.[5,17,25–27]

Long-term care facility

Asymptomatic bacteriuria in the institutionalized population is associated with increased functional impairment, incontinence of bladder and bowel, and cognitive impairment.[1] The most important contributing factors are likely voiding abnormalities accompanying the chronic neurologic diseases that precipitate the need for institutional care, including cerebrovascular disease, Parkinson's disease, and dementia. The determinants of symptomatic urinary infection other than the presence of a chronic indwelling catheter are not well described. Increased postvoid residual urine volumes did not correlate with symptomatic or asymptomatic urinary tract infection in institutionalized men or women.[31,32] Men with continence managed using an external condom catheter have an increased prevalence of bacteriuria and symptomatic urinary infection compared with incontinent men not using these devices.[33]

Microbiology

Community population

E coli is the most frequent species isolated from symptomatic infection.[34,35] Other species, including other Enterobacteriaceae, Enterococcus spp, and nonfermenters such Pseudomonas aeruginosa are isolated less frequently. Coagulase-negative staphylococci may be isolated from asymptomatic men.[8] Candida spp occur in some patients, usually with risk factors of diabetes, indwelling urologic devices, and broad-spectrum antimicrobial therapy.

Bacterial strains isolated from older subjects may have an increased frequency of resistance relative to younger populations. This is attributable to repeated prior antimicrobial courses and health care exposures, including urologic interventions in subjects with complicated infection.[3,36] In a Spanish study of 153 men of mean age 60.7 years with community-acquired febrile urinary infection, age was significantly associated with isolation of fluoroquinolone resistant E coli. However, only previous health care exposure and antimicrobial use in the previous month remained independent predictors of resistance.[37] An American survey reported 60% of tigecycline nonsusceptible carbapenem-resistant Klebsiella pneumoniae in acute care subjects were isolated from urine cultures, with admission from a skilled nursing facility an independent risk factor for tigecycline nonsusceptibility.[38]

Long-term care facility

E coli remains the most common organism isolated from women with urinary tract infection in long-term care facilities, although other Enterobacteriaceae are isolated more frequently than in community subjects.[1] E coli is less common in men, whereas Proteus mirabilis, coagulase-negative staphylococci, and Enterococcus spp occur more frequently. About 10% to 25% of residents without an indwelling catheter have polymicrobial bacteriuria. The urine is a frequent site of isolation of organisms of increased antimicrobial resistance in these facilities.[39,40]

DIAGNOSIS
Clinical Presentations

Community population

Symptomatic urinary tract infection presents with clinical symptoms and signs ranging from minor, irritative lower tract symptoms to septic shock. Elderly individuals in the community usually present with the classic symptoms and signs of urinary tract infection. Cystitis presents with 1 or more lower tract irritative symptoms of frequency, urgency, dysuria, nocturia, suprapubic discomfort and, occasionally, hematuria.

Pyelonephritis presents as costovertebral angle pain or tenderness, often with fever, and with variable lower tract symptoms.

Long-term care facility

Clinical presentations are more difficult to assess in some elderly residents of long-term care facilities because of impaired communication and the frequent presence of chronic symptoms.[41,42] Chronic genitourinary symptoms are not attributable to bacteriuria.[43] Clinical deterioration without localizing genitourinary symptoms is unlikely symptomatic urinary tract infection in the bacteriuric resident.[1,43] Nonlocalizing signs or symptoms and nonspecific changes in clinical status such as increased falls, decreased function, or changes in mental status are frequently attributed to urinary tract infection. Symptoms independently correlated with bacteriuria plus pyuria in women nursing home residents with possible urinary infection were mental status change, change in character of the urine, and dysuria.[44] However, the observation of mental status change is confounded by underlying patient factors. In a further analysis, falls were not associated with bacteriuria.[45] Another cross-sectional study reported no association of urine culture results and nonlocalizing symptoms in men or women.[46]

Changes in character of the urine such as odor, color, or turbidity are correlated with bacteriuria but are usually attributable to alterations such as increased incontinence or dehydration rather than symptomatic infection. These are not sufficient, by themselves, for a diagnosis of infection. The presentation of acute confusion without localizing findings is an important diagnostic problem attributed to a wide variety of infectious and noninfectious causes.[47] Studies that report an association of urinary infection and acute delirium are compromised by a failure to use rigorous diagnostic criteria for urinary infection.[48,49] Symptomatic urinary infection is an unlikely cause of delirium in a resident without a chronic indwelling catheter and with no acute genitourinary findings.[50,51]

Consensus clinical criteria for initiation of empiric antimicrobial therapy for presumed infection in long-term care residents have been developed.[52] The specific clinical presentations are acute dysuria, by itself, or fever, acute confusion, or chills with at least 1 new or worsening genitourinary symptom (urgency, frequency, suprapubic pain, gross hematuria, costovertebral angle tenderness, urinary incontinence). A prospective clinical trial subsequently reported that implementation of these guidelines decreased antimicrobial use compared with standard care and was safe.[53] Current surveillance guidelines also require localizing genitourinary findings for diagnosis of urinary infection.[41,43] When the diagnosis is uncertain, observation and monitoring of residents is recommended.[54] A clinical presentation suggesting severe infection in a patient without localizing findings should be managed as potential sepsis of unknown cause rather than assuming urinary infection.

Laboratory Diagnosis

Urine culture

A urine culture confirms the diagnosis of urinary infection and informs antimicrobial management by identifying the specific infecting organism and susceptibilities. The wide variety of potential infecting organisms and increased likelihood of antimicrobial resistance in older populations means a urine culture is essential for appropriate management.[1,41] An exception to this recommendation is the healthy woman living in the community who experiences recurrent acute cystitis, for whom empirical short-course antimicrobial therapy is usually effective. A urine culture should be obtained from these women, however, if presenting symptoms are atypical, response to empirical therapy is inadequate, or there is early symptomatic recurrence post-therapy, suggesting infection with a resistant organism.

The urine specimen must be collected before initiating antimicrobial therapy, using a technique that minimizes contamination.[42] A voided clean-catch urine specimen is usually appropriate. For women who cannot cooperate for specimen collection, in-and-out catheter collection is recommended. For men, urine specimens may be collected using an external condom catheter after applying a clean condom and leg bag.[42]

The diagnostic bacterial count is greater than or equal to 10^5 colony-forming units (cfu)/mL of a single organism isolated from a urine specimen. When lower bacterial counts or multiple organisms are reported, the culture result is interpreted in the context of the clinical presentation. Lower quantitative counts are isolated from as many as 10% of healthy, postmenopausal women in the community with acute uncomplicated urinary infection.[5] Lower counts may also occur in men or women with cystitis when diuresis or frequency limits urine bladder incubation time. For men, greater than or equal to 10^3 cfu/mL of a uropathogen from a clean-catch voided specimen is suggested to be consistent with symptomatic infection.[55] When specimens are collected from men using an external catheter, greater than or equal to 10^5 cfu/mL is the appropriate criteria.[1] If pyelonephritis is suspected, greater than or equal to 10^4 cfu/mL of a single organism is the proposed quantitative criteria. A quantitative count of greater than or equal to 10^2 cfu/mL is relevant when a specimen is collected by in-and-out catheter.[3]

Other laboratory investigations

Pyuria is a nonspecific finding in older populations.[1,3,41] It is frequently positive in elderly patients without bacteriuria, and for bacteriuric patients does not differentiate asymptomatic or symptomatic infection. The absence of pyuria, however, has a high negative predictive value and is useful to exclude urinary tract infection.[41] When the diagnosis of symptomatic urinary infection is considered in a long-term care facility resident, a urine specimen should be screened for pyuria. If negative, urinary infection is excluded and a urine culture should not be obtained.[41]

A preliminary study in women greater than or equal to 80 years of age suggested elevated levels of urinary cytokines interleukin IL-8 and IL-6, and of leukocyte esterase might discriminate between asymptomatic bacteriuria and acute cystitis.[56] However, although urine IL-6 and IL-8 correlate with bacteriuria, there is substantial inter-resident variation, so these biomarkers do not seem useful for differentiating symptomatic infection from bacteriuria.[57]

Blood cultures are indicated when patients present with severe sepsis or acute confusional states with or without localizing symptoms. Isolation of the same organism from blood and urine usually supports a diagnosis of urosepsis.

ANTIMICROBIAL TREATMENT
Asymptomatic Bacteriuria

Treatment of asymptomatic bacteriuria is not indicated for older populations.[2] Antimicrobial therapy does not decrease the subsequent frequency of symptomatic infection or improve chronic genitourinary symptoms such as incontinence[1,42] but is associated with adverse drug effects and promotes reinfection with more resistant organisms. Recurrent bacteriuria usually occurs early post-treatment. Thus, screening of older individuals for asymptomatic bacteriuria is not indicated. Because treatment of asymptomatic bacteriuria is the most common reason for inappropriate antimicrobial use in older populations, strategies to limit antimicrobial use for asymptomatic bacteriuria should be incorporated into antimicrobial stewardship programs for elderly persons.

Antimicrobial Selection

The antimicrobial regimen is selected considering efficacy, patient tolerance, clinical presentation, renal function, need for parenteral therapy, and cost. There is a predictable decline in creatinine clearance with aging but changes in antimicrobial agent or dose based on age alone are not indicated. When symptoms are mild, initiation of antimicrobial therapy should be delayed until urine culture results are available. This supports optimal antimicrobial selection and limits unnecessary antimicrobial treatment.

First-line oral therapy for cystitis includes trimethoprim/sulfamethoxazole (TMP/SMX) and nitrofurantoin (**Table 3**). Nitrofurantoin is not effective for renal or prostate infection. *K pneumoniae*, *P mirabilis*, and *P aeruginosa* are uniformly resistant to nitrofurantoin but other resistant organisms such as extended-spectrum beta lactamase (ESBL)-producing *E coli* and vancomycin-resistant enterococci usually remain susceptible. The fluoroquinolones (norfloxacin, ciprofloxacin, and levofloxacin) are effective for treatment of susceptible organisms[34,58] but increasing fluoroquinolone-resistance may limit efficacy. These agents should be reserved for empiric treatment of patients with severe presentations such as pyelonephritis, when organisms resistant to other agents are likely, or for patients unable to tolerate other therapies. Oral cephalosporins, fosfomycin, doxycycline, amoxicillin, or amoxicillin/clavulanic acid are effective second-line oral agents for selected patients, depending on antimicrobial susceptibility and tolerance.

Parenteral therapy is indicated for patients who present with hemodynamic instability, are unable to tolerate oral therapy, have uncertain gastrointestinal absorption, or are infected with an organism known or suspected to be resistant to available oral agents. Ceftriaxone or cefotaxime, an aminoglycoside (gentamicin, tobramycin) with or without ampicillin, or a fluoroquinolone (ciprofloxacin or levofloxacin) are recommended, depending on organism susceptibility (see **Table 3**). Parenteral therapy is usually given for the initial 48 to 72 hours, then re-evaluated and changed to oral therapy, if possible, considering the urine culture result and initial clinical response. If more

Table 3
Antimicrobial regimens for treatment of urinary tract infection in older persons with normal renal function

	Oral	Parenteral
First-line	TMP/SMX 160/800 mg bid Nitrofurantoin monohydrate/ macrocrystals 100 mg bid Ciprofloxacin 250–500 mg bid Norfloxacin 400 bid Levofloxacin 250–500 mg od	Ampicillin 2 g q6h ± gentamicin or tobramycin 5–7 mg/kg q24h Ceftriaxone 1–2 g q24h Cefotaxime 1 g q8h Ciprofloxacin 400 mg q12h Levofloxacin 500–750 mg q24h
Other	Amoxicillin 500 mg tid Amoxicillin/clavulanic acid 500 mg tid or 875 mg bid Cephalexin 500 mg qid Cefuroxime axetil 500 mg bid Cefixime 400 mg od Cefpodoxime proxetil 100–1200 mg bid Doxycycline 100 mg bid Fosfomycin 3 g Trimethoprim 100 mg bid	Amikacin 7.5 mg/kg q12h or 15 mg/kg q24h Cefazolin 1 g q8h Ceftazidime 1 g q8h Ceftazidime/avibactam 2.5 g q8h Doripenem 500 mg q6h Ertapenem 1 g od Meropenem 500 mg q6h or 1 g q8h Piperacillin/tazobactam 3.375 g q8h Vancomycin[a] 1 g IV q12h

[a] Gram-positive organisms only.

prolonged (>7 days) aminoglycoside therapy is indicated, monitoring of drug levels and renal function is required.

Duration of Therapy

Older women in the community presenting with acute cystitis should receive short-course antimicrobial therapy. A study in women of mean age 78.5 years reported similar outcomes with 3 or 7 days ciprofloxacin, and significantly fewer adverse effects with the shorter regimen.[34] TMP/SMX is also likely effective as a 3-day regimen, and nitrofurantoin given as a 5-day course. The optimal duration of therapy for women residents in long-term care facilities has not been determined. Treatment of men or women with complicated urinary infection is individualized based on clinical presentations, underlying urologic abnormality, and response to therapy. Seven days is usually sufficient for patients presenting with lower tract symptoms, and 10 to 14 days for renal infection.

PREVENTION

Long-term low-dose prophylactic antimicrobial therapy can prevent frequent recurrent acute uncomplicated urinary infection in older women in the community. First-line regimens are nitrofurantoin 50 or 100 mg daily or TMP/SMX one-half regular strength tablet daily or every other day. An initial course is usually for 6 or 12 months. The strategy of self-treatment with 3 days TMP/SMX or a fluoroquinolone has not been evaluated specifically in older women.

Two small trials of topical vaginal estrogen reported a decreased frequency of urinary infection[23,24,59] in women with frequent symptomatic recurrence but an estrogen-containing pessary was less effective than nitrofurantoin prophylaxis.[60] Thus, the role of topical estrogen for prevention of urinary infection requires further evaluation. Systemic estrogen therapy does not decrease the frequency of urinary infection.[59]

A prospective, cohort study in women ages 55 to 75 years reported no association of use of cranberry products and frequency of infection.[5] Cranberry juice was less effective than prophylactic trimethoprim in preventing urinary infection in older women.[61] A clinical trial enrolling women admitted to an elderly assessment and rehabilitation hospital ward reported no differences in symptomatic infections in women receiving cranberry juice or placebo.[62] Lactobacillus was significantly less effective than TMP/SMX in preventing recurrent infection in postmenopausal women with uncomplicated urinary infection, despite a high prevalence of isolation of TMP/SMX resistant organisms.[63]

Effective interventions to decrease urinary infection in institutionalized populations have not been described. Systemic estrogen therapy[64] and cranberry products[61,62,65,66] are not beneficial. Correction of the underlying genitourinary abnormality in persons with complicated urinary infection, if possible, may limit recurrent infection. Prophylactic antimicrobial therapy does not decrease symptomatic episodes in patients with complicated infection.[42] Long-term suppressive therapy to control frequent recurrent symptomatic episodes is indicated, rarely, when the underlying abnormality cannot be corrected.

Patients with asymptomatic bacteriuria who undergo a genitourinary procedure with a high likelihood of mucosal bleeding (eg, prostate resection, ureteric stent) are at high risk of postprocedure bacteremia and sepsis. A single dose of prophylactic antimicrobial therapy given immediately before the procedure will usually prevent this complication.[2]

CHRONIC INDWELLING CATHETER
Epidemiology

In an American study, 12.6% of long-term care facility residents had an indwelling catheter at admission, and 4.5% at annual review.[67] In 78 Swedish nursing homes, 16% of men and 3% of women used chronic indwelling catheters.[68] Individuals with voiding managed by a chronic indwelling catheter are always bacteriuric.[3] The incidence of infection with a new organism is 3% to 7% per day. There is substantially higher morbidity attributed to symptomatic urinary infection in catheterized residents compared with bacteriuric residents without a catheter (see **Table 1**). In catheterized residents, symptomatic urinary infection occurs 2.2 times more frequently,[69] fever from a urinary source 3 times more frequently,[70] bacteremia from a urinary source 3 to 39 times more frequently,[71,72] and evidence of acute pyelonephritis at autopsy 8 times more frequently.[70] Local suppurative complications such as urethritis, Bartholin gland abscesses, prostatitis, and acute epididymo-orchitis may occur. The increased mortality reported in residents with chronic indwelling catheters is attributed to higher functional impairment and comorbidities rather than urinary infection.[3]

Pathogenesis

Biofilm
An indwelling device in the urinary tract becomes rapidly coated with biofilm.[3] Microorganisms initially adhere to a conditioning layer that forms on the device immediately following insertion, then grow along interior and external surfaces of the catheter within an extracellular polysaccharide substance produced by the organisms. Urine components including Tamm-Horsfall protein and magnesium and calcium ions are incorporated into this biofilm. Organisms grow as microcolonies within the biofilm in a protected environment, which restricts diffusion of antimicrobials and limits access of host defenses such as neutrophils or immunoglobulins. Urease production by some species creates an alkaline urine with precipitation of magnesium and calcium ions, creating a crystalline biofilm, which may lead to catheter encrustation and obstruction.

The determinants of symptomatic infection in these patients are not well described. However, mucosal trauma or catheter obstruction are risk factors for systemic infection.

Microbiology
Individuals with a chronic indwelling urethral catheter have 2 to 5 organisms isolated at any time. A wide spectrum of bacteria is isolated, with E coli, Enterococcus faecalis, and P mirabilis the most frequent.[3,73] Urease-producing bacteria such as P mirabilis, Morganella morganii, K pneumoniae, and Providencia stuartii are particularly common.[74] Bacterial strains persist for variable periods of time. Enterococcus spp persisted for only a few weeks, whereas P mirabilis persisted for several months in 1 study.[74] P mirabilis has unique properties, including producing copious biofilm. About 80% of episodes of catheter obstruction are attributed to P mirabilis colonization and crystalline biofilm formation.[75] Resistant organisms are more common in residents with indwelling catheters.[76]

Diagnosis

Clinical presentation
The most common presentation of symptomatic infection in residents with a chronic indwelling catheter is fever without localizing genitourinary signs or symptoms.[3,43] Localizing signs such as costovertebral angle pain or tenderness, catheter obstruction, or hematuria may occur in some patients. Consensus definitions for clinical

presentations to initiate empiric antimicrobial therapy for residents with a chronic catheter include only the presence of 1 or more of fever, new costovertebral angle tenderness, rigors, or new onset delirium, in the absence of an alternate source.[52]

Laboratory diagnosis

Urine collected through a catheter will sample biofilm as well as bladder urine. A chronic indwelling catheter in place for 2 weeks or more should be replaced before starting antimicrobial therapy, and the urine specimen obtained from the freshly inserted catheter.[77] This samples only bladder urine, so culture results are more relevant for therapeutic decisions. A quantitative count of greater than or equal to 10^5 cfu/mL is appropriate to identify bacteriuria.[42]

The degree of pyuria does not vary between asymptomatic periods and symptomatic episodes, so pyuria is not a useful diagnostic test.[78]

Treatment

Treatment of asymptomatic bacteriuria is not recommended because it does not decrease the frequency of symptomatic episodes but promotes reinfection with more-resistant bacteria.[2] Antimicrobial therapy for symptomatic infection is similar to other presentations of urinary infection (see **Table 3**). The optimal duration of therapy has not been evaluated. If there is a prompt clinical response, 7 days is recommended to minimize the likelihood of reinfection with more resistant organisms.

Catheter replacement before initiating antimicrobial therapy for symptomatic infection improves clinical outcomes, including more rapid defervescence and decreased symptomatic relapse.[53] These clinical benefits are presumed to be attributable to removal of organisms that persist in the biofilm despite antimicrobial therapy.

Prevention

Evidence based guidelines provide comprehensive recommendations for prevention of catheter-acquired urinary infection.[79,80] The most important practices are to limit use of an indwelling catheter and, when a catheter is indicated, discontinue the catheter as soon as possible.[3,42] Use of an external condom catheter for incontinence management may avoid indwelling catheter use in some men and has a lower risk of infection.[81] Clean intermittent catheterization is an option for selected residents.[42] Appropriate catheter care to prevent trauma and identify obstruction promptly will likely limit episodes of systemic infection. Routine catheter change or catheter irrigation, specific catheter type, antimicrobial impregnated catheters, or antiseptics in the drainage bag do not decrease the frequency of symptomatic urinary infection and are not recommended.[42,82] A low incidence of transient bacteremia is observed with catheter replacement but is not associated with harmful outcomes, so antimicrobial prophylaxis is not recommended with catheter change.[42]

SUMMARY

Urinary infection is an important clinical problem for older populations. Asymptomatic bacteriuria is ubiquitous and should not be treated. Variables promoting the high prevalence of asymptomatic bacteriuria in residents of long-term care facilities are not well characterized. Effective strategies to limit inappropriate antimicrobial use for asymptomatic bacteriuria require further characterization. Appropriate management of symptomatic infection for noncatheterized subjects requires diagnosis based on localizing genitourinary signs or symptoms. Further evaluation of urine biomarkers is a potential diagnostic approach to identify symptomatic infection is needed. The efficacy of topical vaginal estrogen replacement for prevention of urinary infection in older women also requires further study. Comparative clinical trials exploring both optimal antimicrobial selection and duration of therapy are needed for all older populations experiencing symptomatic urinary infection. Limiting bacteriuria and urinary infection in residents with chronic indwelling catheters will require advances in development of biofilm-resistant biomaterials.

REFERENCES

1. Nicolle LE. Urinary tract infection in the elderly. Clin Geriatr Med 2009;25:423–36.
2. Nicolle LE, Bradley S, Colgan R, et al. Infectious Diseases Society of America guidelines for the diagnosis and treatment of asymptomatic bacteriuria in adults. Clin Infect Dis 2005;40:643–54.
3. Nicolle LE. Catheter-related urinary tract infection: practical management in the elderly. Drugs Aging 2014;31:1–10.
4. Rodhe N, Lofgren S, Matussek A, et al. Asymptomatic bacteriuria in the elderly: high prevalence and high turnover of strains. Scand J Infect Dis 2008;40:804–10.
5. Jackson SL, Boyko EJ, Scholes D, et al. Predictors of urinary tract infection after menopause: a prospective study. Am J Med 2004;117:903–11.
6. Caljouw MA, den Elzen WP, Cools HJ, et al. Predictive factors of urinary tract infections among the oldest old in the general population: a population-based prospective follow-up study. BMC Med 2011;9:57–64.
7. Foxman B, Klemstine KL, Brown PD. Acute pyelonephritis in US hospitals in 1997: hospitalization and in-hospital mortality. Ann Epidemiol 2003;13:144–50.
8. Mims AD, Norman DC, Yamamura RH, et al. Clinically inapparent (asymptomatic) bacteriuria in ambulatory elderly men: epidemiological, clinical, and microbiological findings. J Am Geriatr Soc 1990;38:1209–14.
9. Griebling TL. Urologic diseases in America project: trends in resource use for urinary tract infections in men. J Urol 2005;173:1288–94.
10. Nicolle LE, Friesen D, Harding GK, et al. Hospitalization from acute pyelonephritis in Manitoba, Canada during the period 1989-1992. Impact of diabetes, pregnancy, and aboriginal origin. Clin Infect Dis 1996;22:1051–6.
11. Stevenson KB, Moore J, Colwell H, et al. Standardized infection surveillance in long-term care: interfacility comparisons from a regional cohort of facilities. Infect Control Hosp Epidemiol 2005;26:231–8.
12. Engelhart ST, Hanses-Derendorf L, Exner M, et al. Prospective surveillance for healthcare-associated infections in German nursing home residents. J Hosp Infect 2005;60:46–50.
13. Esparcia A, Artero A, Eiros JM, et al. Influence of inadequate antimicrobial therapy on prognosis in elderly patients with severe urinary tract infections. Eur J Intern Med 2014;25:523–7.
14. Tal S, Guller V, Levi S, et al. Profile and prognosis of febrile elderly patients with bacteremic urinary tract infection. J Infect 2005;50:296–305.
15. Rotjanapan P, Dosa D, Thomas KS. Potential inappropriate treatment of urinary tract infection in two Rhode Island nursing homes. Arch Intern Med 2011;171:438–43.
16. Mylotte JM, Tayara A, Goodnough S. Epidemiology of bloodstream infection in nursing home residents: evaluation in a large cohort from multiple homes. Clin Infect Dis 2002;35:1484–90.
17. Raz R, Gennesin Y, Wasser J, et al. Recurrent urinary tract infections in postmenopausal women. Clin Infect Dis 2000;30:152–6.

18. Foxman B, Somsel P, Tallman P, et al. Urinary tract infection among women aged 40 to 65: behavioral and sexual risk factors. J Clin Epidemiol 2001;54:710–8.
19. Moore EE, Hawes SE, Scholes D, et al. Sexual intercourse and risk of symptomatic urinary tract infection in post-menopausal women. J Gen Intern Med 2008;23: 595–9.
20. Boyko EJ, Fihn SD, Scholes D, et al. Risk of urinary tract infection and asymptomatic bacteriuria among diabetic and nondiabetic postmenopausal women. Am J Epidemiol 2005;161:557–64.
21. Pabich WL, Fihn SD, Stamm WE, et al. Prevalence and determinants of vaginal flora alterations in postmenopausal women. J Infect Dis 2003;188:1054–8.
22. Burton JP, Reid G. Evaluation of the bacterial vaginal flora of 20 postmenopausal women by direct (Nugent score) and molecular (polymerase chain reaction and denaturing gradient gel electrophoresis) techniques. J Infect Dis 2002;186: 1770–80.
23. Raz R, Stamm WE. A controlled trial of intra-vaginal estriol in post-menopausal women with recurrent urinary tract infections. N Engl J Med 1993;329:753–7.
24. Eriksen B. A randomized, open, parallel group study on the preventive effect of an estriol-releasing vaginal ring (Estring) on recurrent urinary tract infections in postmenopausal women. Am J Obstet Gynecol 1999;180:1072–9.
25. Hu KK, Boyko EJ, Scholes D, et al. Risk factors for urinary tract infections in postmenopausal women. Arch Intern Med 2004;164:989–93.
26. Orlander JD, Jick SS, Dean AD, et al. Urinary tract infections and estrogen use in older women. J Am Geriatr Soc 1992;40:817–20.
27. Rodhe N, Molstad S, Englund L, et al. Asymptomatic bacteriuria in a population of elderly residents living in a community setting: prevalence, characteristics, and associated factors. Fam Pract 2006;23:303–7.
28. Moore EE, Jackson SL, Boyko EJ, et al. Urinary incontinence and urinary tract infection: temporal relationships in post-menopausal women. Obstet Gynecol 2008;111(2 Pt 1):317–23.
29. Stern JA, Hsieh YC, Schaeffer AJ. Residual urine in the elderly female population: novel implications for oral estrogen replacement and impact on recurrent urinary tract infection. J Urol 2004;171(2 Pt 1):768–70.
30. Truzzi JC, Almeida FM, Nunes EC, et al. Residual urinary volume and urinary tract infection—when are they linked? J Urol 2008;180:182–5.
31. Omli R, Skotnes LH, Mykletun A, et al. Residual urine as a risk factor for lower urinary tract infection: a 1-year follow-up study in nursing homes. J Am Geriatr Soc 2008;56:871–4.
32. Barabas G, Molstad S. No association between elevated post-void residual volume and bacteriuria in residents of nursing homes. Scand J Prim Health Care 2005;23:52–6.
33. Ouslander JG, Greengold B, Chen S. External catheter use and urinary tract infection among incontinent male nursing home patients. J Am Geriatr Soc 1987;35:1063–70.
34. Vogel T, Verreault R, Gourdeau M, et al. Optimal duration of antimicrobial therapy for uncomplicated urinary tract infection in older women: a double-blind, randomized controlled trial. CMAJ 2004;170:469–73.
35. Boyko EJ, Fihn SD, Scholes D, et al. Diabetes and the risk of acute urinary tract infection among postmenopausal women. Diabetes Care 2002;25:1778–83.
36. Colodner R, Kometiani I, Chazan B, et al. Risk factors for community-acquired urinary tract infection due to quinolone-resistant E. coli. Infection 2008;36:41–5.

37. Smithson A, Chico C, Ramos J, et al. Prevalence and risk factors for quinolone resistance among *Escherichia coli* strains isolated from males with community febrile urinary tract infection. Eur J Clin Microbiol Infect Dis 2012;31:423–30.

38. van Duin D, Cober E, Richter SS, et al. Residence in skilled nursing facilities is associated with tigecycline non-susceptibility in carbapenem-resistant *Klebsiella pneumoniae*. Infect Control Hosp Epidemiol 2015;36:942–8.

39. Das R, Towle V, Van Ness PH, et al. Adverse outcomes in nursing home residents with increased episodes of observed bacteriuria. Infect Control Hosp Epidemiol 2011;32:84–6.

40. Van der Donk CF, Schols JM, Driessen CJ, et al. Prevalence and spread of multi-drug resistant *Escherichia coli* isolates among nursing home residents in the southern part of The Netherlands. J Am Med Dir Assoc 2013;14:199–203.

41. High KP, Bradley SF, Gravenstein S, et al. Clinical practice guideline for the evaluation of fever and infection in older adult residents of long-term care facilities. Clin Infect Dis 2009;48:149–71.

42. Nicolle LE, SHEA Long-Term-Care-Committee. Urinary tract infections in long-term care facilities. Infect Control Hosp Epidemiol 2001;22:167–75.

43. Stone ND, Ashraf MS, Calder J, et al. Surveillance definitions of infections in long-term care facilities: revisiting the McGeer criteria. Infect Control Hosp Epidemiol 2012;33:965–77.

44. Juthani-Mehta M, Quagliarello V, Perrelli E, et al. Clinical features to identify urinary tract infection in nursing home residents: a cohort study. J Am Geriatr Soc 2009;57:963–70.

45. Rowe T, Towle V, Van Ness PH. Lack of positive association between falls and bacteriuria plus pyuria in older nursing home residents. J Am Geriatr Soc 2013;61:653–4.

46. Sundvall PD, Ulleryd P, Gunnarsson RK. Urine culture doubtful in determining etiology of diffuse symptoms among elderly individuals: a cross-sectional study of 32 nursing homes. BMC Fam Pract 2011;12:36.

47. Laurila JV, Laakkonen ML, Tilvis RS, et al. Predisposing and precipitating factors for delirium in a frail geriatric population. J Psychosom Res 2008;65:249–54.

48. Boockvar K, Signor D, Ramaswamy R, et al. Delirium during acute illness in nursing residents. J Am Med Dir Assoc 2013;14:656–60.

49. Eriksson I, Gustafson Y, Fagerstrom L, et al. Urinary tract infection in very old women is associated with delirium. Int Psychogeriatr 2011;23:496–502.

50. Drinka P. Does urinary infection cause residents' mental status change? J Am Geriatr Soc 2009;57:2387–8.

51. D'Agata E, Loeb MB, Mitchell SL. Challenges in assessing nursing home residents with advanced dementia for suspected urinary tract infections. J Am Geriatr Soc 2013;61:62–6.

52. Loeb M, Bentley DW, Bradley S, et al. Development of minimum criteria for the initiation of antibiotics in residents of long-term-care facilities: results of a consensus conference. Infect Control Hosp Epidemiol 2001;22:120–4.

53. Loeb M, Brazil K, Lohfeld L, et al. Effect of a multifaceted intervention on number of antimicrobial prescriptions for suspected urinary tract infections in residents of nursing homes: cluster randomized controlled trial. BMJ 2005;331(7518):669.

54. Nace DA, Drinka PJ, Crnich CJ. Clinical uncertainties in the approach to long term care residents with possible urinary tract infection. J Am Med Dir Assoc 2014;15:133–9.

55. Lipsky BA. Urinary tract infections in men. Epidemiology, pathophysiology, diagnosis and treatment. Ann Intern Med 1989;110:138–50.

56. Rodhe N, Lofgren S, Strindhall J, et al. Cytokines in urine in elderly subjects with acute cystitis and asymptomatic bacteriuria. Scand J Prim Health Care 2009;27:74–9.

57. Sundvall PD, Elm M, Ulleryd P, et al. Interleukin-6 concentrations in the urine and dipstick analyses were related to bacteriuria but not symptoms in the elderly: a cross sectional study of 421 nursing home residents. BMC Geriatr 2014;14:88.

58. Gomolin IH, Siami PF, Reuning-Scherer J, et al. Efficacy and safety of oral ciprofloxacin suspension versus trimethoprim-sulfamethoxazole oral suspension for treatment of older women with acute urinary tract infection. J Am Geriatr Soc 2001;49:1606–13.

59. Penrotta C, Aznar M, Mejia R, et al. Oestrogens for preventing recurrent urinary tract infections in post-menopausal women. Cochrane Database Syst Rev 2008;(2):CD005131.

60. Raz R, Colodner R, Rohana Y, et al. Effectiveness of estriol-containing vaginal pessaries and nitrofurantoin macrocrystal therapy in the prevention of recurrent urinary tract infection in postmenopausal women. Clin Infect Dis 2003;36:1362–8.

61. McMurdo ME, Argo I, Phillips G, et al. Cranberry or trimethoprim for the prevention of recurrent urinary tract infections? A randomized controlled trial in older women. J Antimicrob Chemother 2009;63:389–95.

62. McMurdo ME, Bissett LY, Price RJ, et al. Does ingestion of cranberry juice reduce symptomatic urinary tract infections in older people in hospital? A double-blind, placebo-controlled trial. Age Ageing 2005;34:256–61.

63. Beerepoot MA, ter Riet G, Nys S, et al. *Lactobacilli* vs antibiotics to prevent urinary tract infections: a randomized double-blind, noninferiority trial in post-menopausal women. Arch Intern Med 2012;172:704–12.

64. Ouslander JG, Greendale GA, Uman G, et al. Effects of oral estrogen and progestin on the lower urinary tract among female nursing home residents. J Am Geriatr Soc 2001;49:803–7.

65. Juthani-Mehta M, Perley L, Chen S, et al. Feasibility of cranberry capsule administration and clean-catch urine collection in long-term care residents. J Am Geriatr Soc 2010;58:2028–9.

66. Bianco L, Perrelli E, Towle V, et al. Pilot randomized controlled dosing study of cranberry capsules for reduction of bacteriuria plus pyuria in female nursing home residents. J Am Geriatr Soc 2012;60:1180–1.

67. Rogers MAM, Mody L, Kaufman SR, et al. Use of urinary collection devices in skilled nursing facilities in five states. J Am Geriatr Soc 2008;56:854–61.

68. Jonsson K, E-son Loft AL, Nasic S, et al. A prospective registration of catheter life and catheter interventions in patients with long-term indwelling urinary catheters. Scand J Urol Nephrol 2011;45:401–5.

69. Wang L, Lansing B, Symons K, et al. Infection rate and colonization with antibiotic-resistant organisms in skilled nursing facility residents with indwelling devices. Eur J Clin Microbiol Infect Dis 2012;31:1797–804.

70. Warren JW. Catheter-associated urinary tract infections. Infect Dis Clin North Am 1997;11:609–22.

71. Muder RR, Brennen C, Wagener MM, et al. Bacteremia in a long-term-care facility: a five-year prospective study of 163 consecutive episodes. Clin Infect Dis 1992;14:647–54.

72. Rudman D, Hontanosas A, Cohen Z, et al. Clinical correlates of bacteremia in a veterans administration extended care facility. J Am Geriatr Soc 1988;36:726–32.

73. Jonsson K, Claesson BE, Hedelin H. Urine cultures from indwelling bladder catheters in nursing home patients: a point prevalence study in a Swedish county. Scand J Urol Nephrol 2011;45:265–9.

74. Warren JW, Tenney JH, Hoopes JM, et al. A prospective microbiologic study of bacteriuria in patients with chronic indwelling urethral catheters. J Infect Dis 1982;146:719–23.

75. Jacobsen SM, Stickler DJ, Mobley HL, et al. Complicated catheter-associated urinary tract infections due to *Escherichia coli* and *Proteus mirabilis*. Clin Microbiol Rev 2008;21:26–59.

76. Han JH, Maslow J, Han X, et al. Risk factors for the development of gastrointestinal colonization with fluoroquinolone-resistant *Escherichia coli* in residents of long-term care facilities. J Infect Dis 2014;209:420–5.

77. Raz R, Schiller D, Nicolle LE. Chronic indwelling catheter replacement prior to antimicrobial therapy for symptomatic urinary infection. J Urol 2000;164:1254–8.

78. Steward DK, Wood GL, Cohen RL, et al. Failure of the urinalysis and quantitative urine culture in diagnosing symptomatic urinary tract infections in patients with long-term urinary catheters. Am J Infect Control 1985;13:154–60.

79. Gould CV, Umscheid CA, Agarwal RK, et al. Guideline for prevention of catheter-associated urinary tract infections 2009. Infect Control Hosp Epidemiol 2010;31:319–26.

80. Lo E, Nicolle LE, Coffin SE, et al. Strategies to prevent catheter-associated urinary tract infections in acute care hospitals: 2014 update. Infect Control Hosp Epidemiol 2014;35(Suppl 2):S32–48.

81. Saint S, Kaufman SR, Rogers MA, et al. Condom versus indwelling urinary catheters: a randomized trial. J Am Geriatr Soc 2006;54:1055–61.

82. Mody L, Saint S, Galecki A, et al. Knowledge of evidence-based urinary catheter care practice recommendations among healthcare workers in nursing homes. J Am Geriatr Soc 2010;58:1532–7.

Herpes Zoster

Kenneth Schmader, MD[a,b,*]

KEYWORDS

- Herpes zoster • Varicella-zoster virus • Postherpetic neuralgia • Elderly • Aged

KEY POINTS

- The strongest risk factors for herpes zoster are aging and suppression of cellular immunity. The increase in the likelihood of herpes zoster with aging starts around 50 to 60 years of age and increases markedly into late life.
- Laboratory diagnostic testing is indicated when differentiating herpes zoster from herpes simplex virus, for suspected organ involvement, and for atypical presentations, particularly in the immunocompromised host. Polymerase chain reaction is the preferred diagnostic test.
- The goal of the treatment of herpes zoster in older adults is to decrease the length of the acute attack and to reduce pain by the use of early antiviral therapy (acyclovir, famciclovir, valacyclovir), scheduled analgesia, and, if the pain is not adequately controlled, adjunctive agents.
- Lidocaine patch 5%, gabapentin, pregabalin, opioids, and tricyclic antidepressants constitute first-line therapies for the management of postherpetic neuralgia.
- The live attenuated zoster vaccine is recommended for all immunocompetent adults 60 years and older by the Advisory Committee on Immunization Practices and the US Centers for Disease Control and Prevention for the prevention of herpes zoster and postherpetic neuralgia.

INTRODUCTION

Herpes zoster is a neurocutaneous disease that is caused by the reactivation of varicella-zoster virus (VZV) from a latent infection of dorsal sensory or cranial nerve ganglia after primary infection with VZV earlier in life. VZV is a double-stranded DNA herpesvirus with a genome that contains at least 70 gene products.[1] VZV expresses gene products and attempts replication throughout life, but cellular immunity is critical

This work was supported by the Durham VA Medical Center Geriatric Research, Education and Clinical Center (GRECC) and Duke Pepper Older Americans Independence Center NIA P30 AG028716.

[a] Division of Geriatrics, Department of Medicine, Center for the Study of Aging and Human Development, Duke University Medical Center, Box 3003, Durham, NC 27705, USA;
[b] Geriatric Research, Education and Clinical Center (GRECC), Durham Veterans Affairs Medical Center, 182 GRECC, Durham, NC 27705, USA
* Durham Veterans Affairs Medical Center, 182 GRECC, Durham, NC.
E-mail address: kenneth.schmader@duke.edu

to containing VZV. With aging-related decline in cellular immunity to VZV, the virus may escape cell-mediated immune containment and spread in the affected ganglia and sensory nerves to the skin.

EPIDEMIOLOGY

The estimated incidence of herpes zoster in persons older than 65 years varies from approximately 10 to 14 cases per 1000 per year.[2–4] The lifetime incidence of herpes zoster is estimated to be about 20% to 30% in the general population, and may be as high as 50% among those surviving to 85 years or higher.[5] Current population figures and herpes zoster incidence data yield estimates of about 1 million new cases of herpes zoster each year in the United States.[6] The incidence of recurrent herpes zoster is not as well established but the frequency of recurrent events is higher in immunocompromised individuals.[7,8] In one study, the frequency of recurrent herpes zoster was 5.7% among immune-competent individuals.[7]

The strongest risk factors for herpes zoster are aging and suppression of cellular immunity. The increase in the likelihood of herpes zoster with aging starts around 50 to 60 years and increases into late life in individuals older than 80 years.[2,3] Immunocompromised patients at risk for herpes zoster include persons with human immunodeficiency virus infection, Hodgkin's disease, non-Hodgkin's lymphomas, leukemia, bone marrow and other organ transplants, systemic lupus erythematosus, rheumatoid arthritis, and those individuals taking immunosuppressive medications, including tumor necrosis factor inhibitors.[5,6,9] Other risk factors include white race, female sex, and physical trauma.[5,10,11] The childhood varicella vaccination program in the United States does not appear to have affected the incidence of herpes zoster.[12]

Patients with herpes zoster who have a vesicular rash may transmit VZV via direct contact, airborne route, or droplet nuclei to seronegative, nonimmune individuals.[13] These individuals may then subsequently have varicella, usually within 10 to 21 days after contact with a case. In one study of school and day care settings, of 290 herpes zoster cases reported, 27 (9%) resulted in 84 secondary varicella cases.[13] If the rash is only maculopapular or crusted, there is no danger of VZV transmission. Important groups at risk for varicella from contact with herpes zoster patients include children who have not received the varicella vaccine or who have had an insufficient response to the vaccine and susceptible health care workers and staff in hospital or in nursing homes particularly if they are pregnant or immunocompromised. The exposure of a latently infected individual to herpes zoster does not cause herpes zoster or varicella. Nearly all older adults are latently infected with VZV.

CLINICAL FEATURES

VZV reactivation and spread in the affected sensory ganglion and peripheral sensory nerve evokes a cellular immune response and neuronal inflammation and destruction.[6] Before VZV reaches the skin, the patient experiences prodromal sensations in the affected dermatome, such as aching, burning, or lancinating pain or itching or tingling. Prodromal symptoms baffle patients and physicians by imitating other painful conditions in older persons (ie, migraine headaches, trigeminal neuralgia, myocardial infarction, cholecystitis, biliary or renal colic, appendicitis, lumbosacral strain, or pulled muscles). One clue to incipient herpes zoster is sensitive skin in the affected dermatome before the rash breaks out. The prodrome usually lasts a few days. VZV may not reach the skin in some patients, which results in a unilateral, dermatomal neuralgia without a rash. This condition is known as *zoster sine herpete*.

Once VZV invades the dermis and epidermis, the rash appears and reveals the reason for the patient's pain or discomfort. The rash is unilateral, dermatomal, red, and maculopapular and usually develops vesicles (**Fig. 1**). It is not uncommon for patients to have lesions in adjacent dermatomes. The rash generally starts crusting over in a week to 10 days and heals within 2 to 4 weeks. Atypical rashes may occur in older persons. The rash may be limited to a small patch located within a dermatome or may remain maculopapular without ever developing vesicles. Conversely, vesicles may form for several days and involve several dermatomes.

VZV-induced acute neuritis produces unilateral dermatomal neuralgic pain in many older adults, although a few patients never have pain, whereas others may experience the delayed onset of pain days or weeks after rash onset. The neuritis is described as burning, deep aching, tingling, itching, or stabbing. A subset of patients may have severe pain, especially those with trigeminal nerve involvement. Acute herpetic neuralgia has a profound negative impact on functional status and quality of life and usually results in substantial health service utilization.[14,15]

In general, the number of older herpes zoster patients with pain decreases over weeks to months from rash onset. Unfortunately, a significant number of older persons with herpes zoster continue to experience pain for months after the acute phase of the illness; therefore, postherpetic neuralgia (PHN) develops. Increasing age is the strongest risk factor for PHN.[16] The PHN patient may suffer from constant pain (burning, aching, throbbing), intermittent pain (stabbing, shooting) and stimulus-evoked pain such as allodynia (tender). Allodynia, the experience of pain after a nonpainful stimulus, is a particularly disabling component of the disease. Patients with allodynia suffer from severe pain after the lightest touch of the affected skin by things as trivial as a cold wind or a piece of clothing. These subtypes of pain may produce chronic fatigue, disordered sleep, depression, anorexia, weight loss, and social isolation. Furthermore, PHN can impair the elderly patient's functional status by interfering with basic activities of daily life such as dressing, bathing and mobility and instrumental activities such as traveling, shopping, cooking, and housework.

Herpes zoster involving the ophthalmic division of the trigeminal nerve may cause serious ocular complications. The likelihood of inflammation of the eye seems to be higher when the rash is on the tip of the nose (nasociliary branch involvement), but in general the appearance and location of the facial rash does not predict the presence or extent of eye involvement. VZV-induced damage to the cornea and uvea and other eye structures can cause corneal anesthesia and ulceration, glaucoma, optic neuritis,

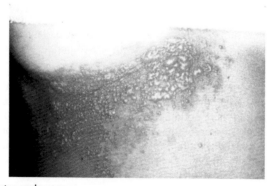

Fig. 1. Herpes zoster rash.

eyelid scarring and retraction, visual impairment, and blindness in patients who did not receive antiviral therapy.

Other less frequent but important complications of herpes zoster in older adults include stroke secondary to granulomatous arteritis of the internal carotid artery in ophthalmic herpes zoster; focal motor paresis in muscles served by nerve roots of the corresponding affected dermatome; disordered balance, hearing, and facial paresis in cranial neuritis (Ramsay-Hunt syndrome); meningoencephalitis; and secondary bacterial infection of the rash.[6]

DIAGNOSIS

Herpes zoster may be diagnosed clinically with high confidence when the characteristic unilateral, dermatomal, vesicular rash and neuralgic pain present in an older patient. The main source of diagnostic error is herpes simplex virus (HSV) infection.[6] Features that may distinguish HSV from herpes zoster include multiple recurrences, especially around the genitals or mouth, and the absence of chronic pain. However, it may be impossible to distinguish the 2 conditions on clinical grounds because HSV presents with a unilateral, red, maculopapular, vesicular rash and acute pain similar to herpes zoster. The differential diagnosis also includes contact dermatitis, burns, and vesicular lesions associated with fungal infections, but the history and examination usually make the distinction clear.

Herpes zoster should be diagnosed using laboratory diagnostic testing when differentiating herpes zoster from HSV infection is difficult, for suspected organ involvement, and for atypical presentations, particularly in the immunocompromised host. The best diagnostic test is polymerase chain reaction because of its very high sensitivity and specificity.[17] Vesicle fluid is the best specimen for polymerase chain reaction analysis. Lacking vesicle fluid, acceptable specimens include lesion scrapings, crusts, tissue biopsy, or cerebrospinal fluid for the first 3 techniques.

TREATMENT
Acute Herpes Zoster

General principles
The main goal of the treatment of herpes zoster in older adults is the reduction or elimination of acute pain and the prevention of PHN. It is important to understand that the impact of herpes zoster on functional status, mood, and quality of life in older adults is directly related to pain intensity. Education and counseling about herpes zoster reduce anxiety and misunderstandings about the disease. Questions about the duration of pain and transmission of VZV are common. Social support, mental and physical activity, adequate nutrition, and a caring attitude help patients cope with the illness. Treatment adherence and response may be altered in older adults who are living alone, cognitively impaired, frail, or coping with recent negative life events.

Antiviral therapy
Acyclovir, famciclovir, and valacyclovir are nucleoside analogues that effectively treat VZV infections (**Table 1**).[6] These agents are phosphorylated by viral thymidine kinase and cellular kinases to a triphosphate form that interferes with viral DNA synthesis by inhibiting viral DNA polymerase. Valacyclovir and famciclovir are prodrugs that are better absorbed than acyclovir after oral administration, which results in much higher blood levels of antiviral activity.

Multiple randomized, controlled trials found that oral acyclovir (800 mg 5 times a day for 7 days), famciclovir (500 mg every 8 hours for 7 days) and valacyclovir (1 g 3 times a

Table 1
Oral anti-VZV medications for herpes zoster (US)

Characteristic	Acyclovir	Valacyclovir	Famciclovir
Structure	Deoxyguanosine analog	Valine ester of acyclovir	Diacetyl 6-deoxy analog of penciclovir, a deoxyguanosine analog
Active agent	Acyclovir	Acyclovir	Penciclovir
Oral bioavailability	10%–20%	54%	77%
Standard dosing	800 mg every 4 h (5 times a day) for 7 d	1 g every 8 h (3 times a day) for 7 d	500 mg every 8 h (3 times a day) for 7 d
Renal dosing	CrCl ≥25 mL/min, no adjustment CrCl 10–24 mL/min: 800 mg every 8 h CrCl <10 mL/min: 800 mg every 12 h	CrCl ≥50 mL/min: no dosage adjustment CrCl 30–49 mL/min: 1 g every 12 h CrCl 10–29 mL/min: 1 g every 24 h CrCl <10 mL/min: 500 mg every 24 h	CrCl ≥60 mL/min: no dosage adjustment CrCl 40–59 mL/min: 500 mg every 12 h CrCl 20–39 mL/min: 500 mg every 24 h CrCl <20 mL/min: 250 mg every 24 h
Benefit: pain median days to resolution, drug vs control[8,11,12]	41 vs 101 (placebo)	38 vs 51 (acyclovir)	63 vs 163 (placebo)
Adverse events	Nausea/vomiting, headache, diarrhea	Nausea/vomiting, headache, diarrhea	Nausea/vomiting, headache, diarrhea
How supplied	200-mg capsules; 200-, 400-, 800-mg tablets; 200 mg/5 mL solution	500 mg, 1-g tablets	125-, 250-, and 500-mg tablets

day for 7 days) reduce acute pain and duration of chronic pain in older herpes zoster patients who are treated within 72 hours of rash onset.[6,18] The most common adverse effects are nausea, vomiting, diarrhea, and headache. No head-to-head study has found superiority of one of these agents over another, so all 3 agents are acceptable. Because of their superior pharmacokinetics and simpler dosing schedule, famciclovir and valacyclovir are preferred to acyclovir for oral therapy for VZV infections. The benefits of treating herpes zoster patients who present more than 72 hours after rash onset are unknown. Some experts recommend antiviral therapy for patients presenting more than 72 hours after rash onset with continued new vesicle formation or when there are cutaneous, motor, neurologic, or ocular complications. Unfortunately, 20% to 30% of treated patients in antiviral trials had pain 6 months from herpes zoster onset. These data indicate that even optimally treated patients can subsequently have PHN.

Ophthalmic herpes zoster is important in older patients because of the risk of visual impairment or blindness in persons who may already have compromised vision from other age-related conditions such as glaucoma, macular degeneration, cataracts or diabetic neuropathy. Oral acyclovir, famciclovir, and valacyclovir are effective for the prevention of ocular complications from ophthalmic herpes zoster. Ophthalmologist consultation is recommended in older patients with ophthalmic herpes zoster to determine the presence and extent of ocular involvement and to determine the utility of local treatments such as mydriatics, glucocorticoids, or topical antivirals.

Analgesics

Acute herpes zoster pain management requires the same principles as managing any pain: use of standardized pain measures, scheduled analgesia, and consistent and frequent follow-up to adjust dosing to the needs of the patient. The choice of treatment will be contingent on the patient's comorbidities, concurrent medications, pain intensity, and preferences.

Patients with mild pain may be treated with acetaminophen or nonsteroidal agents. Patients with moderate-to-severe pain usually require treatment with a strong opioid analgesic (eg, oxycodone).[19] There are several approaches to using short- or long-acting opioids in the treatment of herpes zoster pain. One commonly used approach is to start with a short-acting medication at an oxycodone equianalgesic dose of 5 mg 4 times daily and titrating the dose until pain is reduced or the adverse effects become intolerable.[19] If an effective and tolerable dose is found, then treatment can be switched from a short-acting to a long-acting medication depending on cost and patient preference. Long-acting medications are more convenient and may also provide a more consistent level of pain relief. Rescue doses of a short-acting opioid can be used for exacerbations of pain as needed with the long-acting opioid. Opioids have multiple adverse effects including nausea, constipation, and sedation, which may be intolerable in some older adults. In most cases, constipation should be anticipated and managed with laxative therapy.

Corticosteroids

Randomized, controlled trials of corticosteroids versus placebo or acyclovir with or without corticosteroids in older herpes zoster patients showed equal rates of PHN.[20–22] These findings argue against the routine use of corticosteroids in older herpes zoster patients. In most trials, corticosteroids reduced acute herpes zoster pain, although that beneficial effect was not sustained. In the a trial of acyclovir and prednisone, time to uninterrupted sleep, return to daily activity, and cessation of analgesic therapy was significantly accelerated in patients who received corticosteroids.[22] However, the patients in the trial had an average age of 60 years and no relative contraindications to corticosteroids such as hypertension, diabetes mellitus, or osteoporosis. In the trial, prednisone was administered orally at 60 mg/d for days 1 to 7, 30 mg/d for days 8 to 14, and 15 mg/d for days 15 to 21. The most common adverse effects of short-term prednisone use are gastrointestinal symptoms (dyspepsia, nausea, vomiting), edema, and granulocytosis. Some clinicians use corticosteroids for VZV-induced facial paralysis and cranial polyneuritis to improve motor outcomes, reduce peripheral nerve damage from foraminal compression, and reduce pain. If corticosteroid treatment is considered, it should always be used with antiviral therapy.

Adjuvant agents

If moderate-to-severe herpes zoster pain is inadequately relieved by antiviral agents in combination with oral analgesic medications or corticosteroids, then other therapies to consider include gabapentin or pregabalin or neural blockade. None of these approaches are found to prevent PHN, but they may be useful in reducing acute pain.

A single 900-mg dose of gabapentin was found to reduce acute herpes zoster pain over a 6-hour period.[23] However, neither gabapentin nor pregabalin were found to prevent PHN or provide significant acute herpes zoster pain relief in randomized, controlled trials.[19] If used, it should be recognized that gabapentin and pregabalin can cause sedation, dizziness, ataxia, and peripheral edema. It is best to give starting doses at bedtime and carefully increase subsequent doses to 3 times daily for gabapentin and twice daily for pregabalin.

If pain control from antiviral agents and analgesics with or without any of the adjuvant drugs noted above is inadequate, then anesthetic nerve blocks should be considered. This intervention will require referral to a pain specialist. A randomized, controlled trial of antiviral therapy, oral analgesics, and a single epidural block with bupivacaine and methylprednisolone compared with antiviral therapy and oral analgesics alone showed that neural blockade reduces acute pain but does not prevent PHN.[24]

Postherpetic Neuralgia

General principles
The main goal of the treatment of PHN in older adults is the reduction of pain and associated symptoms including depression, insomnia, fatigue, and functional impairment. No one treatment is uniformly and completely effective in all older PHN patients. Therefore, it is important to set realistic goals with the patient. Specifically, the patient needs to know that it is unlikely that any single intervention will take the pain away completely, but some interventions are likely to reduce pain while balancing the risk of potential adverse effects. Persons affected by PHN need to understand that the natural history of PHN is one of improvement over weeks, months, and even years, regardless of the underlying treatment in many patients. The same comments in the section on herpes zoster treatment regarding pain management apply to the PHN patient as do comments regarding social support, mental and physical activity, adequate nutrition, and a caring attitude.

Pharmacotherapy
The topical lidocaine patch, gabapentin, pregabalin, opioids, tricyclic antidepressants (TCAs), tramadol, and topical capsaicin are considered evidence-based therapies because one or more randomized, controlled trials found efficacy and relative safety with these agents.[25] Gabapentin, pregabalin, the topical lidocaine patch 5%, and topical capsaicin patch 8% are approved by the US Food and Drug Administration (FDA) for the treatment of PHN. Opioids and TCAs are not approved by the FDA partly because the manufacturers of these products have not sought FDA approval. Pharmacotherapy for neuropathic pain, including PHN, is discussed in more detail in recently published summaries.[25–27] In general, these agents produce clinically significant reduction in pain in about 30% to 60% of patients. Unfortunately, there is no good way to predict which patient will respond or not respond to a given drug. Furthermore, there are few head-to-head comparisons of these drugs, so it is unknown if one agent is clearly superior in efficacy to another. Clinical information about these drugs is summarized in **Table 2**. Remember that starting doses and maximum doses of drugs are generally lower in frail older adults. The upward titration of drug doses often needs to be slower in frail older adults as well.

The initial choice of agent depends on the patient's comorbidities and preferences as well as cost and formulary restrictions. The topical lidocaine patches, gabapentin and pregabalin, are generally better tolerated than opioids and TCAs in older adults. The topical lidocaine patch is easy to use, gives initial pain relief in hours to days when effective (2 weeks for an adequate trial) but can produce a skin rash that prevents use of the patch. Gabapentin has few drug interactions and gives initial pain relief in days to weeks when effective (adequate trial requires 3–8 weeks for titration plus 1–2 weeks at maximum tolerated dosage) but can produce somnolence, dizziness, and peripheral edema. These adverse effects require monitoring and possibly dosage

Table 2
Medications for PHN

Characteristic	Lidocaine Patch	Gabapentin	Nortriptyline	Opioids	Pregabalin	Tramadol
Structure	Amino amide anesthetic	Gamma-aminobutyric acid analog	Dibenzocycloheptene tricyclic antidepressant	Mu opioid receptor agonist	Gamma-aminobutyric acid analog	Mu opioid agonist and serotonin and norepinephrine reuptake inhibitor
Kinetics	Very little systemic absorption	Renal elimination; prolonged half-life with renal impairment	Hepatic metabolism; higher levels of active metabolites in the elderly	Hepatic metabolism and renal elimination	Renal elimination; prolonged half-life with renal impairment	Hepatic metabolism and renal elimination
Standard dosing	Up to 3 patches applied over the affected area for 12 h/d	Start at 100–300 mg at night; increase by 100–300 mg/d every 1–7 d as tolerated in 3× a day dosing; maximum dose 3600 mg/d	Start 10 mg at night; increase by 10 mg every 4–7 d by the same amount until reduction in pain; maximum dose 75–150 mg/d	In morphine equivalents start 2.5–15 mg every 4 h; after 1–2 wk, convert total daily dosage to long-acting opioid analgesic and continue short-acting medication as needed	150 mg/d given in 2 or 3 divided doses; may increase to 300 mg/d, given in 2 or 3 divided doses, within 1 wk; maximum dosage 600 mg/d	Start 50 mg once daily; increase by 50 mg daily in divided doses every 3–7 d as tolerated; maximum dose 400 mg daily; in patients >75 y, 300 mg daily in divided doses
Benefit: % significant improvement	≥50% reduction in pain scores: 31% lidocaine patch vs 8% placebo patch	Moderate or much pain improvement: 41%–43% gabapentin vs 12%–23% placebo	Moderate to good pain relief: 44%–67% TCAs vs 5%–19% placebo or control drug	Masked preference: 67% oxycodone vs 11% placebo	≥50% reduction in pain scores: 50% pregabalin vs 20% placebo	≥50% reduction in pain scores; 77% tramadol vs 56% placebo

Adverse events	Skin redness or rash	Somnolence, dizziness, ataxia, peripheral edema	Arrhythmia, cardiac conduction block, orthostatic hypotension, urinary retention, constipation, cognitive impairment	Constipation, sedation, nausea/vomiting, respiratory depression, nervous system symptoms, pruritis	Somnolence, dizziness, ataxia, peripheral edema	Constipation, sedation, nausea/vomiting, respiratory depression, nervous system symptoms, seizures
Main drug-drug interactions	Class I antiarrythmics	Opioids	Antipsychotics, anticholinergics, SSRIs, sedative-hypnotics, antiarrhythmics, monoamine oxidase inhibitors	Anticholinergics, sedative-hypnotics, anxiolytics, CYP2D6 inhibitors, TCAs, muscle relaxants	Opioids	Anticholinergics, sedative-hypnotics, anxiolytics, CYP2D6 inhibitors, SSRIs, TCAs, muscle relaxants
Main drug-disease interactions	None	Dementia, ataxia, falls	Myocardial infarction, QT prolongation, AV block, bundle branch block, ileus, prostatic hypertrophy, seizure disorder, glaucoma, dementia	Ileus, chronic obstructive pulmonary disease, dementia, prostatic hypertrophy	Dementia, ataxia, falls	Ileus, chronic obstructive pulmonary disease, dementia, prostatic hypertrophy, seizure disorder
How supplied	10- × 14-cm lidocaine patch contains 5% lidocaine base on polyester backing	100-mg, 300-mg, 400-mg capsules; 600-mg, 800-mg tablets	10-mg, 25-mg, 50-mg, 75-mg capsules; 10 mg/5 mL solution	Multiple drugs and dosage forms	25-mg, 50-mg, 75-mg, 100-mg, 150-mg, 200-mg, 225-mg, 300-mg capsules	50-mg tablet

adjustment but usually not treatment discontinuation. Gabapentin may cause or exacerbate gait and balance problems and cognitive impairment in the frail elderly, which can require discontinuation of therapy. Pregabalin has few drug interactions, has a more rapid onset of action than gabapentin, and gives initial pain relief within one to 2 days when effective but also produces the same adverse effects as gabapentin.

Opioids give initial pain relief in hours to days when effective (adequate trial requires 4 weeks) but the well-known adverse effects of opioids will preclude their use in some older adults. Opioid analgesics must be used cautiously in patients with a history of substance abuse. The risk that substance abuse will develop in patients who do not have a history of substance abuse is thought to be low in the older patient with PHN. Tramadol gives initial pain relief in hours to days when effective (adequate trial requires 4 weeks) but has similar adverse effects as opioids because a major metabolite is a mu opioid agonist. Tramadol is associated with an increased risk of seizures in patients who have a history of seizures or use drugs that can reduce the seizure threshold and serotonin syndrome in patients who use serotonergic medications, especially selective serotonin reuptake inhibitors (SSRIs).

Nortriptyline gives initial pain relief in several days to weeks when effective (adequate trial requires 6–8 weeks with at least 1–2 weeks at maximum tolerated dosage) but has several potentially significant anticholinergic and cardiac adverse effects in older adults. A screening electrocardiogram to check for cardiac conduction abnormalities is recommended before beginning any TCA treatment in the elderly. TCAs are contraindicated in patients with QT prolongation or familial histories of long-QT syndromes, with atrioventricular block or bundle-branch block, and with a recent acute myocardial infarction. Although amitriptyline was tested in many PHN trials, it is often poorly tolerated in older adults because of its much higher anticholinergic activity. Nortriptyline has equivalent efficacy compared with amitriptyline in PHN but is better tolerated.[28] Desipramine is a reasonable alternative to nortriptyline. In a crossover study of PHN comparing opioid analgesics, TCAs, and placebo, controlled-release morphine and TCAs provided significant benefits on pain.[29] In this trial, patients preferred treatment with opioid analgesics compared with TCAs and placebo but there was a greater incidence of adverse effects and dropouts during opioid treatment.

Topical capsaicin is available in creams, gels, or lotions in concentrations of 0.025%, 0.075%, and 0.25% and as an 8% patch. The burning from capsaicin makes it difficult to tolerate for many patients. Nonetheless, topical capsaicin may be considered as a back-up therapeutic option in PHN because there may be some individuals who tolerate it. The patch requires application in a clinic by personnel who are trained on how to properly apply and monitor it.

Nonresponse to single-drug therapy often leads to combination therapy with one or more of the above agents, but there are few data regarding the additive or synergistic benefits of combination treatment. The potential advantages of combination therapy include augmentation of a partial response to a single drug, more rapid effect when a medication that requires titration to reach an effective dosage is also being used, and better analgesia at lower doses of drug. The potential disadvantages of combination therapy in older adults include an increased risk of adverse effects as the number of medications is increased, the difficulty determining which medication is responsible for adverse effects, and increased cost. In a randomized, controlled trial of the effects of morphine alone, gabapentin alone, or a morphine-gabapentin combination on neuropathic pain that included patients with PHN, gabapentin and morphine combined achieved modestly better pain relief at lower doses of each drug than either as a single agent.[30] However, the combination was associated with higher levels of sedation, dry mouth, and cognitive dysfunction than the maximal tolerated dose of each single agent. In a similar randomized, controlled trial of the effects of nortriptyline alone, gabapentin alone or a nortriptyline-gabapentin combination on neuropathic pain that included patients with PHN, gabapentin and nortriptyline combined achieved modestly better pain relief at lower doses of each drug than either as a single agent. However, the combination was associated with higher levels of dry mouth than the maximal-tolerated dose of each single agent.[31]

Other treatments

Some older patients with PHN will not have an adequate response to any of the front-line medications. For these patients, other drug and nondrug treatments deserve consideration. Patients who require complex drug combinations, risky second-line medications, or invasive treatments should be referred to a pain management center. A detailed review of these interventions is beyond the scope of this article, but nondrug noninvasive and invasive treatments are briefly summarized.

Noninvasive treatments include physical modalities such as cold application or transcutaneous electrical nerve stimulation, percutaneous electrical nerve stimulation, psychological treatments, and acupuncture. These interventions have little risk and may be useful in some patients, but whether they are effective in a population of patients with PHN is unknown and needs to be tested in controlled clinical trials. Some PHN patients may have associated myofascial pain in addition to neuropathic pain.[32] The presence of myofascial pathology is indicated by taut muscle bands (ie, a group of tense muscle fibers extending from a trigger point to the muscle attachments) and trigger point(s) (ie, a hyperirritable spot in skeletal muscle that is painful on compression) in the affected dermatome. These patients are good candidates for a trial of percutaneous electrical nerve stimulation.

Invasive treatments may be considered when patients do not obtain adequate relief from noninvasive treatment approaches. Invasive treatments include peripheral and central neural blockade, central nervous system drug delivery, spinal cord stimulation, and neurosurgical techniques. Neural blockade techniques include sensory nerve, plexus, and sympathetic nerve blocks as well as epidural and intrathecal blockade with lidocainelike drugs or corticosteroids. Many PHN patients note initial relief of pain with nerve blocks, but few experience long lasting relief. Central nervous system drug delivery attempts to place drug (eg, morphine) as close as possible to central pain receptors in the spinal cord corresponding to the affected dermatome(s). Spinal cord stimulation requires implantation of an electrode in the thoracic or lumbar epidural space and the placement of a percutaneous electrical stimulator. These interventions represent rational approaches to pain relief, but they have not been proven effective in controlled trials, partly because the design and conduct of such trials are difficult, and they carry procedural risks in the elderly. In general, these interventions have a limited role in PHN treatment and should be contemplated in patients who have not responded to all other treatments and continue to have disabling pain.

PREVENTION
Live Attenuated Zoster Vaccine

The live attenuated zoster vaccine significantly boosts VZV-specific cellular immunity in older adults, which provides the scientific rationale for using the vaccine because cellular immunity to VZV declines with age.[4] The clinical rationale for the zoster vaccine lies in the facts that herpes zoster causes substantial morbidity, antiviral therapy does not prevent PHN and must be initiated within 72 hours of rash onset for maximum benefit, and PHN treatments are incompletely effective and often poorly tolerated by older adults.

The efficacy of the live attenuated zoster vaccine in reducing the incidence and severity of herpes zoster in older adults was demonstrated in the Shingles Prevention Study.[4] The Shingles Prevention Study was a randomized, double-blind, placebo-controlled trial involving 38,546 community-dwelling persons $\geq$60 years old who were followed up for herpes zoster and adverse events for a median of 3 years after receiving vaccine or placebo. The vaccine reduced incidence of herpes zoster from 11.12 to 5.42 cases (51.3%) per 1000 person-years for a number needed to treat of 59 over the 3.12 years of the study. The vaccine reduced the incidence PHN from 1.38 to 0.46 cases (66.5%) per 1000 person years for a number needed to treat of 362 over the duration of the study. The zoster vaccine also reduced the pain burden of illness (a pain severity by duration measure) caused by herpes zoster by 61.1%. Two large cohort studies of the use of zoster vaccine in real-world practice settings showed similar results for vaccine efficacy for incidence of herpes zoster.[33,34] The zoster vaccine also reduces interference with herpes zoster–related functional impairments and health-related quality of life.[35] In addition, the zoster vaccine seems to reduce the incidence of herpes zoster in patients who later undergo chemotherapy.[36] Reactions at the injection site are more frequent among vaccine recipients but are generally mild. The results of pre- and postlicensure studies indicate that the vaccine is generally safe and well tolerated.[37,38]

The Advisory Committee on Immunization Practices (ACIP) of the Centers for Disease Control and Prevention recommends the live attenuated zoster vaccine for the prevention of herpes zoster and PHN in immunocompetent adults 60 years of age and older.[5] Anaphylactic reactions to gelatin or neomycin; in those with leukemia, lymphomas, or other malignant neoplasms affecting the bone marrow or lymphatic system; those on immunosuppressive therapy, including high-dose corticosteroids ($\geq$20 mg/d of prednisone or equivalent) lasting 2 or more weeks; those with AIDS or other clinical manifestations of human immunodeficiency virus, including persons with CD4^{+} T-lymphocyte values $\leq$200 per cubic millimeter undergoing hematopoietic stem cell transplantation or receiving recombinant human immune mediators and immune modulators are contraindications to the live attenuated zoster vaccine. The live attenuated zoster vaccine can be given simultaneously with other inactivated vaccines including influenza, pneumococcal polysaccharide, and pneumococcal conjugate vaccines.[5]

The exact duration of the protection against herpes zoster by the zoster vaccine is unknown. In the Short Term Persistence Substudy of the Shingles Prevention Study, 7320 vaccine and 6950 placebo recipients were followed up through year 7 after vaccination.[39] Vaccine efficacy for herpes zoster and pain burden persisted through year 5 after vaccination. In the Long Term Persistence Substudy of the Shingles Prevention Study, 6867 subjects were followed up for 11 years after vaccination and compared with historical controls. Vaccine efficacy for herpes zoster and pain burden persisted through year 8 after vaccination.[40] Currently, there is no recommendation for a booster dose of the vaccine.

The efficacy of the live attenuated zoster vaccine in 50- to 59-year-old individuals was demonstrated in a large randomized, placebo-controlled trial that showed vaccine efficacy of 69.8%.[41] The FDA licensed the vaccine for use in immunocompetent adults 50 years of age and greater based on the results of this trial. However, The ACIP retained the recommendation to vaccinate at 60 years of age and older because zoster vaccine administration should be timed to achieve the greatest reduction in burden of herpes zoster and its complications, which is in persons older than 60 years.[42] Given that there is insufficient evidence for long-term protection offered by the herpes zoster vaccine, persons vaccinated at younger than 60 years may not be protected when the incidence of herpes zoster and its complications are highest. Conversely, neither the

FDA nor the ACIP set an upper age limit on the use of the vaccine. These individuals are at highest risk for herpes zoster and PHN and reduction of herpes zoster pain severity and duration occurs in the "old–old" even when herpes zoster is not prevented.

The efficacy of the zoster vaccine in individuals who have already had herpes zoster is unknown. However, older adults with prior herpes zoster ask for the vaccine because they don't want to experience zoster again, and herpes zoster recurs in immune competent individuals. The ACIP recommends the zoster vaccine for persons older than 60 years regardless of whether they report a prior episode of herpes zoster.

Subunit Adjuvanted Zoster Vaccine

A recently developed subunit zoster vaccine containing VZV glycoprotein E and the AS01 B adjuvant system (called *HZ/su*) showed a strong immune response and a clinically acceptable safety profile in phase I and II studies.[43] VZV glycoprotein E is an important antigen target in the cellular immune response to VZV, and it plays a role in VZV replication and spread. The AS01 B adjuvant system stimulates CD4$^+$ T-cell and humoral immune responses against recombinant proteins.

The subunit adjuvanted zoster vaccine was tested for efficacy against herpes zoster in a multisite randomized, placebo-controlled trial called the Zoster Efficacy Study in Adults 50 Years of Age or Older (ZOE-50).[43] A total of 15,411 participants received the vaccine (n = 7698) or placebo (n = 7713). The participants were stratified by age groups (50–59, 60–69, and ≥70 years). The intervention was 2 intramuscular doses of the vaccine or placebo 2 months apart. The mean follow-up was 3.2 years. The results showed that the subunit adjuvanted vaccine reduced the incidence of herpes zoster in this age group by 97.2% with an adequate safety profile. The results of a similar study with individuals 70 years and older is pending. This vaccine is not yet licensed by the FDA but looks to be an exciting addition to our interventions against herpes zoster.

SUMMARY

Most herpes zoster cases occur among older adults because the incidence of herpes zoster and PHN increases markedly with aging, which is related to an age-related decline in the cellular immune response to VZV. Acute herpes zoster pain, other herpes zoster complications (eg, ophthalmic zoster), and PHN may profoundly affect physical, psychological, and social health and reduce quality of life in older people. Clinicians have several tools to prevent and treat herpes zoster and PHN. Those tools include the zoster vaccines, early antiviral therapy, careful acute pain management, and several neuropathic pain treatments. The thoughtful use of these interventions will markedly reduce the suffering of older adults from herpes zoster and PHN.

REFERENCES

1. Cohen JI. The varicella-zoster virus genome. Curr Top Microbiol Immunol 2010; 342:1–14.
2. Yawn BP, Saddier P, Wollan PC, et al. A population-based study of the incidence and complication rates of herpes zoster before zoster vaccine introduction. Mayo Clin Proc 2007;82:1341–9.
3. Pinchinat S, Cebrian-Cuenca AM, Bricout H, et al. Similar herpes zoster incidence across Europe: results from a systematic literature review. BMC Infect Dis 2013;13:170.
4. Oxman MN, Levin MJ, Johnson GR, et al, For the Shingles Prevention Study Group. A vaccine to prevent herpes zoster and postherpetic neuralgia in older adults. N Engl J Med 2005;352:2271–84.

5. Harpaz R, Ortega-Sanchez IR, Seward JF, et al, Advisory Committee on Immunization Practices (ACIP) Centers for Disease Control and Prevention (CDC). Prevention of herpes zoster: recommendations of the advisory committee on immunization practices (ACIP). MMWR Recomm Rep 2008;57(RR-5):1–30.

6. Cohen JI. Herpes zoster. N Engl J Med 2013;369:255–63.

7. Yawn BP, Wollan PC, Kurland MJ, et al. Herpes zoster recurrences more frequent than previously reported. Mayo Clin Proc 2011;86:88–93.

8. Tseng HF, Chi M, Smith N, et al. Herpes zoster vaccine and the incidence of recurrent herpes zoster in an immunocompetent elderly population. J Infect Dis 2012;206:190–6.

9. Winthrop KL, Baddley JW, Chen L, et al. Association between the initiation of anti-tumor necrosis factor therapy and the risk of herpes zoster. JAMA 2013;309:887–95.

10. Schmader KE, George LK, Hamilton JD. Racial differences in the occurrence of herpes zoster. J Infect Dis 1995;171:701–5.

11. Zhang JX, Joesoef RM, Bialek S, et al. Association of physical trauma with risk of herpes zoster among Medicare beneficiaries in the United States. J Infect Dis 2013;207:1007–11.

12. Hales CM, Harpaz R, Joesoef MR, et al. Examination of links between herpes zoster incidence and childhood varicella vaccination. Ann Intern Med 2013;159:739–45.

13. Viner K, Perella D, Lopez A, et al. Transmission of varicella zoster virus from individuals with herpes zoster or varicella in school and day care settings. J Infect Dis 2012;205:1336–41.

14. Katz J, Cooper EM, Walther RR, et al. Acute pain in herpes zoster and its impact on health-related quality of life. Clin Infect Dis 2004;39:342–8.

15. Schmader KE, Sloane R, Pieper C, et al. The impact of acute herpes zoster pain and discomfort on functional status and quality of life in older adults. Clin J Pain 2007;23:490–7.

16. Jung BF, Johnson RW, Griffin DR, et al. Risk factors for postherpetic neuralgia in patients with herpes zoster. Neurology 2004;62:1545–51.

17. Harbecke R, Oxman MN, Arnold BA, et al. A real-time PCR assay to identify and discriminate among wild-type and vaccine strains of varicella-zoster virus and herpes simplex virus in clinical specimens, and comparison with the clinical diagnoses. J Med Virol 2009;81:1310–22.

18. Dworkin RH, Johnson RW, Breuer J, et al. Recommendations for the management of herpes zoster. Clin Infect Dis 2007;44:S1–26.

19. Dworkin RH, Barbano RL, Tyring SK, et al. A randomized, placebo-controlled trial of oxycodone and of gabapentin for acute pain in herpes zoster. Pain 2009;142:209–17.

20. Esmann V, Geil JP, Kroon S, et al. Prednisolone does not prevent postherpetic neuralgia. Lancet 1987;2:126–9.

21. Wood MJ, Johnson RW, McKendrick MW, et al. A randomized trial of acyclovir for 7 days or 21 days with and without prednisolone for treatment of acute herpes zoster. N Engl J Med 1994;330:896–900.

22. Whitley RJ, Weiss H, Gnann JW, et al. Acyclovir with and without prednisone for the treatment of herpes zoster: a randomized, placebo-controlled trial. Ann Intern Med 1996;125:376–83.

23. Berry JD, Petersen KL. A single dose of gabapentin reduces acute pain and allodynia in patients with herpes zoster. Neurology 2005;65:444–7.

24. van Wijck AJM, Opstelten W, Moons KG, et al. The PINE study of epidural ste-roids and local anaesthetics to prevent postherpetic neuralgia: a randomised controlled trial. Lancet 2006;367:219–24.
25. Johnson RW, Rice AS. Postherpetic neuralgia. N Engl J Med 2014;371:1526–33.
26. NICE clinical guideline 173. Neuropathic pain—pharmacological management: the pharmacological management of neuropathic pain in adults in non-specialist settings. London: National Institute for Health and Care Excellence; 2013. Available at: http://guidance.nice.org.uk/CG173.
27. Dworkin RH, O'Connor AB, Audette J, et al. Recommendations for the pharmaco-logical management of neuropathic pain: an overview and literature update. Mayo Clin Proc 2010;85(Suppl):S3–14.
28. Watson CPN, Vernich L, Chipman M, et al. Nortriptyline versus amitriptyline in postherpetic neuralgia: a randomized trial. Neurology 1998;51:1166–71.
29. Raja SN, Haythornthwaite JA, Pappagallo M, et al. Opioids versus antidepres-sants in postherpetic neuralgia: a randomized, placebo-controlled trial. Neurology 2002;59:1015–21.
30. Gilron I, Bailey JM, Tu D, et al. Morphine, gabapentin, or their combination for neuropathic pain. N Engl J Med 2005;352:1324–34.
31. Gilron I, Bailey JM, Tu D, et al. Nortriptyline and gabapentin, alone and in combi-nation for neuropathic pain: a double-blind, randomised controlled crossover trial. Lancet 2009;374:1252–61.
32. Weiner DK, Schmader KE. Postherpetic pain: more than sensory neuralgia? Pain Med 2006;7:243–9.
33. Tseng HF, Smith N, Harpaz R, et al. Herpes zoster vaccine in older adults and the risk of subsequent herpes zoster disease. JAMA 2011;305:160–6.
34. Langan SM, Smeeth L, Margolis D, et al. Herpes zoster vaccine effectiveness against incident herpes zoster and post-herpetic neuralgia in an older US popu-lation: a cohort study. PLoS Med 2013;10(4):e1001420.
35. Schmader KE, Johnson GR, Saddier P, et al. Effect of a zoster vaccine on herpes zoster-related interference with functional status and health-related quality of life measures in older adults. J Am Geriatr Soc 2010;58:1634–41.
36. Tseng HF, Tartof S, Harpaz R, et al. Vaccination against zoster remains effective in older adults who later undergo chemotherapy. Clin Infect Dis 2014;59:913–9.
37. Simberkoff MS, Arbeit RD, Johnson GR, et al, For the Shingles Prevention Study Group. Safety of the herpes zoster vaccine in the Shingles Prevention Study: a randomized trial. Ann Intern Med 2010;152:545–54.
38. Tseng HF, Liu A, Sy L, et al. Safety of zoster vaccine in adults from a large managed-care cohort: a Vaccine Safety Datalink study. J Intern Med 2012;271: 510–20.
39. Schmader KE, Oxman MN, Levin MJ, et al, For the Shingles Prevention Study Group. Persistence of the efficacy of zoster vaccine in the shingles prevention study and the short-term persistence substudy. Clin Infect Dis 2012;55:1320–8.
40. Morrison VA, Oxman MN, Johnson G, et al. Long-term persistence of zoster vac-cine efficacy. Clin Infect Dis 2015;60:900–9.
41. Schmader KE, Levin MJ, Gnann JW, et al. Efficacy, safety, tolerability of herpes zoster vaccine in persons 50-59 years of age. Clin Infect Dis 2012;54:922–8.
42. Hales CM, Harpaz R, Ortega-Sanchez I, et al. Update on recommendations for use of herpes zoster vaccine. MMWR Morb Mortal Wkly Rep 2014;63(33):729–31.
43. Lal H, Cunningham AL, Godeaux O, et al. Efficacy of an adjuvanted herpes zoster subunit vaccine in older adults. N Engl J Med 2015;372(22):2087–96.

Bone and Joint Infections in Older Adults

Simon C. Mears, MD, PhD*, Paul K. Edwards, MD

KEYWORDS

- Prosthetic joint infection • Osteomyelitis • Septic joint • Antibiotics • Frailty • Biofilm

KEY POINTS

- Septic native joints are treated with aspiration or irrigation and debridement and antibiotics depending on the size and location of the joint.
- Osteomyelitis is treated with surgical debridement and antibiotics. Depending on the type and location of osteomyelitis secondary reconstruction may be required.
- Prosthetic joint infection can be difficult to diagnose. Any painful joint can be infected. Inflammatory markers are the first step in diagnosis and if elevated joint aspiration should be performed.
- Acute infections of prosthetic joints may be treated with surgical washout, polyethylene exchange, and intravenous antibiotics.
- Chronic infections of prosthetic joints are most commonly treated with implant removal and spacer placement. After a course of intravenous antibiotics, a second prosthetic joint may be placed.

INTRODUCTION

Bone and joint infections are difficult to manage and cause serious morbidity and mortality in the older adult. These range from native joint infections, to osteomyelitis, to prosthetic joint infections (PJI). Because the number of prosthetic joints is increasing, PJIs are an increasing medical problem with great cost and morbidity. Treatment of bone and joint infections is made troublesome by the poor host status of a frail elderly patient and by the ability of bacteria to create biofilm. Frailty makes it harder for patients to tolerate surgery and biofilm allows bacteria to become inactive and more difficult to eradicate. Native joint infections are treated with either aspiration or surgical debridement, and antibiotics. Osteomyelitis can either be suppressed or surgically excised and treated with antibiotics. PJI is most commonly treated with implant

Neither author has commercial or financial conflict of interest, or funding sources for this article.
Department of Orthopaedic Surgery, University of Arkansas for Medical Services, 4301 West Markham Street, Little Rock, AR 72207, USA
* Corresponding author.
E-mail address: scmears@uams.edu

removal and two-stage reconstruction and a 6-week course of intravenous antibiotics. The need for multiple surgeries makes the treatment of a frail elderly patient with infection challenging. Careful coordination between the surgeon and infectious disease expert is important to improve results. Treatment with long-term intravenous antibiotics is usually required, which may have additional side effects in the elderly patient who is already on multiple medications. Often this results in long-term hospitalization or nursing care at great cost. This article concentrates on the treatment of bone and joint infections in the elderly patient.

HOST FACTORS IN ELDERLY PATIENTS

Risk factors for joint and bone infections include diabetes mellitus, rheumatoid arthritis, intravenous drug use, other infections, and immunosuppression. The notion of the type of host is important in the treatment of bone infections. The Cierny/Mader classification looks at the host type and the anatomic type of osteomyelitis.[1] The host type involves systemic and local factors. Hosts are rated as an A, B, or C: type A hosts are healthy, type B hosts have comorbidities that affect their response to infection, and type C hosts have more comorbidities making the risks of treatment outweigh the benefits.

Type C hosts by definition are treated with suppression of infection and not treatment for cure. Unfortunately many of elderly patients may fall in to the type C host category. Although no studies have examined the relationship of frailty and the host classification of Cierny there is much in common. Type C hosts are most often frail with poor resistance to disease and with local factors, such as venous stasis, that make wound healing more difficult.

Frailty is a syndrome that affects at least 15% of elderly patients.[2] The frail patient is more likely to be a poor host and more difficult to cure of a bone infection. Frailty can be assessed and measured and puts surgical patients at risk for poor outcomes.[3] Because frailty affects all systems of the body, many aspects of infection care are made more difficult. With worsening of the musculoskeletal system and sarcopenia, recovery from joint surgery is more difficult.[4] Because infection surgery may make a patient non–weight bearing, mobilization can be difficult. Lack of mobility increases the risk for pressure ulcers in the decubitus region and on the skin when braces or casts become necessary. Frailty also affects the neurologic system, putting the patient at higher risk for delirium after surgery.[5] The cardiac and renal systems are also affected in the frail patient and these may make surgery and the use of intravenous antibiotics more likely to have serious side effects.

Older patients are more likely to have an infection in a joint with pre-existing osteoarthritis. The changes associated with osteoarthritis make debridement more difficult and more likely to fail. The cartilage loss and associated osteophytes create cracks and crevices that allow bacteria to hide and evade removal (**Fig. 1**). Often there are pouches of fluid, such as those that form behind the knee and are difficult to access. The popliteal or Baker cyst is a common example. The popliteal cyst is created by a one-way valve that forms because of a tear in the posterior aspect of the meniscus.[6] The meniscal tear is a degenerative tear that occurs as part of the arthritic process. Synovial fluid can escape through the tear or one-way valve to the back of the knee creating a swelling termed a popliteal cyst. This process is common with knee arthritis and allows infection to escape into the back of the knee.[7] With standard aspiration or arthroscopic debridement of the knee this posterior region may not be washed out and the infection is not eradicated. In some cases, an open arthrotomy is required to washout the infection. In the worst cases, resection of the bone and cement spacer

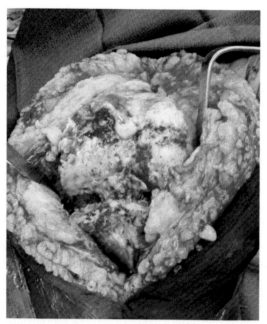

Fig. 1. Intraoperative photograph of a septic arthritic knee. Note the roughened and irregular joint surfaces.

should be considered. A knee replacement can then be placed after treating the infection.

The ability of microorganisms to produce a biofilm is important to understand in the treatment of bone and joint infections. Biofilm is formed by the bacteria and changes the response to antibiotics and to the host immune system. The bacteria that form biofilm may go dormant and hide for long periods of time. In particular *Staphylococcus aureus* creates biofilm[8] and is the most common type of bone and joint infection.

Biofilm is a polysaccharide/protein matrix produced by microbial colonies. It functions to prevent the host immune system and systemic antibiotics from attacking the bacteria. The biofilm is a relatively impermeable barrier to antibiotics. It also causes the bacteria within to change to a more inactive state lowering the susceptibility of antibiotics by up to 10^3.[9]

Biofilm is extremely difficult to eradicate and must be surgically excised to allow for cure. Debridement of the bone to healthy tissue is considered the gold standard. This is known by the visualization of punctate bleeding of healthy bone. Future work is examining different prosthetic joint surfaces that may be resistant to biofilm formation.

NATIVE JOINT INFECTIONS

Native joints may become infected by direct inoculation, by hematogenous seeding, or by invasion from a neighboring infection. Elderly patients have a higher rate of underlying osteoarthritis, which may make treatment of the infection more difficult. Risk factors include diabetes and immunosuppression. The most common causes of infection are staphylococci, followed by streptococci and gram-negative bacilli.[10]

Any joint in the body can become infected including the knee, shoulder, wrist, elbow, ankle, hip, and sternoclavicular joints. The onset is usually acute pain, difficulty moving the joint, and erythema. Systemic signs of sepsis may develop, such as fever and mental changes or dehydration. Usually the infection is monoarticular in presentation. If more than one joint is infected, seeding from a hematogenous source, such as an infected heart valve, should be considered. Immunosuppression is a risk factor for infection and this may make diagnosis more difficult.[11] Intravenous drug use is a risk factor, more commonly in younger patients. Diagnosis is by clinical examination and subsequent joint aspiration. Inflammatory markers can help in the diagnosis of septic joint[12] but analysis of joint fluid and culture is the gold standard for diagnosis.

In the differential diagnosis of a painful joint, it is important to rule out acute joint injury or fracture and gout, pseudogout, or a flare of osteoarthritis. Generally, an injury presents acutely with a specific history; however, in the confused or demented patient this may be difficult to ascertain. Gout is difficult to distinguish from infection. More often gout is polyarticular in nature or the patient may have a history of prior attacks. A radiograph should be obtained to rule out fracture. In some cases further imaging is of value. MRI is more sensitive for injury or stress fracture. It also shows if there is a joint effusion or if there is a soft tissue abscess.

Blood testing for inflammatory markers is helpful in diagnosing infection. Infection raises the C-reactive protein (CRP) and erythrocyte sedimentation rate (ESR). Unfortunately, patients with septic arthritis can also have normal laboratory test values.[13] The white blood cell (WBC) count may be normal unless the patient is septic. Gout may raise the uric acid level, which should be checked.

If initial clinical examination gives a high suspicion for joint infection, the next step is joint aspiration. With most joints this is attempted at bedside. If fluid is unable to be obtained then radiologic guidance either with fluoroscopy or ultrasound should be used. The hip is a deep joint that requires radiologic-guided aspiration. Some deep areas, such as the spine or sacroiliac joints, may require computer tomography–guided aspiration.

Analysis of joint fluid should include a WBC count and differential. The synovial fluid WBC count and the percentage of polymorphonuclear cell (PMN) are predictive of infection. However, there is no absolute value that proves infection. The higher the WBC count, the more likely septic arthritis is the cause.[14] A PMN count of 90% or more is predictive of infection.[15] Crystal analysis should be performed to look for gout. Fluid should also be sent for aerobic and anaerobic culture. Fungal and mycobacteria require separate cultures and should be considered.

The decision to get surgical (usually orthopedic) consultation is at the preference of the treating physician. If the treating physician is not comfortable with joint aspiration then consultation should be obtained. The "shotgun" approach of starting antibiotics without aspirating the joint should be avoided. Starting antibiotics before aspirating the joint may make the culture less likely to grow bacteria.[16] The best treatment is performed when knowing precisely what organism is the causative agent. Gout is very common and may resemble an infection. Gout does not get better with antibiotics and antibiotics may have harmful side effects. The only scenario in which antibiotics should be started without cultures is a very unstable patient with sepsis where delay of starting antibiotics cannot be tolerated.

After cultures have been obtained, broad-spectrum antibiotics should be started if there is concern for a septic joint. Treatment of a native joint infection depends on the location of the joint. Some joints can be treated with serial aspiration and intravenous antibiotics. The decision to operate is complex. The data supporting joint washout versus aspiration are poor and only two studies have evaluated this to date. Goldenberg and colleagues[17] in 1975 showed better results with medical treatment when compared with surgical treatment. A subsequent study also did not show better results with surgical treatment.[18] Prompt treatment, initiated within 48 hours of diagnosis, seems to give the best results.[19] However, regardless of treatment, results of septic arthritis are poor in 25% to 50% of elderly patients.[20]

Decision making is particularly difficult in the frail patient. If surgical treatment is selected, this may be arthroscopic or open. In the wrist, arthroscopic treatment has been shown to require fewer procedures and less days in hospital with similar results to open treatment.[21] Arthroscopic treatment has proven effective in many joints including the shoulder,[22] ankle,[23] elbow,[24,25] and knee.[26]

The condition of the joint is important. Arthritic joints have irregular surfaces, osteophytes, and cartilage loss. Debridement is more difficult in the arthritic joint. In the worst of cases, surgical excision of the joint with placement of a spacer may be considered. A later second-stage joint replacement may be considered after the infection is eradicated.

If joint aspiration with subsequent antibiotic treatment does not improve the symptoms, consideration for further surgery should be made. Further imaging, such as an MRI, may be helpful, especially in the knee, where a popliteal bursa posterior to the knee may be concomitantly infected. Imaging should be considered especially if an infection is not getting better. This may reveal other soft tissue abscesses or osteomyelitis. Repeat debridement may be needed if the clinical condition is not improving. Risk factors for repeat debridement include history of an inflammatory arthritis, large joint infection, diabetes mellitus, *S aureus* infection, or synovial fluid nucleated cell count of greater than 85.0×10^9 cells/L on joint aspiration.[27] The length of intravenous antibiotic treatment is debated, although usually a 6-week course is given.

There are limited papers published on outcomes of joint infections in elderly patients. There is a high rate of poor results especially if the infection is not identified and treated quickly. In one study of elderly patients 25% to 50% were believed to have irreversible loss of function in the joint.[20] Late treatment of septic joints is with arthroplasty.[28]

OSTEOMYELITIS

Spontaneous osteomyelitis is not common in the elderly patient. Hematogenous spread is more likely in pediatric patients who have a more vigorous blood supply to the bones. Older patients are more likely to have chronic osteomyelitis from previous injuries, wounds, or from diabetic infections. It is possible for osteomyelitis to linger and be dormant for 20 or more years. The bacteria form a biofilm and remain inactive. Spontaneous drainage may occur years later as the bacteria reactivate (**Fig. 2**). Old open fractures or gunshot wounds are an example. Diabetic foot infections are the most common cause of osteomyelitis. Lack of protective sensation leads to neuropathy and subsequent ulceration over a pressure spot. Subsequent infection

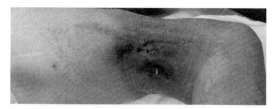

Fig. 2. Chronic osteomyelitis with a draining sinus tract from the lateral femur.

of the toe or foot occurs. The rate of diabetic foot infections is estimated to be 0.3% per year.[29]

The rate of osteomyelitis may be increasing. In a study from Olmsted County in Minnesota, the annual incidence was 2.8 cases per 100,000 person-years. This has increased from 11.4 cases per 100,000 person-years from 1969 to 1979 to 24.4 cases per 100,000 person-years from 2000 to 2009.[30] The reasons for this increase are unclear but may be caused by diabetes. The most common locations of osteomyelitis are in the foot (43%) followed by the femur and tibia (20%).

Bone can be infected by many different organisms. The most common is *S aureus* (42%) followed by streptococci species (25%) and *Staphylococcus epidermidis* (22%). *Pseudomonas* species, anaerobic organisms, and *Escherichia coli* are other less common causative organisms.[30]

The Cierny/Mader classification system is used to classify osteomyelitis.[1]

- Type I or intramedullary osteomyelitis refers to a nidus of infection inside the bone. This makes up about 2% of cases.
- Type 2 or superficial osteomyelitis refers to infection in the cortex of the bone that extends through the soft tissue. Most commonly this is seen in a pressure ulcer.
- Type 3 of localized osteomyelitis has a full-thickness cortical sequestrum. Removal of the sequestrum still allows for continuity of the bone. Hardware may be present.
- Type 4 or diffuse osteomyelitis has the components of types 1, 2, and 3 osteomyelitis but either the bone is unstable or debridement of the infection leads to instability.

Treatment of osteomyelitis is either suppressive or curative and is guided by both the host and infection classification. Critical to both treatments is identification of the specific microorganism involved to select appropriate antibiotic management. Cultures of the bone should be obtained when the patient is off of antibiotics to have the most likelihood of a positive culture. Suppressive treatment with antibiotics does not eradicate the bone infection but may suppress it. The patient may have a chronically draining wound that is manageable with dressing care. Suppressive treatment is considered for those patients who are extremely poor hosts (type C) and may not tolerate surgery whether from a local wound healing perspective or from systemic risk factors.

Type 1 or medullary osteomyelitis is treated surgically by opening the bone and debriding the nidus of infection. A course of intravenous antibiotics is also given after the debridement. Type 2 osteomyelitis is also treated with excision; however, the soft tissue defect must be covered using plastics surgical techniques. Surgical treatment may be difficult and have worse outcomes requiring multistage surgery or even amputation. Type 3 osteomyelitis requires excision of the infection but leaves the bone in continuity (**Fig. 3**). Reconstruction must include dead space management and soft tissue reconstruction. In type 4 osteomyelitis the bone is unstable and must be reconstructed. Options include bone transport or vascularized bone grafts.[31–33]

After surgical debridement, a prolonged course of intravenous antibiotics is typically recommended for 4 to 6 weeks. There is little literature to support the exact length of antibiotic treatment needed.[34]

Treatment of diabetic foot infections is complex and involves a multidisciplinary approach.[35] Improved control of blood glucose levels is critical to success. In addition, excellent foot care combined with shoes designed to offload foot pressure points decreases plantar ulcers. In cases of deformity, realignment surgery may be required to offload the ulcer. If ulceration or osteomyelitis has developed, surgery may be

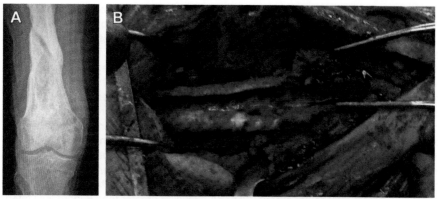

Fig. 3. (*A*) Anteroposterior (AP) radiograph of the femur showing intramedullary osteomyelitis. There is evidence of a lucency or sinus tract from the canal and extensive cortical changes. (*B*) Intraoperative photograph showing a corticotomy or opening of the lateral cortex of the femur to debride intramedullary osteomyelitis.

required. Most typically this is a limited amputation. If the infection is severe, further amputation may be necessary. It is important to get vascular studies to make sure there is enough blood flow for limb healing. If not, a vascular surgeon should be involved to determine if vascular flow can be improved or if higher amputation should be considered.

As the type of osteomyelitis becomes more complex, the chances of success decrease. Outcomes are also affected by the host classification: Type A hosts have better chance of success than type B hosts for all types of osteomyelitis.[33] One of the strengths of the Cierny/Mader classification system is the correlation between grade, host, and outcomes. As the type of osteomyelitis and the host becomes more complex, the risk of recurrence of infection increases.

Treatment decisions in the elderly patient become more difficult. If the patient does not tolerate multiple debridement surgeries with subsequent reconstruction then other options should be considered. In Cierny classification these patients are termed type C hosts. Either further suppressive care or amputation could be considered.

A rare complication of chronic osteomyelitis is malignant transformation. Most typically this occurs in a chronic wound or sinus tract after several years of treatment.[36] Squamous cell carcinoma is the most common type of cancer that occurs as a result of malignant transformation and it is treated with wide resection of the tumor.

PROSTHETIC JOINT INFECTIONS

PJIs are currently the biggest challenge in joint replacement surgery. Infections cause long-term morbidity and are expensive to treat. In the elderly patient, treatment of PJI is even more difficult and expensive because long-term nursing home stays are typically necessary.

Infections occur in 2% to 2.4% of patients after knee and hip replacement and this number is increasing with time.[37] Infection is the number one cause of revision surgery for knee replacements[38] and number three for hip replacements.[39,40] Infection may occur immediately after replacement surgery and is likely caused by bacterial contamination at the time of surgery. PJI may also occur later during the patient's life at a rate of 0.7% per year.[41]

Risk factors for infection have been termed modifiable or nonmodifiable. Modifiable risks include operating time, elevated body mass index, tobacco use, and S aureus colonization.[42] Operating time should be reduced and outcomes of joint replacements are found to be better in high-volume centers.[43] A 9% increase in infection rates is thought to occur for every 15 minutes extra spent in the operating room for knee replacement.[44] Obesity has shown an increased risk for PJI. A maximum body mass index of 40 has been suggested to help decrease risk of infection.[45,46] Cigarette smoking increases the risk of infection and patients should be enrolled in a cessation program before joint replacement. Even former smokers have increased risk of infection after arthroplasty.[47] S aureus colonization can be tested with nasal culture. If positive, a decolonization program with intranasal mupirocin or povidone should be instituted.[48] Vancomycin should also be added to the preoperative antibiotic for methicillin-resistant S aureus (MRSA) positive patients. Diabetes should be well controlled before joint replacement. A HGBA$_{1c}$ level of greater than 8 increases infection risks.[49] Diabetic control should be improved before joint replacement.

Nonmodifiable conditions that increase the risk of infection are often present in the elderly population and include rheumatologic disease, coagulopathy, cirrhosis, and preoperative anemia.[50,51]

Infections may be bacterial, fungal, atypical mycobacteria, and possibly viral. The most common bacterial organisms are S aureus and coagulase-negative staphylococci, which cause about 60% of infections.[52] The rates of MRSA differ by geographic location.[53] Streptococci and gram-negative bacilli, such as Pseudomonas aeruginosa, enterococci, and Klebsiella pneumoniae are the next most common isolates. In some cases, an organism cannot be identified despite signs of obvious infection.[54] In 20% of cases, infections occur from multiple organisms.[55] Fungal infections are particularly difficult to eradicate.

In the shoulder, another common cause of infection is Propionibacterium acnes.[56] This organism is endemic to the skin of the shoulder region and is the most causative organism in about half of infected shoulder arthroplasties.[57]

Diagnosis of PJI may be difficult. Clinical practice guidelines have been published by the Infectious Diseases Society of America.[58] The usual presentation of an infected joint replacement is pain of the joint. It may also be warm, swollen, or stiff. In immediate postoperative infections, the wound may not heal or may continue to drain. In late infection, a sinus tract may form. Rarely a patient may present with sepsis and bacteremia from the infected joint replacement. Any painful joint replacement may potentially be infected. The evaluation for PJI is an algorithm and is described in the American Academy of Orthopedic Surgeons guideline.[59]

After physical examination, plain radiographs of the joint should obtained. Signs of chronic infection include loosening of the prosthesis and erosive bone changes around the implants (**Fig. 4**). Serum inflammatory markers including CRP and ESR should be checked. Rarely is the WBC count elevated and this is not a good screening test for infection.[60] If both the CRP and ESR are normal, it is very unlikely that the joint replacement is infected. If either or both are elevated infection cannot be ruled out. Inflammatory markers can be elevated from other processes in the body including rheumatoid arthritis or other injuries or infections.

The next step in the evaluation is joint aspiration. If either the CRP or ESR is elevated, aspiration should be performed. Fluid from the joint should be sent for cell count with differential, and aerobic and anerobic cultures. In the knee, a WBC count higher than 27,800 cells/μL in the first 6 weeks after surgery strongly suggests infection.[61] In knees implanted longer than 6 weeks, WBC count greater than 1700 or PMN percentage greater than 60 strongly suggests infection.[62] In the hip, these numbers

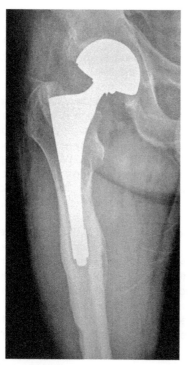

Fig. 4. AP radiograph of the hip showing an infected hip replacement. There is cortical remodeling and lucencies around the stem.

are slightly higher, WBC greater than 12,800 and PMN percentage greater than 89.[60] Newer tests are now available that may help in diagnosis of infection including the synovial fluid CRP,[63] the alpha-defensin level,[64] and the use of polymerase chain reaction to detect specific bacteria.[65] Nuclear medicine tests, such as bone scan and ^{18}F-labeled fluorodeoxyglucose-PET, may also be useful in diagnosis.

When a joint replacement has been diagnosed as infected there are several possible treatments. It is important to know the length of time that the symptoms have been present and the time interval for the joint replacement surgery. If the joint replacement has been performed within the last 3 weeks and the symptoms are less than 2 weeks old, consideration can be given to saving the prosthesis with surgical washout.[66] At the time of surgery a capsulectomy is performed and the plastic liner changed. This allows the surgeon to clean the implants behind the plastic liner. The patient is then treated with 6 weeks of intravenous antibiotics. Washout and implant retention is controversial. There is some evidence that outcomes are worse if a washout is performed and some authors advocate a more aggressive approach.[67]

If the infection is deemed chronic, then a washout has very little chance of success. If washout is performed the patient is likely to have a worse outcome.[67] This is often a result of the growth of biofilm on the implant surface. The biofilm allows bacteria to become dormant and very resistant to antibiotics treatment. The biofilm itself is difficult to remove from the implant surface making debridement much harder.

Treatment of chronic PJI is usually operative and involves the removal of the infected joint replacement. There is a limited role for suppressive antibiotics for chronically infected joint replacement. These patients need to know that antibiotics alone will not eradicate their infection. The goal of suppressive therapy is to prevent sepsis and bacteremia. These patients often have a chronically draining wound or sinus tract requiring dressing care. In the very elderly or infirm patient, chronic treatment with antibiotics may be reasonable if an operative approach cannot be tolerated or desired.[68]

Operative treatment can be in the form of a one- or two-stage approach. It is currently unclear which approach is better and both have advantages and disadvantages.[69,70] This is particularly true for the elderly and infirm patient. In the two-stage approach the goal for the first surgical stage is to remove all of the infected joint replacement and any infected bone or tissue. Any cement used for the replacement must also be removed. In some cases this may require cutting the bone or performing an osteotomy to gain access to the implants. Well-fixed implants can be difficult to remove. After the bones have been completely debrided, a cement spacer is then placed. Choices are available with the spacer. This may be articulating or not articulating. The nonarticulating spacer is a block of cement (**Fig. 5**). Antibiotics are added to the cement so that it elutes into the joint space after surgery. An articulating spacer is often an implant that is cheaply obtained (**Fig. 6**).[71] This is then loosely cemented into the bone. This does allow some motion, which may facilitate the second surgery. No differences in outcomes have been found between spacer types.[72] Patients with large bone defects require static (nonarticulating) spacers to keep tissue length. Patients with MRSA infections and infections in which bacteria are not cultured have worse rates of successful eradication of infection.[73]

After the spacer is placed, the patient is typically treated with 6 weeks of intravenous antibiotics. The antibiotics are then stopped. If the wound remains healed the second

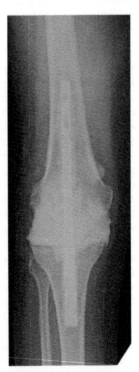

Fig. 5. AP radiograph of a knee with a static spacer. The cement fills the space between the femur and the tibia and a metal bar is used as rebar.

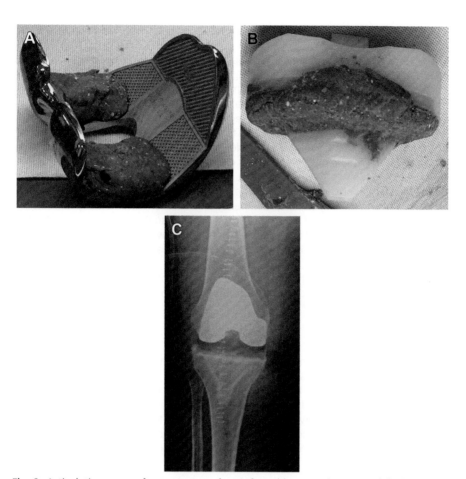

Fig. 6. Articulating spacer for treatment of an infected knee replacement. (*A*) Photograph of the femoral prosthesis with cement with added antibiotics and methylene blue for visibility. (*B*) For the tibial implant a one-piece all plastic implant is used that is less expensive. (*C*). AP radiograph of the spacer in place. The patient can weight bear and bend the knee with this temporary prosthesis.

stage is conducted and the spacer is removed and a new implant is placed. Typically revision implants are used for the reimplantation.

In the single-stage approach the debridement and the reimplantation are carried out in one operation. Excellent results have been published using this approach.[74,75] With the one-stage approach there are different options for antibiotic delivery. One option is 6 weeks of intravenous antibiotics. Another option is the delivery of the antibiotics through a catheter into the joint itself.[76,77]

The single-stage approach may have some advantages in the elderly patient in whom a second operation may be difficult or not tolerated well. It is thought that eradication of the infection is higher using the two-stage approach and this has been suggested as the gold standard of care.[78] The two-stage approach offers an 85% chance of success.[79,80] There been no prospective randomized trials to help determine if the one-stage or the two-stage approach are better.

Other possible treatments of PJI include joint fusion in the knee (see **Fig. 6**), permanent joint resection, or amputation. Although these options are not as functional as revision knee replacement, these salvage procedures may be necessary in cases where the host is poor or when a two-stage approach has already failed.

Soft tissue defects can also make treatment much more difficult. Defects are more common around the knee where the tissue over the tibial tubercle has thin subcutaneous tissue. A chronic sinus tract in that region may necessitate soft tissue coverage either with a muscle rotational flap or with free tissue transfer. This is particularly difficult in the elderly patient. Serious discussion needs to be taken whether limb salvage is a viable option in this patient subgroup or whether amputation is a better option.

Successful outcomes for the treatment of infected joints are around 80%. Clearly after several surgeries the overall outcome of the joint in terms of motion and function is less than after a primary joint replacement. Poor function is particularly hard on the elderly patient. The chance of a successful outcome is also thought to be related to the type of organism. MRSA and nonidentified organisms have a higher failure rate with a two-stage approach.[73] Morbid obesity and lymphedema[79] are other risk factors for failure of treatment.

After reimplantation it is unknown whether further antibiotics may help. A recent study has suggested that lifelong oral antibiotics may improve the results and increase the eradication of infection.[81]

SUMMARY

Infections of the bone and joint in the elderly population include infections of the native joint, osteomyelitis, and PJIs. Because of pre-existing arthritis, comorbidities, and frailty these are difficult to treat. Typically treatment is debridement of infection and intravenous antibiotics. Infections of prosthetic joints are increasingly common and are particularly expensive and difficult diagnoses to treat. The most common treatment is a two-stage process with removal of implants, treatment with intravenous antibiotics, and subsequent reimplantation of a second joint replacement.

REFERENCES

1. Cierny G 3rd, Mader JT, Penninck JJ. A clinical staging system for adult osteomyelitis. Clin Orthop Relat Res 2003;(414):7–24.
2. Bandeen-Roche K, Seplaki CL, Huang J, et al. Frailty in older adults: a nationally representative profile in the United States. J Gerontol A Biol Sci Med Sci 2015; 70(11):1427–34.
3. Makary MA, Segev DL, Pronovost PJ, et al. Frailty as a predictor of surgical outcomes in older patients. J Am Coll Surg 2010;210(6):901–8.
4. Higuera CA, Elsharkawy K, Klika AK, et al. 2010 Mid-America Orthopaedic Association Physician in Training Award: predictors of early adverse outcomes after knee and hip arthroplasty in geriatric patients. Clin Orthop Relat Res 2011; 469(5):1391–400.
5. Eeles EM, White SV, O'Mahony SM, et al. The impact of frailty and delirium on mortality in older inpatients. Age Ageing 2012;41(3):412–6.
6. Frush TJ, Noyes FR. Baker's cyst: diagnostic and surgical considerations. Sports Health 2015;7(4):359–65.
7. Papadopoulos A, Karachalios TS, Malizos CN, et al. Complicated septic arthritis after knee arthroscopy in a 75-year-old man with osteoarthritis and a popliteal cyst. BMJ Case Rep 2015;2015 [pii:bcr2014207394].

8. Cassat JE, Smeltzer MS, Lee CY. Investigation of biofilm formation in clinical isolates of *Staphylococcus aureus*. Methods Mol Biol 2014;1085:195–211.

9. Gbejuade HO, Lovering AM, Webb JC. The role of microbial biofilms in prosthetic joint infections. Acta Orthop 2015;86(2):147–58.

10. Dubost JJ, Couderc M, Tatar Z, et al. Three-decade trends in the distribution of organisms causing septic arthritis in native joints: single-center study of 374 cases. Joint Bone Spine 2014;81(5):438–40.

11. Salar O, Baker B, Kurien T, et al. Septic arthritis in the era of immunosuppressive treatments. Ann R Coll Surg Engl 2014;96(2):e11–2.

12. Roberts J, Schaefer E, Gallo RA. Indicators for detection of septic arthritis in the acutely swollen joint cohort of those without joint prostheses. Orthopedics 2014; 37(2):e98–102.

13. Li SF, Henderson J, Dickman E, et al. Laboratory tests in adults with monoarticular arthritis: can they rule out a septic joint? Acad Emerg Med 2004;11(3):276–80.

14. Carpenter CR, Schuur JD, Everett WW, et al. Evidence-based diagnostics: adult septic arthritis. Acad Emerg Med 2011;18(8):781–96.

15. Margaretten ME, Kohlwes J, Moore D, et al. Does this adult patient have septic arthritis? JAMA 2007;297(13):1478–88.

16. Hindle P, Davidson E, Biant LC. Septic arthritis of the knee: the use and effect of antibiotics prior to diagnostic aspiration. Ann R Coll Surg Engl 2012;94(5):351–5.

17. Goldenberg DL, Brandt KD, Cohen AS, et al. Treatment of septic arthritis: comparison of needle aspiration and surgery as initial modes of joint drainage. Arthritis Rheum 1975;18(1):83–90.

18. Ravindran V, Logan I, Bourke BE. Medical vs surgical treatment for the native joint in septic arthritis: a 6-year, single UK academic centre experience. Rheumatology (Oxford) 2009;48(10):1320–2.

19. Kodumuri P, Geutjens G, Kerr HL. Time delay between diagnosis and arthroscopic lavage in septic arthritis. Does it matter? Int Orthop 2012;36(8):1727–31.

20. Chen CM, Lin HH, Hung SC, et al. Surgical treatment for septic arthritis of the knee joint in elderly patients: a 10-year retrospective clinical study. Orthopedics 2013;36(4):e434–43.

21. Sammer DM, Shin AY. Comparison of arthroscopic and open treatment of septic arthritis of the wrist. J Bone Joint Surg Am 2009;91(6):1387–93.

22. Abdel MP, Perry KI, Morrey ME, et al. Arthroscopic management of native shoulder septic arthritis. J Shoulder Elbow Surg 2013;22(3):418–21.

23. Mankovecky MR, Roukis TS. Arthroscopic synovectomy, irrigation, and debridement for treatment of septic ankle arthrosis: a systematic review and case series. J Foot Ankle Surg 2014;53(5):615–9.

24. Moon JG, Biraris S, Jeong WK, et al. Clinical results after arthroscopic treatment for septic arthritis of the elbow joint. Arthroscopy 2014;30(6):673–8.

25. van den Ende KI, Steinmann SP. Arthroscopic treatment of septic arthritis of the elbow. J Shoulder Elbow Surg 2012;21(8):1001–5.

26. Balabaud L, Gaudias J, Boeri C, et al. Results of treatment of septic knee arthritis: a retrospective series of 40 cases. Knee Surg Sports Traumatol Arthrosc 2007; 15(4):387–92.

27. Hunter JG, Gross JM, Dahl JD, et al. Risk factors for failure of a single surgical debridement in adults with acute septic arthritis. J Bone Joint Surg Am 2015; 97(7):558–64.

28. Lee GC, Pagnano MW, Hanssen AD. Total knee arthroplasty after prior bone or joint sepsis about the knee. Clin Orthop Relat Res 2002;(404):226–31.

29. Peters EJ, Lipsky BA. Diagnosis and management of infection in the diabetic foot. Med Clin North Am 2013;97(5):911–46.

30. Kremers HM, Nwojo ME, Ransom JE, et al. Trends in the epidemiology of osteomyelitis: a population-based study, 1969 to 2009. J Bone Joint Surg Am 2015; 97(10):837–45.

31. Cierny G 3rd, DiPasquale D. Treatment of chronic infection. J Am Acad Orthop Surg 2006;14(10 Spec No.):S105–10.

32. Cierny G 3rd. Surgical treatment of osteomyelitis. Plast Reconstr Surg 2011; 127(Suppl 1):190S–204S.

33. Forsberg JA, Potter BK, Cierny G 3rd, et al. Diagnosis and management of chronic infection. J Am Acad Orthop Surg 2011;19(Suppl 1):S8–19.

34. Haidar R, Der Boghossian A, Atiyeh B. Duration of post-surgical antibiotics in chronic osteomyelitis: empiric or evidence-based? Int J Infect Dis 2010;14(9): e752–8.

35. Lindbloom BJ, James ER, McGarvey WC. Osteomyelitis of the foot and ankle: diagnosis, epidemiology, and treatment. Foot Ankle Clin 2014;19(3):569–88.

36. Panteli M, Puttaswamaiah R, Lowenberg DW, et al. Malignant transformation in chronic osteomyelitis: recognition and principles of management. J Am Acad Orthop Surg 2014;22(9):586–94.

37. Kurtz SM, Lau E, Watson H, et al. Economic burden of periprosthetic joint infection in the United States. J Arthroplasty 2012;27(8 Suppl):61–5.e1.

38. Bozic KJ, Kurtz SM, Lau E, et al. The epidemiology of revision total knee arthroplasty in the United States. Clin Orthop Relat Res 2010;468(1):45–51.

39. Bozic KJ, Kurtz SM, Lau E, et al. The epidemiology of revision total hip arthroplasty in the United States. J Bone Joint Surg Am 2009;91(1):128–33.

40. Kamath AF, Ong KL, Lau E, et al. Quantifying the burden of revision total joint arthroplasty for periprosthetic infection. J Arthroplasty 2015;30(9):1492–7.

41. Huotari K, Peltola M, Jamsen E. The incidence of late prosthetic joint infections: a registry-based study of 112,708 primary hip and knee replacements. Acta Orthop 2015;86(3):321–5.

42. Maoz G, Phillips M, Bosco J, et al. The Otto Aufranc Award: modifiable versus nonmodifiable risk factors for infection after hip arthroplasty. Clin Orthop Relat Res 2015;473(2):453–9.

43. Muilwijk J, van den Hof S, Wille JC. Associations between surgical site infection risk and hospital operation volume and surgeon operation volume among hospitals in the Dutch nosocomial infection surveillance network. Infect Control Hosp Epidemiol 2007;28(5):557–63.

44. Namba RS, Inacio MC, Paxton EW. Risk factors associated with deep surgical site infections after primary total knee arthroplasty: an analysis of 56,216 knees. J Bone Joint Surg Am 2013;95(9):775–82.

45. Friedman RJ, Hess S, Berkowitz SD, et al. Complication rates after hip or knee arthroplasty in morbidly obese patients. Clin Orthop Relat Res 2013;471(10): 3358–66.

46. McElroy MJ, Pivec R, Issa K, et al. The effects of obesity and morbid obesity on outcomes in TKA. J Knee Surg 2013;26(2):83–8.

47. Duchman KR, Gao Y, Pugely AJ, et al. The effect of smoking on short-term complications following total hip and knee arthroplasty. J Bone Joint Surg Am 2015; 97(13):1049–58.

48. Rao N, Cannella BA, Crossett LS, et al. Preoperative screening/decolonization for Staphylococcus aureus to prevent orthopedic surgical site infection: prospective cohort study with 2-year follow-up. J Arthroplasty 2011;26(8):1501–7.

49. Marchant MH Jr, Viens NA, Cook C, et al. The impact of glycemic control and diabetes mellitus on perioperative outcomes after total joint arthroplasty. J Bone Joint Surg Am 2009;91(7):1621–9.

50. Bozic KJ, Lau E, Kurtz S, et al. Patient-related risk factors for periprosthetic joint infection and postoperative mortality following total hip arthroplasty in Medicare patients. J Bone Joint Surg Am 2012;94(9):794–800.

51. Jiang SL, Schairer WW, Bozic KJ. Increased rates of periprosthetic joint infection in patients with cirrhosis undergoing total joint arthroplasty. Clin Orthop Relat Res 2014;472(8):2483–91.

52. Peel TN, Cheng AC, Buising KL, et al. Microbiological aetiology, epidemiology, and clinical profile of prosthetic joint infections: are current antibiotic prophylaxis guidelines effective? Antimicrob Agents Chemother 2012;56(5):2386–91.

53. Moran E, Masters S, Berendt AR, et al. Guiding empirical antibiotic therapy in orthopaedics: the microbiology of prosthetic joint infection managed by debridement, irrigation and prosthesis retention. J Infect 2007;55(1):1–7.

54. Berbari EF, Marculescu C, Sia I, et al. Culture-negative prosthetic joint infection. Clin Infect Dis 2007;45(9):1113–9.

55. Marculescu CE, Cantey JR. Polymicrobial prosthetic joint infections: risk factors and outcome. Clin Orthop Relat Res 2008;466(6):1397–404.

56. Richards J, Inacio MC, Beckett M, et al. Patient and procedure-specific risk factors for deep infection after primary shoulder arthroplasty. Clin Orthop Relat Res 2014;472(9):2809–15.

57. Pottinger P, Butler-Wu S, Neradilek MB, et al. Prognostic factors for bacterial cultures positive for *Propionibacterium acnes* and other organisms in a large series of revision shoulder arthroplasties performed for stiffness, pain, or loosening. J Bone Joint Surg Am 2012;94(22):2075–83.

58. Osmon DR, Berbari EF, Berendt AR, et al. Diagnosis and management of prosthetic joint infection: clinical practice guidelines by the Infectious Diseases Society of America. Clin Infect Dis 2013;56(1):e1–25.

59. Della Valle C, Parvizi J, Bauer TW, et al. American Academy of Orthopaedic Surgeons clinical practice guideline on: the diagnosis of periprosthetic joint infections of the hip and knee. J Bone Joint Surg Am 2011;93(14):1355–7.

60. Yi PH, Cross MB, Moric M, et al. The 2013 Frank Stinchfield Award: diagnosis of infection in the early postoperative period after total hip arthroplasty. Clin Orthop Relat Res 2014;472(2):424–9.

61. Bedair H, Ting N, Jacovides C, et al. The Mark Coventry Award: diagnosis of early postoperative TKA infection using synovial fluid analysis. Clin Orthop Relat Res 2011;469(1):34–40.

62. Ghanem E, Parvizi J, Burnett RS, et al. Cell count and differential of aspirated fluid in the diagnosis of infection at the site of total knee arthroplasty. J Bone Joint Surg Am 2008;90(8):1637–43.

63. Omar M, Ettinger M, Reichling M, et al. Synovial C-reactive protein as a marker for chronic periprosthetic infection in total hip arthroplasty. Bone Joint J 2015; 97-B(2):173–6.

64. Deirmengian C, Kardos K, Kilmartin P, et al. Combined measurement of synovial fluid alpha-Defensin and C-reactive protein levels: highly accurate for diagnosing periprosthetic joint infection. J Bone Joint Surg Am 2014;96(17):1439–45.

65. Moojen DJ, Spijkers SN, Schot CS, et al. Identification of orthopaedic infections using broad-range polymerase chain reaction and reverse line blot hybridization. J Bone Joint Surg Am 2007;89(6):1298–305.

66. Kuiper JW, Willink RT, Moojen DJ, et al. Treatment of acute periprosthetic infections with prosthesis retention: review of current concepts. World J Orthop 2014;5(5):667–76.

67. Sherrell JC, Fehring TK, Odum S, et al. The Chitranjan Ranawat Award: fate of two-stage reimplantation after failed irrigation and debridement for periprosthetic knee infection. Clin Orthop Relat Res 2011;469(1):18–25.

68. Prendki V, Zeller V, Passeron D, et al. Outcome of patients over 80 years of age on prolonged suppressive antibiotic therapy for at least 6 months for prosthetic joint infection. Int J Infect Dis 2014;29:184–9.

69. Leonard HA, Liddle AD, Burke O, et al. Single- or two-stage revision for infected total hip arthroplasty? a systematic review of the literature. Clin Orthop Relat Res 2014;472(3):1036–42.

70. Masters JP, Smith NA, Foguet P, et al. A systematic review of the evidence for single stage and two stage revision of infected knee replacement. BMC Musculoskelet Disord 2013;14:222.

71. Shaikh AA, Ha CW, Park YG, et al. Two-stage approach to primary TKA in infected arthritic knees using intraoperatively molded articulating cement spacers. Clin Orthop Relat Res 2014;472(7):2201–7.

72. Voleti PB, Baldwin KD, Lee GC. Use of static or articulating spacers for infection following total knee arthroplasty: a systematic literature review. J Bone Joint Surg Am 2013;95(17):1594–9.

73. Mortazavi SM, Vegari D, Ho A, et al. Two-stage exchange arthroplasty for infected total knee arthroplasty: predictors of failure. Clin Orthop Relat Res 2011;469(11):3049–54.

74. Gehrke T, Zahar A, Kendoff D. One-stage exchange: it all began here. Bone Joint J 2013;95-B(11 Suppl A):77–83.

75. Haddad FS, Sukeik M, Alazzawi S. Is single-stage revision according to a strict protocol effective in treatment of chronic knee arthroplasty infections? Clin Orthop Relat Res 2015;473(1):8–14.

76. Whiteside LA, Peppers M, Nayfeh TA, et al. Methicillin-resistant *Staphylococcus aureus* in TKA treated with revision and direct intra-articular antibiotic infusion. Clin Orthop Relat Res 2011;469(1):26–33.

77. Antony SJ, Westbrook RS, Jackson JS, et al. Efficacy of single-stage revision with aggressive debridement using intra-articular antibiotics in the treatment of infected joint prosthesis. Infect Dis (Auckl) 2015;8:17–23.

78. Parvizi J, Adeli B, Zmistowski B, et al. Management of periprosthetic joint infection: the current knowledge: AAOS exhibit selection. J Bone Joint Surg Am 2012;94(14):e104.

79. Kubista B, Hartzler RU, Wood CM, et al. Reinfection after two-stage revision for periprosthetic infection of total knee arthroplasty. Int Orthop 2012;36(1):65–71.

80. Mahmud T, Lyons MC, Naudie DD, et al. Assessing the gold standard: a review of 253 two-stage revisions for infected TKA. Clin Orthop Relat Res 2012;470(10):2730–6.

81. Siqueira MB, Saleh A, Klika AK, et al. Chronic suppression of periprosthetic joint infections with oral antibiotics increases infection-free survivorship. J Bone Joint Surg Am 2015;97(15):1220–32.

Human Immunodeficiency Virus/Acquired Immunodeficiency Syndrome in Older Adults

Jake Scott, MD, Matthew Bidwell Goetz, MD*

KEYWORDS

- Human immunodeficiency virus • Acquired immunodeficiency syndrome
- Antiretroviral therapy • Immunocompromised host • Epidemiology

KEY POINTS

- The population of older human immunodeficiency virus (HIV)–infected patients is increasing. By 2020, more than 50% of HIV-infected persons in the United States will be older than 50 years of age.
- Untreated older HIV-infected patients progress more rapidly to AIDS with higher mortality rates.
- Patients up to age 64 should be routinely offered HIV testing; testing up to age 75 is recommended for adults who might transmit HIV to others.
- The occurrence of comorbidities not traditionally associated with HIV infection now exceeds that of AIDS-related events and are especially relevant to older patients.
- Antiretroviral therapy should be offered to all HIV-infected patients regardless of age, symptoms, CD4+ cell count, or HIV viral load. Early treatment is especially important in older patients.

INTRODUCTION

The development of better tolerated and more efficacious combined antiretroviral therapy (ART) has transformed what was once an inexorably progressive illness into a manageable chronic disease for which life expectancy has begun to approach that of the general population. This substantial increase in survival has led to a steady increase in the number of HIV-infected individuals who are older than 50 years of age. This demographic change is coupled with substantial clinical issues unique to older

Disclosures: None.

Infectious Diseases Section, Department of Medicine, VA Greater Los Angeles Healthcare System, David Geffen School of Medicine at UCLA, 11301 Wilshire Boulevard, Los Angeles, CA 90073, USA

* Corresponding author. Infectious Diseases, VA Greater Los Angeles Healthcare System, 111-F, 11301 Wilshire Boulevard, Los Angeles, CA 90073.

E-mail address: Matthew.Goetz@va.gov

Clin Geriatr Med 32 (2016) 571–583
http://dx.doi.org/10.1016/j.cger.2016.02.010
0749-0690/16/$ – see front matter Published by Elsevier Inc.

geriatric.theclinics.com

human immunodeficiency virus (HIV)–infected persons and provides important challenges to clinicians caring for older patients.

EPIDEMIOLOGY

In 2012, 40% of all HIV-infected persons in the United States were 50 years of age or older; by 2020, more than 50% of HIV-infected persons will have reached this age.[1,2] Aging of the HIV-infected population is not unique to the developed world. The World Health Organization estimates that as of 2014, there were 4.2 million people in the world living with HIV who were older than age 50; most of these people are in Sub-Saharan Africa (**Fig. 1**).[3]

NATURAL HISTORY OF HUMAN IMMUNODEFICIENCY VIRUS INFECTION IN OLDER PATIENTS

After infection, initial plasma HIV-1 RNA levels (viral load) are higher and CD4+ cell counts are lower in older patients than in younger patients. Subsequently, the rate of decline of CD4+ cells is greater in older patients, resulting in a more rapid progression to AIDS and death. Although the major complications of HIV infection generally occur after the CD4+ count decreases to less than 200 cells/µL, older individuals have higher rates of AIDS-defining events than do younger individuals at any given CD4+ cell count.[4]

DIAGNOSIS OF HUMAN IMMUNODEFICIENCY VIRUS INFECTION AND CASE IDENTIFICATION

The US Preventive Services Task Force recommends that all patients aged 13 to 64 be offered HIV testing at least once per lifetime as a part of routine medical care and regardless of known or perceived risk.[5] An exception to the recommendation was made for populations in which the prevalence of undiagnosed HIV infection is known to be less than 0.1%. Furthermore, the American College of Physicians (ACP) recommends offering testing up to age 75 for persons who might, if infected, transmit HIV to others.[6]

In addition to once-per-lifetime testing, high-risk individuals, such as men who have sex with men, injection-drug users, and sex partners of HIV-infected persons, should have annual or more frequent testing. Targeted testing is also indicated for patients with a potential recent high-risk event or with unexplained symptoms consistent with HIV infection, including weight loss, unexplained dementia, mucosal candidiasis, or AIDS-defining opportunistic infections or malignancies.

As of 2012, 13% of the estimated 1.2 million persons infected with HIV in the United States remained unaware of their diagnosis; 5% of the undiagnosed population was 55 years of age or older.[7] Among HIV-infected individuals over the age of 50 to 55, the median duration of infection before diagnosis is estimated to be 6.8 years.[8]

Delayed testing for HIV infection in older patients stems from several different factors. Because of a lack of awareness, older individuals are less likely to request HIV testing, and health care providers are less likely to offer routine testing. Finally, targeted testing is often delayed because older HIV-infected individuals often present with nonspecific manifestations, such as gradually worsening weight loss and fatigue that mimics other maladies.[9]

Delays in testing contribute to the fact that older HIV-infected patients are more likely to have progressed to full-blown AIDS when they are diagnosed (**Fig. 2**) and are much more likely to die within 1 to 3 years of their diagnosis than are younger adults (**Fig. 3**).[2]

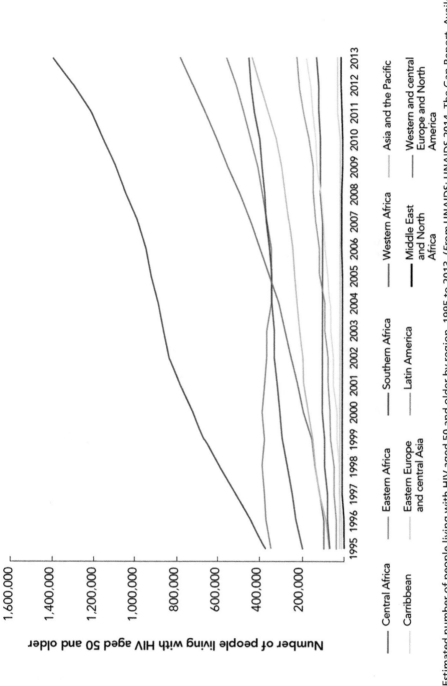

Fig. 1. Estimated number of people living with HIV aged 50 and older by region, 1995 to 2013. (*From* UNAIDS: UNAIDS 2014. The Gap Report. Available at: http://www.unaids.org/node/42898. Accessed October 24, 2015.)

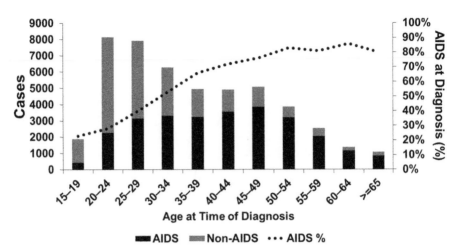

Fig. 2. Clinical status at time of diagnosis USA, 2013. Bars show the number of cases in each age strata who at the time of diagnosis of HIV infection who did (*black bar*) or did not (*gray bar*) have an AIDS-defining diagnosis. The dotted line shows the percentage of patients who had an AIDS-defining diagnosis. (*Data from* Centers for Disease Control and Prevention. HIV Surveillance Report, 2013. Available at: http://www.cdc.gov/hiv/library/reports/surveillance/2013/surveillance_Report_vol_25.html. Accessed August 9, 2015.)

TREATMENT

Combination ART has led to decreased rates of the opportunistic infections and malignancies traditionally associated with HIV infection as well as to decreases in the incidence of HIV-associated non-AIDS (HANA) comorbidities such as cardiovascular disease, the metabolic syndrome, diabetes mellitus, liver disease, kidney disease, neurologic disease, and non-AIDS-related malignancies.[10,11] ART achieves these goals by suppressing HIV replication, thereby restoring immunologic function. Of great

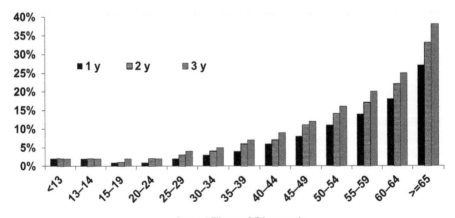

Fig. 3. Mortality after diagnosis of HIV infection in the United States, 2004–2009. Bars show the mortality at 1 (*black bar*), 2 (*horizontal dashes bar*), and 3 (*gray bar*) years after a diagnosis of HIV infection stratified by age. (*Data from* Centers for Disease Control and Prevention. HIV Surveillance Report, 2013. Available at: http://www.cdc.gov/hiv/library/reports/surveillance/2013/surveillance_Report_vol_25.html. Accessed August 9, 2015.)

societal importance is effective ART, also markedly decreasing the risk of HIV transmission by infected individuals.[10]

Timing of Initiation of Antiretroviral Therapy

Clinical trials have led to a long-standing strong recommendation that ART should be initiated in asymptomatic HIV-infected persons with less than 350 CD4+ cells/μL or with a history of an AIDS-defining illness. Although recommendations for starting therapy at higher CD4+ cells have been more moderate, recent clinical trials have now conclusively demonstrated that ART reduces HIV-related and overall morbidity and mortality regardless of the CD4+ cell count or viral load when therapy is initiated.[12] In particular, the recently concluded Strategic Timing of AntiRetroviral Treatment (START) study demonstrated that immediate initiation of ART in patients with CD4+ cell counts greater than 500 cells/μL is superior to the deferral of ART until the CD4+ cell count declines to less than 350 cells/μL.[11] The benefits of the immediate therapy include lower rates of serious AIDS-related and serious non-AIDS-related events (ie, HANA); the benefits did not differ according to age, sex, race, CD4+ cell count, viral load, or risk factors for serious non-AIDS diseases. Although only 25% of the subjects were older than 44 years of age, it is highly unlikely that any future randomized control trial data will be available for still older patients.

Based on these trial results, updated authoritative guidelines now strongly recommend that ART be initiated in all individuals who are willing and ready to start therapy regardless of their CD4+ cell count or age.[12] The guidelines specifically advocate for universal ART in HIV-infected persons older than age 50, regardless of their immune status, because "the risk of non-AIDS related complications may increase and the immunologic response to ART may be reduced in older HIV-infected patients".[10]

Consequently, although taking into consideration comorbidities, drug-drug interactions, polypharmacy, patient preference, and readiness to be adherent to therapy, providers should now offer ART to all patients regardless of age or CD4+ cell count. Deferrals of therapy, such as for patients who require a change in their baseline medications due to clinically significant drug-drug interactions with ART or for persons with serious barriers to adherence, should be brief, especially in persons with less than 200 CD4+ cells/μL.[10]

Selection of Therapy

Although the 6 classes of antiretroviral agents include more than 2 dozen individual agents, only 5 regimens are recommended for initial therapy (**Box 1**). Based on safety and efficacy, regimens containing a nonnucleoside reverse transcriptase inhibitor (NNRTI) or a protease inhibitor (PI) other than darunavir are no longer regarded as first-line regimens for ART-treatment-naïve patients.[10]

The choice of the antiretroviral regimen should take into consideration the patient's existing viral load, CD4+ cell count and resistance testing results, and the agent's virologic efficacy, toxicity, pill burden, dosing frequency, and potential for drug-drug interactions. In addition, it is important to consider the adverse effects of antiretroviral agents on any pre-existing comorbidities (**Table 1**).[10]

Response to Therapy

When started on effective therapy, adherent patients achieve at least a 90% (one-log) reduction in the plasma HIV-1 RNA concentration (viral load) within 1 month of initiating therapy. The viral load should decrease to less than 400 HIV-1 RNA copies/mL in 3 months. A viral load persistently less than 200 HIV-1 RNA copies/mL represents treatment success; this is should be achieved within 6 months of treatment initiation. Failure

---

Box 1
Recommended regimens for ART-naïve patients

Integrase strand transfer inhibitor (INBSTI)–based regimens:

- Dolutegravir/abacavir/lamivudine (given as the fixed combination pill Triumeq): *only* for patients who are HLA-B*5701-negative

- Dolutegravir plus TDF/emtricitabine (given as the fixed combination pill Truvada)

- Elvitegravir/cobicistat/TDF/emtricitabine (given as the fixed combination pill Stribild): *only* for patients with pre-ART CrCl greater than 70 mL/min

- Raltegravir plus TDF/emtricitabine (given as the fixed combination pill Truvada)

Protease inhibitor (PI)–based regimens:

- Darunavir/ritonavir plus TDF/emtricitabine

For more detailed recommendations, readers are encouraged to refer to the most up-to-date DHHS guideline (http://aidsinfo.nih.gov/guidelines).
Abbreviations: ART, antiretroviral therapy; HLA, human leukocyte antigen.

---

to achieve these virologic outcomes represents treatment failure due to nonadherence or antiretroviral resistance. Management of patients with treatment failure should be in coordination with a specialist in HIV care and is beyond the scope of this review. Comprehensive treatment recommendations are available at http://aidsinfo.nih.gov/guidelines.

PATHOPHYSIOLOGIC EFFECTS OF LONG-TERM HUMAN IMMUNODEFICIENCY VIRUS INFECTION

Compared with uninfected individuals, even patients with excellent virologic and immunologic responses to treatment remain at increased risk for a wide variety of HANA complications.[10,13] Indeed, the overall morbidity and mortality related to comorbidities now exceed those of AIDS-related events.[14]

Although increased rates of cigarette, alcohol, and recreational drug use are important contributors to the occurrence of HANA comorbidities, the contribution of HIV-related immune activation and inflammation has become increasingly apparent as elevated levels of inflammatory and coagulation biomarkers such as C-reactive protein, interleukin-6 and D-dimer are associated with increased risk of all-cause mortality and non-AIDS-defining events. Although the highest levels of immune activation and inflammation are seen among individuals with uncontrolled HIV replication, these phenomena persist, albeit at generally lower levels, and predict the occurrence of poor clinical outcomes despite effective viral suppression.[13]

HUMAN IMMUNODEFICIENCY VIRUS–ASSOCIATED, NON-ACQUIRED IMMUNODEFICIENCY SYNDROME COMPLICATIONS

Cardiovascular disease is a particularly important and complex issue affecting HIV-infected patients. Although various ART regimens have been associated with metabolic disturbances that increase the risk of cardiovascular disease, effective ART lowers the risk of cardiovascular disease.[15] Nonetheless, even with effective ART, the risk of cardiovascular disease is approximately 50% higher in HIV-infected persons than in uninfected control populations.[16] Importantly, the increased risk of myocardial infarction is not fully accounted for by other comorbidities, substance use, or by the Framingham or other risk calculators.[16] In addition, HIV-infected

Table 1
Common adverse effects of frequently used antiretroviral agents

Agent	Associated Potential Adverse Effects[a]
NRTIs	
All NRTIs	Lactic acidosis and hepatic steatosis (rare but high mortality, highest incidence with stavudine, didanosine, and to a lesser extent zidovudine) Lipodystrophy (mostly with stavudine and zidovudine)
Abacavir	Hypersensitivity (in patients positive for HLA-B*5701) Possible increased risk of MI
Emtricitabine, lamivudine	In persons coinfected with HBV coinfection, exacerbation of hepatitis if discontinued
TDF	Renal impairment (concurrent PI use may increase risk) Decrease in bone mineral density In persons coinfected with HBV coinfection, exacerbation of hepatitis if discontinued Headache, GI intolerance
Zidovudine	Bone marrow suppression Hyperlipidemia Insulin resistance Headache, GI intolerance Myopathy
NNRTIs	
All NNRTIs	Rash (including Stevens-Johnson syndrome) Hepatotoxicity (especially NVP) Drug-drug interactions
Efavirenz	Neuropsychiatric Sleep disturbance Hyperlipidemia
Rilpivirine	Depression Insomnia Headache
PIs	
All PIs	Hyperlipidemia Lipodystrophy Hepatotoxicity GI intolerance Drug-drug interactions
Atazanavir	Hyperbilirubinemia PR prolongation on electrocardiogram Nephrolithiasis, cholelithiasis Renal insufficiency
Darunavir	Rash Hepatotoxicity
Lopinavir/ritonavir	GI intolerance Diabetes/insulin resistance Possible increased risk of MI PR and QT prolongation on electrocardiogram

(continued on next page)

Table 1 (continued)	
Agent	**Associated Potential Adverse Effects[a]**
INSTIs	
All INSTIs	Minimal toxicity and generally well-tolerated
Dolutegravir	Headache Insomnia Rash, hypersensitivity
Elvitegravir	Nausea, diarrhea
Raltegravir	Rash, hypersensitivity Nausea Headache Diarrhea CPK elevation, myopathy, rhabdomyolysis
Other	
Cobicstat and ritonavir	Drug-drug interactions Increased serum creatinine (cobicistat) GI intolerance and hepatitis (ritonavir)

Abbreviations: CPK, creatine phosphokinase; GI, gastrointestinal; HLA, human leukocyte antigen; MI, myocardial infarction; NVP, nevirapine.

[a] This list includes key toxicities for the most commonly used antiretroviral agents but is not all-inclusive. An additional comprehensive list of drug interactions can be found at http://www.hiv-druginteractions.org/. Further information about drug adverse effects is available within the DHHS guidelines.[10]

patients have increased rates of hypertension, heart failure, sudden death, and cerebrovascular events.

The causes and mechanisms leading to increased risk of cardiovascular disease in HIV-infected patients represent a complex interplay between pre-existing cardiovascular risk factors, HIV infection, chronic inflammation, and ART. Some PIs (eg, lopinavir-ritonavir and indinavir) but not others (atazanavir) are independently associated with increased risk of myocardial infarction.[17] Although not shown in randomized, controlled clinical trials done in low-risk, relatively young patients,[18] retrospective studies done in older patients have found that abacavir, a commonly used nucleoside reverse transcriptase inhibitor (NRTI), is associated with an increased cardiovascular disease risk.[19]

The adjusted rate of incident diabetes mellitus has been reported to be 4-fold higher among HIV-infected men receiving ART than among uninfected men. Implicated agents include NRTIs and PIs that are now less commonly used, for example, stavudine, didanosine, zidovudine, indinavir, and lopinavir/ritonavir.[20] Whether there is an association between newer ART agents or between HIV infection per se and increased risk of diabetes remains unclear.[20]

Fat redistribution, that is, lipoatrophy (loss of subcutaneous fat) and lipohypertrophy (visceral fat accumulation), commonly affects those infected with HIV and has been associated with insulin resistance, abnormal lipid metabolism, hypertension, and increased mortality.[21] Mitochondrial DNA toxicity associated with NRTIs, especially with drugs used more often in prior years such as didanosine, stavudine and zidovudine, has been proposed as a cause of lipoatrophy.[22]

Untreated HIV infection is associated with increased triglycerides and decreased high-density and low-density lipoproteins, that can improve after the initiation of ART, particularly among persons with a normal baseline body mass index (BMI).[23]

However, some commonly used antiretroviral drugs are associated with hyperlipidemia, including selected ritonavir-boosted PIs, efavirenz, and elvitegravir/cobicistat-containing regimens; other NNRTIs, integrase strand transfer inhibitors (INSTIs), and tenofovir are associated with less deleterious effects.[10]

Approximately 25% of HIV-infected patients have been reported to have the metabolic syndrome, that is, abdominal obesity, dyslipidemia, hypertension, and insulin resistance.[20] Risk factors include the use of PIs, particularly lopinavir/ritonavir, stavudine, and didanosine, and unsuppressed HIV replication.[24]

Liver disease is a significant cause of mortality in patients with HIV. Risk factors for liver disease include low CD4+ cell counts, uncontrolled HIV infection, and intravenous drug use, as well as active hepatitis B or C virus (HBV and HCV, respectively) infection.[25] HBV and HCV are particularly important given their high prevalence in HIV-infected patients. Effective treatment for both HIV and HCV decreases the rates of liver-related mortality and death in coinfected patients, whereas HBV coinfection is an important consideration in the selection of ART.[10] In addition, life-threatening hepatotoxicity reactions can occur as a consequence of hypersensitivity reactions (ie, nevirapine) or as a consequence of lactic acidosis and steatosis (eg, with use of stavudine, didanosine, and zidovudine).

HIV-infected patients are at high risk for chronic kidney disease and end-stage renal disease.[26] Risk factors for kidney injury that are specific for HIV include ART-related nephrotoxicities, HCV coinfection, lower CD4+ cell count, and higher HIV RNA levels.[27] HIV medications that are particularly associated with kidney injury include specific PIs (ie, indinavir, lopinavir/ritonavir, and atazanavir) and tenofovir disoproxil fumarate (TDF). HIV-infected African Americans are at particular risk for developing advanced kidney disease due to their susceptibility to HIV-related nephropathy.[26] When choosing combination ART for patients with chronic kidney disease, use of the older formulation of tenofovir (TDF), especially in combination with a PI, should be avoided if possible. Of note, tenofovir alafenamide, a new formulation of tenofovir, is associated with lower rates of nephrotoxicity.[28]

The incidence of AIDS-defining cancers has decreased since the beginning of the AIDS epidemic. However, the incidences of many non-AIDS-defining cancers (eg, lung, liver, colorectal, melanoma, anal, head, and neck cancers, and Hodgkin lymphoma) have increased since the introduction of ART.[29] Some cancers (mainly anal cancer, liver cancer, and Hodgkin lymphoma) occur at younger ages in those infected with HIV compared with those without HIV.[30]

Osteoporosis and fragility-related fractures occur more often in HIV-infected persons. Factors shown to contribute to higher rates of bone disease in people with HIV infection include the use of TDF and possibly PIs (particularly lopinavir/ritonavir), lifestyle differences such as tobacco smoking, alcohol or substance abuse, low BMI, coinfection with HCV, use of proton pump inhibitors, diabetes mellitus, vascular disease, and older age.[31] Tenofovir alafenamide is associated with lower rates of bone demineralization than is TDF.[28]

Neurocognitive deficits are significantly more common in HIV-infected individuals and range from asymptomatic neurocognitive impairment to HIV-associated dementia (HAD). HAD typically manifests as impaired attention and concentration, apathy, and impaired motor skills.[32] Although neurocognitive deficits predominate in untreated patients with advanced HIV/AIDS, mild cognitive deficits frequently occur in patients with well-controlled HIV. Of critical importance is that HIV-related neurocognitive disorders can dramatically respond to effective antiretroviral therapy and are often the presenting manifestations of HIV infection, especially among older patients.

HIV infection is independently associated with increased rates of chronic obstructive pulmonary disease, emphysema, bacterial pneumonia, and pulmonary hypertension and accelerates the rate of complications seen with smoking.[33] Risk factors for pulmonary dysfunction among HIV-infected individuals include more advanced HIV infection and elevated soluble CD14 levels, a measure of immune activation.[34]

Finally, an accelerated rate of frailty, characterized by weight loss, weakness, exhaustion, low physical activity, and slowness, has been observed in people with HIV infection compared with HIV-uninfected individuals. Factors associated with increased rates of frailty in persons with HIV infection include CD4+ cell count, HIV RNA level, increased age, and low BMI.[35]

PREVENTION OF HUMAN IMMUNODEFICIENCY VIRUS INFECTION

Older individuals often fail to see themselves at risk for HIV, a misperception that is unfortunately shared by many clinicians. In general, public educational messages and intervention strategies about HIV prevention focus more on the younger population. Moreover, older adults may be reluctant to talk about sex, and institutions frequented by older adults, such as churches, senior centers, and retirement communities, may also have reservations around discussing sex. Some older heterosexual individuals may misperceive HIV/AIDS as merely a "gay disease" that does not affect them. Because preventing pregnancy is usually not a concern in couples older than 50, they are less likely to use barrier methods (condoms). Discussions between physicians and older patients around risk reduction and safe sex practices can be challenging for many of these reasons. Targeted HIV prevention education for those at risk, and the integration of sexual health into the promotion of general well-being, however, can be invaluable.[9] Counseling is especially relevant for men being treated for erectile dysfunction because higher rates of sexually transmitted diseases and HIV infection occur in this group.[36]

Finally, although pre-exposure prophylaxis with daily TDF plus emtricitabine has been shown to be highly effective in preventing HIV infection among adherent, high-risk younger patients, the balance between risks and benefits of this intervention are less favorable among older patients with increased comorbidities.[37]

SUMMARY

The increasing survival into old age of those infected with HIV reflects an extraordinary achievement in modern medicine. However, the benefits of treatment can only be reaped by HIV-infected patients who are made aware of their condition through diagnostic testing and who are linked to and retained in care for their condition.

The poor survival and high rates of AIDS when HIV is diagnosed among older individuals are in large part the result of inadequate screening and the underrecognition of those with disease. Both the Centers for Disease Control and Prevention and US Preventive Services Task Force recommend routine screening at least once per lifetime for individuals up to age 64, regardless of risk factors, and annually for those who are at significant risk, whereas the ACP recommends testing up to age 75 for persons who might transmit HIV to others.

Once diagnosed, ART is strongly recommended for all patients regardless of CD4+ cell count or age.[10,12] Although recommended for all patients regardless of age, early initiation of therapy is especially important for older patients because they are less likely to recover immunologic function after CD4+ cell loss. Lower CD4+ counts and viral replication place older patients not only at increased risk for HIV-related complications but also for a myriad of comorbidities, including non-AIDS defining malignancies, cardiovascular disease, and neurologic disorders.

The management of HIV infection in older patients requires careful monitoring for bone, kidney, metabolic, cardiovascular, and liver health as well as careful attention to issues related to polypharmacy (eg, drug-drug interactions and adverse effects) and the global care of an increasingly frail population that often suffers from stigma and limited social support. The impact of non-AIDS events underscores the importance of clinicians focusing on modifiable risk factors considered in traditional primary care in addition to optimizing HIV therapy. As the HIV patient population ages, the skills of geriatricians will increasingly be needed to manage these complex patients with multiple morbid conditions.

REFERENCES

1. Brooks JT, Buchacz K, Gebo KA, et al. HIV infection and older Americans: the public health perspective. Am J Public Health 2012;102:1516–26.
2. Centers for Disease Control and Prevention. HIV Surveillance Report, 2013. Available at: http://www.cdc.gov/hiv/library/reports/surveillance/2013/surveillance_Report_vol_25.html. Accessed August 9, 2015.
3. UNAIDS Gap Report. Available at: http://www.unaids.org/node/42898. Accessed October 24, 2015.
4. Collaboration of Observational HIV Epidemiological Research Europe (COHERE) Study Group, Sabin CA, Smith CJ, d'Arminio Monforte A, et al. Response to combination antiretroviral therapy: variation by age. AIDS 2008; 22:1463–73.
5. Moyer VA. Screening for HIV: U.S. Preventive Services Task Force recommendation statement. Ann Intern Med 2013;159:51–60.
6. Qaseem A, Snow V, Shekelle P, et al. Screening for HIV in health care settings: a guidance statement from the American College of Physicians and HIV Medicine Association. Ann Intern Med 2009;150:125–31.
7. Centers for Disease Control and Prevention. Monitoring selected national HIV prevention and care objectives by using HIV surveillance data—United States and 6 dependent areas—2012. HIV Surveillance Supplemental Report 2014;19(No. 3). Available at: http://www.cdc.gov/hiv/library/reports/surveillance/. Accessed August 2, 2015.
8. Hall HI, Song R, Szwarcwald CL, et al. Brief report: time from infection with the human immunodeficiency virus to diagnosis, United States. J Acquir Immune Defic Syndr 2015;69:248–51.
9. Centers for Disease Control and Prevention. HIV Among people aged 50 and over. Available at: http://www.cdc.gov/hiv/group/age/olderamericans/index.html. Accessed October 31, 2015.
10. Panel on Antiretroviral Guidelines for Adults and Adolescents. Guidelines for the use of antiretroviral agents in HIV-infected adults and adolescents. Available at: http://aidsinfo.nih.gov/ContentFiles/AdultandAdolescentGL.pdf. Accessed October 23, 2015.
11. INSIGHT START Study Group, Lundgren JD, Babiker AG, Gordin F, et al. Initiation of antiretroviral therapy in early asymptomatic HIV Infection. N Engl J Med 2015; 373:795–807.
12. HHS Panel on Antiretroviral Guidelines for Adults and Adolescents. Statement by the HHS Panel on Antiretroviral Guidelines for adults and adolescents

regarding results from the START and TEMPRANO Trials. Available at: https://aidsinfo.nih.gov/news/1592/statement-from-adult-arv-guideline-panel–start-and-temprano-trials. Accessed November 11, 2015.

13. Miller CJ, Baker JV, Bormann AM, et al. Adjudicated morbidity and mortality outcomes by age among individuals with HIV infection on suppressive antiretroviral therapy. PLoS One 2014;9:e95061.

14. Smith CJ, Ryom L, Weber R, et al. Trends in underlying causes of death in people with HIV from 1999 to 2011 (D:A:D): a multicohort collaboration. Lancet 2014;384: 241–8.

15. Kuller LH, Tracy R, Belloso W, et al. Inflammatory and coagulation biomarkers and mortality in patients with HIV infection. PLoS Med 2008;5:e203.

16. Freiberg MS, Chang CC, Kuller LH, et al. HIV infection and the risk of acute myocardial infarction. JAMA Intern Med 2013;173:614–22.

17. Monforte A, Reiss P, Ryom L, et al. Atazanavir is not associated with an increased risk of cardio- or cerebrovascular disease events. AIDS 2013;27:407–15.

18. Ding X, Andraca-Carrera E, Cooper C, et al. No association of abacavir use with myocardial infarction: findings of an FDA meta-analysis. J Acquir Immune Defic Syndr 2012;61(4):441–7.

19. Desai M, Joyce V, Bendavid E, et al. Risk of cardiovascular events associated with current exposure to HIV antiretroviral therapies in a US veteran population. Clin Infect Dis 2015;61:445–52.

20. Nix LM, Tien PC. Metabolic syndrome, diabetes, and cardiovascular risk in HIV. Curr HIV/AIDS Rep 2014;11:271–8.

21. Scherzer R, Heymsfield SB, Lee D, et al. Decreased limb muscle and increased central adiposity are associated with 5-year all-cause mortality in HIV infection. AIDS 2011;25:1405–14.

22. Samaras K. Prevalence and pathogenesis of diabetes mellitus in HIV-1 infection treated with combined antiretroviral therapy. J Acquir Immune Defic Syndr 2009; 50:499–505.

23. Krishnan S, Schouten JT, Atkinson B, et al. Changes in metabolic syndrome status after initiation of antiretroviral therapy. J Acquir Immune Defic Syndr 2015;68: 73–80.

24. Krishnan S, Schouten JT, Atkinson B, et al. Metabolic syndrome before and after initiation of antiretroviral therapy in treatment-naive HIV-infected individuals. J Acquir Immune Defic Syndr 2012;61:381–9.

25. Lo RV III, Kallan MJ, Tate JP, et al. Hepatic decompensation in antiretroviral-treated patients co-infected with HIV and hepatitis C virus compared with hepatitis C virus-monoinfected patients: a cohort study. Ann Intern Med 2014;160: 369–79.

26. Lucas GM, Ross MJ, Stock PG, et al. Clinical practice guideline for the management of chronic kidney disease in patients infected with HIV: 2014 update by the HIV Medicine Association of the Infectious Diseases Society of America. Clin Infect Dis 2014;59:e96–138.

27. Mocroft A, Lundgren JD, Ross M, et al. Development and validation of a risk score for chronic kidney disease in HIV infection using prospective cohort data from the D:A:D study. PLoS Med 2015;12:e1001809.

28. Sax PE, Wohl D, Yin MT, et al. Tenofovir alafenamide versus tenofovir disoproxil fumarate, coformulated with elvitegravir, cobicistat, and emtricitabine, for initial treatment of HIV-1 infection: two randomised, double-blind, phase 3, non-inferiority trials. Lancet 2015;385:2606–15.

29. Robbins HA, Pfeiffer RM, Shiels MS, et al. Excess cancers among HIV-infected people in the United States. J Natl Cancer Inst 2015;107(4):dju503.

30. Shiels MS, Pfeiffer RM, Engels EA. Age at cancer diagnosis among persons with AIDS in the United States. Ann Intern Med 2010;153:452–60.

31. Brown TT, Hoy J, Borderi M, et al. Recommendations for evaluation and management of bone disease in HIV. Clin Infect Dis 2015;60:1242–51.

32. Gallego L, Barreiro P, Lopez-Ibor JJ. Diagnosis and clinical features of major neuropsychiatric disorders in HIV infection. AIDS Rev 2011;13:171–9.

33. Crothers K, Huang L, Goulet JL, et al. HIV infection and risk for incident pulmonary diseases in the combination antiretroviral therapy era. Am J Respir Crit Care Med 2011;183:388–95.

34. Attia EF, Akgun KM, Wongtrakool C, et al. Increased risk of radiographic emphysema in HIV is associated with elevated soluble CD14 and nadir CD4. Chest 2014;146:1543–53.

35. Greene M, Covinsky KE, Valcour V, et al. Geriatric syndromes in older HIV-infected adults. J Acquir Immune Defic Syndr 2015;69:161–7.

36. Jena AB, Goldman DP, Kamdar A, et al. Sexually transmitted diseases among users of erectile dysfunction drugs: analysis of claims data. Ann Intern Med 2010;153:1–7.

37. Grant RM, Lama JR, Anderson PL, et al. Preexposure chemoprophylaxis for HIV prevention in men who have sex with men. N Engl J Med 2010;363:2587–99.

Infections in Nursing Homes

Epidemiology and Prevention Programs

Ana Montoya, MD[a], Marco Cassone, MD, PhD[a],
Lona Mody, MD, MSc[a,b],*

KEYWORDS

- Nursing home • Infection control • Infection prevention
- Multidrug-resistant organisms • Epidemiology • Hand hygiene

KEY POINTS

- Nursing homes (NHs) are unique environments with challenges for infection control and prevention. Risk factors for infection in NH residents include resident-level, environmental/institutional-level, and therapy-related factors.
- There are between 1.6 and 3 million infections in NH residents every year; the most common are urinary tract infections, lower respiratory tract infections, skin and soft tissue infections, and gastroenteritis.
- Antibiotic stewardship programs complement national diagnostic and therapeutic guidelines toward the goal of preventing antibiotic overuse and decreasing the rate of multidrug-resistant organism (MDRO) infections.
- The infection control preventionist is essential to enforce compliance with hand hygiene, device care, and increase awareness of MDROs.
- Multimodal interventions including barrier precautions, active surveillance for MDROs and infections, and NH staff education have been proven to be effective.

INTRODUCTION

Nursing homes (NHs) provide health care to people who are unable to manage independently in the community, in 2 different circumstances: for chronic care management and for short-term rehabilitative services after an acute care hospital stay. In the United States, there are presently more people in NHs than in acute care hospitals. Many of these patients are recovering from very serious events and are at high risk for

a Division of Geriatric and Palliative Medicine, University of Michigan Medical School, 300 North Ingalls Street, Room 905, Ann Arbor, MI 48109, USA; b Geriatrics Research Education and Clinical Center, VA Ann Arbor Healthcare System, 2215 Fuller Drive, 11G GRECC, Ann Arbor, MI 48105, USA
* Corresponding author. Division of Geriatric and Palliative Care Medicine, University of Michigan Medical School, 300 North Ingalls Street, Room 905, Ann Arbor, MI 48109.
E-mail address: lonamody@umich.edu

Clin Geriatr Med 32 (2016) 585–607
http://dx.doi.org/10.1016/j.cger.2016.02.004 **geriatric.theclinics.com**
0749-0690/16/$ – see front matter © 2016 Elsevier Inc. All rights reserved.

complications, including infections. Infections cause an important share of morbidity and mortality in NH residents, despite being preventable.[1,2] Urinary tract infections (UTIs), lower respiratory tract infections (LRTIs), skin and soft tissue infections (SSTIs), and gastroenteritis (GE) are the most common infections in this setting, and their diagnosis can be delayed owing to inadequate fever response, lack of specific symptoms and signs, and sampling and testing difficulties. These factors may combine in leading to prolonged and unnecessary antibiotic therapy.

NH residents are more likely to receive antibiotics than any other individual class of drugs[3] and account for at least 20% of all adverse drug reactions experienced.[4] Multidrug-resistant organisms (MDROs) are increasing and colonize about 35% of residents, but their prevalence varies greatly depending on geographic location and characteristics of the resident population.[5] For this reason, it is imperative to customize prevention strategies to the characteristics and local epidemiology of the facility. For example, a facility with an unacceptably high rate of UTIs may benefit more from UTI prevention programs than a facility with high methicillin-resistant *Staphylococcus aureus* (MRSA) colonization rates. Integral to developing an intervention is the recognition of common infections and MDROs epidemiology within the facility. Knowledge of general and specific risk factors for infections is necessary to choose appropriate surveillance protocols capable of defining infection rates.

RISK FACTORS FOR INFECTION IN NURSING HOMES

Older adults are at greater risk for infections owing to their frailty, comorbidities, and prolonged stay in an institutional setting where medical supervision from physicians and physician extenders is generally lower and use of common spaces within the facility is higher, compared with hospital settings. Risk factors can be difficult to recognize and manage in NHs because of the lack of availability of state-of-the-art diagnostics. Risk factors for infection in NH residents can be broadly categorized as resident-level, environmental/institutional-level, and therapy-related factors, such as in the use of antibiotics.

Resident-level Risk Factors

Older age predisposes residents to infection for many reasons, such as senescence of the immune system, loss of integrity of the physical barriers to entry of microorganisms, and difficulty in performing hygiene. When the need for medical care arises, close physical interactions with caregivers may facilitate transmission of pathogens. Moreover, because infections present with atypical or nonspecific symptoms, diagnosis and ensuing therapy may be delayed, leading to poor outcomes and increased hospital transfers.[6] *Immunosenescence* describes key alterations in innate and adaptive immunity that develop with aging.[7] Not only does this affect the response to infections, including latent chronic infections (eg, tuberculosis, herpes zoster), it also affects response to immunization to infection (eg, pneumococcal or influenza vaccination).[8] Some key indicators of immunosenescence are the inversion of the CD4/CD8 ratio and reduced cytotoxicity of natural killer cells with a compensatory increase in quantity. There is some evidence of gender differences and impact of latent viral infections, such as cytomegalovirus infection, on the rate of development of immunosenescence.[9]

The ability of the skin and mucous membranes to act as barriers to systemic infections is compromised by aging owing to biochemical and cell signaling changes. In the intestinal mucosa, for example, a single layer of cells is exposed constantly to a high burden of microorganisms. Its functional integrity depends on a very complex network of signaling and interactions. Small and large molecules are sorted for blocking, filtering, or downstream processing. It is not surprising, thus, that many events directly or indirectly related to aging can impair this delicate balance.[10] In the case of the skin, both permeability and the ability to quickly mount an adequate response to pathogens and autoantigens and alloantigens is impaired in older adults,[11] even when the skin integrity is apparently well-preserved. In addition to a higher susceptibility to skin infections, older adults are more likely to experience progression to systemic infection and sepsis once skin infections are present.[12] Corticosteroids and other sex hormones also play a role in mucosal and skin homeostasis, and differences in the healing ability of the skin, intestinal, gastric, and urogenital mucosae have been reported between males and premenopausal females in several studies.[13] Comorbidities increase with age and make older adults more susceptible to infections. Also, they limit therapeutic options because of toxicity concerns or reduced clearance of the drug. Moreover, for some antibiotics such as aminoglycosides and isoniazide, the risk of toxicity is age dependent.[14]

A delay in recognizing infections may occur owing to presentation with atypical symptoms because of an inadequate mounting of fever response and a preponderance of nonspecific symptoms such as confusion and fatigue over site-specific complaints.[6] In addition, symptoms such as confusion can also be caused by many noninfectious conditions, such as neurologic disease, electrolyte imbalances, or the effect of medications, which can delay proper diagnosis. Cognitive impairment is an important risk and prognostic factor because of the increased need for caregiver contact, which increases the likelihood of exposure to infectious agents, and impairs the residents' ability to describe symptoms and other information useful for diagnosis.[15]

Functional disability increases the likelihood of asymptomatic colonization and infection owing to the need for extensive health care worker (HCW) physical contact and support. Close interactions with HCWs predispose to acquire pathogens. Because the resident–HCW ratio is higher in NH than in acute care settings, each HCW could potentially be a vehicle for pathogens to spread to a large number of residents. Many scoring indexes have been developed to estimate the overall level of dependence in the elderly adult, such as the Lawton–Brody Physical Self-Maintenance Scale, which scores residents ability to perform 6 activities of daily living (bathing, toileting, dressing, feeding, walking, and grooming), with a score ranging from 6 (independent in all 6 categories), to 30 (needs full assistance for all 6).[16] A recent study evaluating the Physical Self-Maintenance Scale as a risk factor for MDRO colonization in NH residents found an increased level of colonization in residents with a higher score, and showed that impairment in selected activities of daily living requiring frequent contact with HCWs had a shorter time to acquisition of MRSA and vancomycin-resistant enterococci.[17] A high Physical Self-Maintenance Scale score has also been indicated as a risk factor for surgical site MRSA infections in hospitalized older adults.[18]

Environmental-level and Institutional-level Risk Factors

NHs represent a different environment than acute care hospitals in many ways, and some of those ways can be linked to specific routes of transmission of pathogens. NHs are often centered around a common core of spaces and activity rooms that are essential to the primary function of the institution, such as rehabilitation rooms and gyms, but also dining and common halls. Thus, there are a number of spaces that are populated with many residents at the same time, offering opportunities for social and pathogen exchange. Additionally, NHs are often slower to implement infection prevention measures that are recommended but not mandatory. For example, in our experience placing alcohol-based hand rub dispensers at multiple strategic, easily accessible locations is standard practice in most hospitals, but is not as widely adopted in NHs.

Structural differences in the way NHs operate might also lead to a higher risk of infections. HCWs training in NH may not be as effective as desired.[19] Upon hire, HCWs typically receive 1 initial training session on infection prevention practices, and may not follow a national standardized curriculum. Training might not be repeated at regular time intervals, and the knowledge gained from the training is infrequently assessed. Additionally, the high turnover and high proportion of part-time staff makes it difficult to maintain a uniform optimal level of competence. Furthermore, staff is given fewer opportunities for "on-the-job" informal learning from experienced and knowledgeable senior staff and physicians. All of these factors contribute to most NHs being challenged to maintain well-trained and knowledgeable staff on current and effective measures to prevent infections.

Inappropriate Use of Antibiotics

The overuse of antibiotics or use of inappropriate regimens such as wide-spectrum antibiotics is a main risk factor for subsequent infections with antimicrobial-resistant organisms, *Clostridium difficile* GE, and fungal infections. Some of these risks are shared by the whole community, and not just the resident receiving the antimicrobial regimen. Evidence is accumulating that residents of NHs where antibiotics are overused are at higher risk for related morbidity even if they have not received antibiotics themselves.[20,21] The burden of antimicrobial resistance has reached the critical mass for spreading independent of antibiotic treatment, thus complicating targeted prevention efforts. Twenty years ago, investigations of epidemics of MDROs in NHs would have shown incoming carriers from acute care facilities as the case zero.[22] Presently, NHs and other long-term care facilities have become a reservoir. Numerous studies report that a recent residence in a NH is an independent risk factor for colonization with MDROs.[23-25] A systematic metaanalysis of factors associated with MRSA colonization at time of hospital admission in 77,000 patients showed that recent NH exposure was at least as important as recent hospitalization.[23]

Use of empirical and prophylactic antibiotics remains high and varies by geographic location. For example, it has been shown that prescribing of empirical and prophylactic antibiotics together account for 80% of all treatments in European NHs.[26] In a report by Latour and colleagues,[26] empirical treatments were most common (54% of all antimicrobial therapies), followed by prophylactic (29%). Only a minority of treatment regimens were microbiologically documented (16%). Although prescribing practices varied widely across countries, the authors identified clinical conditions for which antibiotic prophylaxis should be reduced, among which bacteriuria was the most important.

Reduction of antibiotic use in NHs may be accomplished by the use of standardized definitions of infections to reserve therapy in cases when the diagnosis of infection is likely or confirmed. In particular, the use of Loeb's minimum criteria for initiation of antibiotics should be used to achieve this goal (**Table 1**).[27] Additionally, innovative educational strategies should be used to inform prescribing physicians about currently recommended antibiotic therapy regimens to promote the appropriate use of antimicrobial agents.[28]

EPIDEMIOLOGY OF COMMON INFECTIONS
Burden of Infections in Nursing Homes and the Importance of Colonization

Conservative estimates of the number of infections occurring in the approximately 1.5 million of US NH residents range between 1.6 to 3 million cases every year.[2] As many

Table 1
Minimum criteria to initiate antibiotics in long-term care residents

Infection	Criteria
Urinary tract infection	A. For residents without a urinary catheter, must have 1 or 2 below: 　1. Acute dysuria 　2. Fever (≥37.9°C [100°F] or 1.5°C [2.4°F] increase above baseline temp) and ≥1 of the following: 　　a. New or worsening urgency 　　b. Frequency 　　c. Suprapubic pain 　　d. Gross hematuria 　　d. Costovertebral angle tenderness 　　f. Urinary incontinence B. For residents with a urinary catheter, must have ≥1 of the following: 　1. Fever (temperature ≥ 37.9°C [100°F] or 1.5°C [2.4°F] increase above baseline temperature) 　2. New costovertebral tenderness 　3. Rigors (shaking chills) with or without identified cause 　4. New onset of delirium
Respiratory tract infection	A. Febrile resident 　1. If resident with temperature >38.9°C (102°F), ≥1 of the following: 　　a. Respiratory rate >25 breaths/min 　　b. Productive cough 　2. If resident with temperature >37.9°C (100°F; or a 1.5°C [2.4°F] increase above baseline temperature) but ≤38.9°C (102°F), must include presence of cough, and ≥1 of the following: 　　a. Pulse >100 beats/min 　　b. Delirium 　　c. Rigors (shaking chills) 　　d. Respiratory rate >25 breaths/min B. Afebrile resident 　1. If afebrile resident has COPD, must include new/increased cough with purulent sputum 　2. If afebrile resident does not have COPD, must have presence of new cough with purulent sputum production and ≥1 of the following: 　　a. Respiratory rate >25 breaths/min 　　b. Delirium C. In the setting of a new infiltrate on chest radiograph thought to represent pneumonia, any 1 of the following symptoms or signs would constitute appropriate minimum criteria: 　1. Respiratory rate >25 breaths/min 　2. Productive cough 　3. Fever (temperature >37.9°C [100°F] or 1.5°C [2.4°F] increase above baseline temperature)
Skin and soft tissue infection	A. Must have either 1 or 2 below: 　1. New/increasing purulent drainage at a wound, skin or soft tissue site 　2. At least 2 of the following signs and symptoms: 　　a. Fever (temperature >37.9°C [100°F] or an increase of 1.5°C [2.4°F] above baseline temperature) 　　b. Redness 　　c. Tenderness 　　d. Warmth 　　e. New or increasing swelling at the affected site.

Abbreviation: COPD, chronic obstructive pulmonary disease

Adapted from Loeb M, Bentley DW, Bradley S, et al. Development of minimum criteria for the initiation of antibiotics in residents of long-term-care facilities: results of a consensus conference. Infect Control Hosp Epidemiol 2001;22:120–4; with permission.

as 10% or more of residents are treated for an infection on any given day,[29] and the incidence of new infections vary between 4 and 5 clinically defined infections per 1000 resident days[30,31] to 11 infections per 1000 device days in residents with indwelling devices.[32] In addition to the prolonged length of stay, economic burden, and suffering, infections cause hundreds of thousands of deaths each year.[2,33] Many infections may become difficult to diagnose or treat because of changes in etiologic agents or development of antimicrobial resistance, and some are emerging or reemerging as an important cause of morbidity and mortality in NHs.[34]

The most common infections in NHs are UTIs; LRTIs, including pneumonia, bronchitis and influenza; SSTIs; and GE, among which *C difficile* pseudomembranous enterocolitis and norovirus GE are the most common. Both major causes of GE in NH residents are closely related to the institutional environment, and less so to residents' specific risk factors. Norovirus outbreaks stem from the presence of many susceptible individuals in close proximity to each other, and a less than optimal adoption of proper cleaning practices, whereas *C difficile* stems from use (and often overuse) of antibiotics.

Although UTIs are generally considered the most prevalent infections, followed closely by LRTIs and SSTIs, rates vary greatly between facilities underscoring the importance of local surveillance and facility-specific prevention strategies. When focusing on mortality, LRTIs are responsible for more death and transfer to acute care hospitals than any other infection.[35] Indeed, pneumonia is associated with an increased risk of mortality independent of comorbidities.[36] However, other metrics, in addition to mortality, can be used to evaluate the adverse impact of infections, including antibiotic use, which is often greater for UTIs.[37]

Urinary tract infections

The presence of a urinary catheter, urinary incontinence, urinary retention, or urinary obstruction are specific risk factors for UTIs. It has been estimated that more than 50% of NH residents with a urinary catheter are colonized with an MDRO.[38] Although urinary catheters are only present in a minority of NH residents (5%–10%), varying degrees of urinary incontinence and/or obstruction are very common in this population. Virtually all residents with long-term catheterization and about 25% of those without urinary catheters have bacteriuria. In several studies, including a recent multinational study, asymptomatic bacteriuria was a consistent cause of antibiotic overuse.[26] In the NH setting, management of UTIs can be difficult because of the increased risk of antibiotic adverse effects, higher rate of pyelonephritis, and greater risk for systemic infections. It has been estimated that at least one-half of all episodes of sepsis and 30% of hospital readmissions in NH residents originate from UTIs.[36] In residents with and without catheters, UTI diagnosis must be based clinically on presence of the minimum criteria for infection, and not simply from results of a urinalysis.[39] In symptomatic infections arising from chronic indwelling catheters, it is suggested to change the catheter and collect a bladder specimen for testing, which is more likely to harbor the actual infecting organism, before starting antimicrobial therapy. This practice improves diagnostic accuracy and the treatment outcome.[40]

Almost all UTIs in NHs are preceded by bacterial colonization, and a high percentage of colonizing organisms are MDROs. Prevalence and resistance patterns vary depending on type and location of the facility, with the overall MDRO prevalence rates averaging 20%,[41] but as high as 50% or more in some facilities. Fisch and colleagues[42] observed a prevalence rate exceeding 50% for ciprofloxacin-resistant gram-negative bacilli in NH residents with indwelling devices.

Data on individual organisms, their susceptibility patterns, and their mechanism of resistance are not as widely available for NHs as for acute care hospitals, but available studies demonstrate significant rates of antimicrobial resistance in this institutional environment.[43] The latest PanEuropean Survey of antimicrobial resistance in NHs showed that resistance to third-generation cephalosporins averages 20% for *Escherichia coli* and *Klebsiella* and 30% for *Proteus*. Additionally, 24% of *Pseudomonas aeruginosa* isolates were carbapenem resistant or intermediate.[44]

Lower respiratory tract infections

Older adults in NHs are up to 30 times more likely to develop LRTIs than their counterparts living in the community.[45] Common risk factors for LRTIs include cognitive impairment with altered cough reflex and deglutition, oral hygiene and changes in oral flora, neurologic conditions, chronic obstructive pulmonary disease, heart disease, poor functional status, presence of feeding tubes, and living in close quarters. Clinical presentation of LRTIs, including pneumonia, can be atypical in older adults, often with few respiratory symptoms. *Streptococcus pneumoniae*, *Haemophilus influenzae*, and *S aureus* are among the most common single species causes of LRTI, but gram-negative bacilli are also major causative agents. Unlike in UTIs, important differences in the etiologic mix of LRTIs have been reported between NH and elderly community residents; however, it is unclear if this reflects a biologic difference or a difference in diagnostic testing between the two groups.[46,47]

Vaccination of HCWs is an important strategy to prevent influenza infection. Unfortunately, both influenza and pneumococcal vaccination are less effective in the older adult. However, because higher HCW vaccination rates have resulted in substantial decreases in resident mortality,[48] they are recommended by the Centers for Disease Control and Prevention (CDC).

Skin and soft tissue infections

The most common SSTIs in NHs are cellulitis and pressure ulcer infections. Pressure ulcers are common in both short stay and long stay residents and prevention remains the key. In US NHs, MRSA is now the predominant causative agent of SSTI, likely owing to a high colonization prevalence in NH residents[49] and their immediate environment. In different regions of the United States, methicillin resistance among NH *S aureus* isolates is 30%, with rates as high as 60%. Overall, 8% to 10% of all NH residents are colonized with MRSA.[32,50–53] The likelihood of acquiring new MRSA colonization may be influenced by the type of care received, with NH residents receiving rehabilitation care four times more likely to acquire MRSA compared with those receiving residential care.[54]

CHALLENGES IN INFECTION RECOGNITION AND ROLE OF ANTIMICROBIAL STEWARDSHIP PROGRAMS

Definitions of Infection and Adherence to Guidelines

Recognizing the atypical manifestation of infections in older adults and the limited diagnostic interactions generally available in NHs, specific criteria for the diagnosis of infection were developed in 1991.[55] Since then, the epidemiology of long-term care infections has changed along with a growing short stay patient population. Thus, the original diagnostic criteria have been recently modified,[56] building on a larger body of scientific evidence and improved availability of laboratory diagnostics. In addition, Loeb minimum criteria provides guidance for initiating antibiotic therapy for suspected infection.[27] However, several studies show that adherence to these criteria is inconsistent. In a recent study in North Carolina, only 12.7% of antibiotic prescriptions met the minimum criteria.[57] Adherence varied by facility (5%–22%) and infection site, with 43% of SSTIs, 10% of UTIs, and 2% of respiratory infections meeting criteria. Similarly, in another study in Southeastern Michigan, less than 1 in 5 diagnosed UTIs or pneumonias met the minimum criteria.[32]

Special Challenges in Diagnosing Infection in Older Adults

Many factors that increase the risk of infections in older adults are also responsible for diagnostic difficulties. Specific examples include cognitive deficits that prevent the resident from asking for help and describing symptoms properly, to challenges in the differential diagnosis of precipitating factors of weakness and confusion in residents with chronic heart, liver, respiratory, or kidney disease. Even in residents without comorbidities, the diagnosis of infection is often difficult because older adults may not mount an adequate fever response or show site-specific signs and symptoms (See Norman DC: Clinical Features of Infection in Older Adults, in this issue). In NHs, sampling difficulties and limited timely access to technology such as chest radiographs, blood tests, and microbiology tests may delay the diagnosis.

Another factor that may delay diagnosis and therapy is communication with clinical providers who are often off site. Notably, this leads to an increased reliance on nursing staff for resident assessment, which may encourage providers into "risk-aversion" mode. Those diagnostic uncertainties and laboratory delays, coupled with the urge to "stabilize" frail residents, lead to prolonged administration of empirical antibiotic therapy. Overuse of antibiotics then results in a vicious cycle of selection of MDROs leading in time to further overuse of empiric wide-spectrum antibiotics.[58]

Antibiotic Stewardship Programs

Antibiotic stewardship programs are an effective complement to national diagnostic and therapeutic guidelines toward the goal of preventing antibiotic overuse and decreasing the rate of MDRO infections, because they can be customized specifically to the needs of each facility. Because the antibiotic prescribing process in NHs is different than in acute care hospitals, an increasing body of research is being devoted to improvement of prescribing algorithms specifically in this setting. Crnich and colleagues[58] recently reviewed the need for antibiotic stewardship programs in NHs. Their observations can be summarized as follows: (i) even in the 50% of cases when antibiotics are indicated, they are often administered for a longer time than necessary, and the choice of the agent is often more broad spectrum than is needed; (ii) unnecessary urinary cultures are a major source of inappropriate antibiotic prescriptions in NHs and strategies to improve urine testing and standardize communication between providers and nurses significantly lowers antibiotic prescribing; and (iii) educational interventions have better outcomes when both providers and nurses are engaged.

INFECTION PREVENTION AND CONTROL PROGRAMS

The Federal Nursing Home Reform Act from the Omnibus Budget Reconciliation Act of 1987 mandated the formation of an infection control committee, to evaluate infection rates, implement infection control programs and review policies and procedures. Even though this mandate was removed at the federal level, some states still require them. The Centers for Medicare and Medicaid Services has published requirements for long-term care facilities that apply to NHs accepting Medicare or Medicaid residents; these requirements address the need for an infection control program that includes surveillance of infections; implementation of methods for preventing the spread of infections, including use of appropriate isolation measures, employee health protocols, and hand hygiene practices; and appropriate handling, processing, and storage of linens.

Several guidelines have been published to facilitate infection prevention and control programs in NHs. Among those include the "SHEA/APIC Guideline: Infection Prevention and Control in the Long-Term Care Facility" published in 2008 by the Society for Healthcare Epidemiology of America (SHEA) and Association of Professionals in Infection Control and Epidemiology (APIC),[59] "Common Infections in the LTC Setting" published in 2011 by the American Medical Directors Association,[60] and "Infection Preventionist's Guide to Long Term Care" published in 2013 by the Association for Professionals in Infection Control and Epidemiology.[61] Despite the availability of these guidelines, the consistency of their use in NHs is unknown.

Infection Control Committee

The infection control committee is designed to provide oversight of the infection prevention and control program; its core members are an infection control practitioner, facility administrator, a nursing representative, and the medical director. Participation of other departments such as food services, maintenance, housekeeping, laundry services, clinical services, resident activities, and employee health should also be considered. It is recommended that the infection control committee meet at least quarterly throughout the year and on an emergent basis as needed.

The infection control practitioner is the person assigned the responsibility of implementing, monitoring and evaluating the infection prevention and control program in the NH. The infection control practitioner should have sufficient knowledge of infection prevention and control programs to assume these responsibilities, and be familiar with federal, state, and local regulations related to infection prevention and control program.

To maintain compliance with regulations, NHs have increased the rate of employment of IPs. In Maryland, a survey reported a 5-fold increase in the rate of NH infection control practitioner employment from 8.1% in 2003% to 44% in 2008.[62] Despite the increasing number of IPs in NH, they commonly have responsibilities other than infection control, such as employee health or staff education.[59] In 2005, a Michigan survey reported that only 50% of NHs had a full-time infection control practitioner.[63] Infection control practitioners frequently use external resources like the CDC website and their local Department of Health to guide infection prevention and control practices. The importance of formal training in infection prevention and control program for infection control practitioners has been recognized; however, currently many infection control practitioners in NHs receive no formal infection prevention and control training.[64] Evidence-based infection prevention core competencies have been identified by the Board of Infection Control and Epidemiology, and include identification of an infectious process, surveillance, prevention of transmissions, employee health, communication with management, and education of staff.[65]

Overview of Key Elements of an Infection Control Program

The elements of an infection prevention and control program in NHs include surveillance, outbreak control, isolation precautions, infection control policies and procedures, education, resident and employee health programs, antibiotic stewardship, disease reporting to public health authorities, facility management, performance improvement, and preparedness planning (**Table 2**).[59]

Surveillance is an essential tool used to identify single patients or a cluster of patients who are infected or colonized. *Surveillance* is the ongoing, systematic collection, analysis, and interpretation of health data essential to the planning,

Table 2
Infection control program: Elements

Elements	Components
Surveillance	Using surveillance infection definitions: • Loeb minimum criteria • CDC/NHSN criteria Calculating infection rates
Outbreak management	Disease specific (influenza, tuberculosis, viral gastroenteritis, scabies)
Implementation of routine infection control policies and procedures	Hand hygiene Isolation precautions MDROs Device care
Communication with management	Sharing information and obtaining support for changes in policies and procedures
Disease reporting	Information transfer during care transitions Reporting to public health authorities
Antibiotic stewardship	Review of antimicrobial usage
Resident health programs	Immunizations Tuberculin testing Hand hygiene Oral care
Employee health programs	Immunizations Occupational exposure to infectious organisms
Facility management	Food preparation Laundry services Infectious waste collection and disposal Housekeeping (cleaning, disinfection)

Abbreviations: CDC/NHSN, Centers for Disease Control/National Healthcare Safety Network; MDROs, multidrug-resistant organisms.

implementation, and evaluation of public health practice, closely integrated with timely dissemination of these data to those who need to know. To conduct surveillance correctly, definitions of infections must be adopted.

Several definitions of infections in NHs have been published, the most commonly used are Loeb minimum criteria[27] and the CDC's National Healthcare Safety Network criteria,[56] based on the revised McGeer criteria.[56] The Loeb minimum criteria are proposed standards for the initiation of antibiotics in NHs, based on assessment of symptoms and signs for UTI, respiratory infections, SSTI, and fever of unknown origin. In 2012, the National Healthcare Safety Network updated surveillance definitions for all specific types of infections, particularly UTI, and gastrointestinal infections caused by norovirus and *C difficile*. Infection rates are generally calculated as number of infections as the numerator and resident days as the denominator. It is important that infection rates be shared with infection control committee and be used to allocate efforts for infection prevention and control program initiatives and HCW education.

Surveillance data should be used to detect and prevent outbreaks in NHs. An outbreak should be considered when the number of cases exceeds the normal baseline. Early identification and containment of the outbreak is important. To achieve this, policies and procedures to prevent and reduce exposure and transmission of organisms should be implemented, which may include additional focus on resident screening, hand hygiene, use of personal protective equipment, and HCW education.[66]

Residents in NHs are at increased risk for transmission of infections owing to person-to-person spread of pathogens; NHs focus on preserving quality of life through socialization, group activities, and the use of common areas like dining rooms, as well as increased exposure to contaminated areas such as activities rooms, shared bathrooms, and physical therapy equipment. Resident-to-resident transmission of MDROs has been demonstrated in NHs.[67]

Isolation precautions have 2 tiers of precautions: standard precautions and transmission-based isolation precautions.[68] Standard precautions include measures applied to all patients regardless of their infection status. The main elements of standard precautions include hand hygiene, use of personal protective equipment (eg, gloves, gowns, facemask, eye protection, or face shield), respiratory hygiene/cough etiquette, and safe injection practices to avoid contact with blood, body fluids, secretions, excretions, and mucous membranes.

Transmission-based precautions are used for residents with documented or suspected infection or colonization with highly transmissible or epidemiologically important pathogens. There are 3 main types of transmission-based precautions: contact precautions, droplet precautions, and airborne precautions (**Table 3**). Contact precautions are recommended for residents with MDROs who are ill, depend on HCW for help with daily care, or whose secretions or drainage cannot be contained. Single rooms are preferred for these residents if available. In the case of MRSA, when single patient rooms are not available, and cohorting patients with MRSA is not possible, colonized patients are to be placed in rooms with patients who are at low risk for acquisition of MRSA and associated adverse outcomes from infection (not immunosuppressed, not on antibiotics, without open wounds or devices), and are likely to have a short duration of stay.[68]

Resident health programs should address immunizations, tuberculin testing, and other resident care practices like hand hygiene and oral care. The Centers for Medicare and Medicaid Services final rule requires NHs to offer annual immunization against influenza and lifetime immunization against pneumococcal disease to all residents (See Gnanasekaran G, Biedenbender R, Davidson HE, et al: Vaccinations for the Older Adult, in this issue). It is also important to be aware of the potential benefits of new pneumococcal vaccine formulations covering additional pneumococcal serotypes, and consider offering those in patients vaccinated with previous formulations. Standing orders for these two vaccinations have improved vaccination rates in NHs.[69] The Tdap vaccination is also recommended, given the potential for outbreaks of pertussis among older adults in NHs. Residents should receive a tuberculin skin test on admission, followed by a chest radiograph if the test is positive (See Rajagopalan: Tuberculosis in Older Adults, in this issue).

HCW have the potential for exposure to patients and infectious materials, including body substances, contaminated medical supplies and equipment, contaminated environmental surfaces, or contaminated air. All new employees should undergo a baseline health assessment, review of history of infectious diseases, and immunization status at the time of hire and on a regular basis. HCW are recommended to maintain vaccination against hepatitis B, influenza, measles, mumps, rubella, pertussis, and varicella as indicated per guidelines. Employee immunization records should reflect immunity status for indicated vaccinations and those administered during employment, and should be accessible in the event of an outbreak situation.[70]

HCWs with potentially communicable diseases or infected skin lesions should not provide direct resident contact or become in contact with resident's food. Policies and procedures should be in place to address follow-up and postexposure

Table 3
Transmission-based precautions

Action	Standard Precautions	Contact Precautions	Droplet Precautions	Airborne Precautions
Single room	No	Yes or cohort	Yes or cohort	Yes
Negative air pressure	No	No	No	Yes
Hand hygiene	Nonantimicrobial soap and water or antimicrobial soap and water or ABHR.	Antimicrobial liquid soap or ABHR for MDROs. Hand washing with antimicrobial soap and water is recommended after care of residents with acute diarrhea (eg, *Clostridium difficile* infection).	Nonantimicrobial soap and water or antimicrobial soap and water or ABHR.	Nonantimicrobial soap and water or antimicrobial soap and water or ABHR.
Gloves	When anticipate touching blood, body fluids, secretions, excretions, or nonintact skin.	Before contact with resident or environment, and must remove and dispose before leaving patient room and then perform hand hygiene.	When anticipate touching blood, body fluids, secretions, excretions, or nonintact skin.	When anticipate touching blood, body fluids, secretions, excretions, or nonintact skin.
Gown	When anticipate contact with blood, body fluids, secretions or excretions.	Before contact with patient or environment, and must remove and dispose before leaving patient room.	When anticipate contact with blood, body fluids, secretions or excretions.	When anticipate contact with blood, body fluids, secretions or excretions.
Mask	When anticipate splashes or sprays of blood, body fluids, secretions, or excretions.	When anticipate splashes or sprays of blood, body fluids, secretions, or excretions.	Surgical mask when entering patient's room, and remove at exit to the room. Handle by ties or ear loops.	Particulate N95 respirator when entering patient room, and remove outside the room.
Goggles/ face shield	When anticipate splashes or sprays of blood, body fluids, secretions, or excretions.	When anticipate splashes or sprays of blood, body fluids, secretions, or excretions.	When anticipate splashes or sprays of blood, body fluids, secretions, or excretions.	When anticipate splashes or sprays of blood, body fluids, secretions, or excretions.

Abbreviations: ABHR, alcohol-based hand rub; MDRO, multidrug-resistant organisms.

prophylaxis for human immunodeficiency virus, hepatitis B, hepatitis C, tuberculosis, or scabies. It is recommended that environmental surfaces be disinfected on a regular basis and when visibly soiled, and spills of blood and potentially infectious materials be decontaminated promptly with Environmental Protection Agency–registered germicides.[71] Periodic environmental rounds should be performed to identify deficiencies in cleaning and disinfection practices.

Hand Hygiene: Central to an Infection Prevention Program

Hand hygiene is the most effective infection control measure in NHs; however, compliance with hand hygiene across all health care settings remains low.[59] The World Health Organization global campaign to improve hand hygiene among HCWs, "SAVE LIVES: Clean Your Hands" is a major component of the "Clean Care is Safer Care" program.[72] It advocates the need to improve and sustain hand hygiene practices of HCW at the right times and in the right way to help reduce the spread of potentially life-threatening infections in health care facilities. A systematic review of 56 studies suggested that hand hygiene helped to decrease the infection risk in NHs, with major impacts on respiratory infections and influenza (80%) and gram-positive bacterial infections (76%), and a lower impact on gram-negative bacterial infections (44%).[73] In a recent survey, it was noted that although hand hygiene was an important focus of infection prevention and control programs, formal policies regarding monitoring of staff compliance were lacking.[64]

Hand hygiene refers to both hand washing with soap and water and the use of alcohol-based products. Alcohol-based hand rub for hand hygiene when hands are not visibly soiled is recommended.[72,74,75] Alcohol-based hand rub has been shown to increase compliance with hand hygiene among HCW in NHs.[76] Its use as part of a comprehensive hand hygiene program for NH staff and residents can decrease infection rates in NHs.[77] Residents' ability to comply with hand hygiene may be affected by cognitive and functional impairments in NHs, and therefore encouragement and assistance is important.

Efforts to increase hand hygiene compliance should be implemented, and facilities and product supplies should be available and conveniently located for residents and HCWs. NHs should be aware when installing alcohol-based hand rub dispensers that given that alcohol is flammable, there are potential fire safety concerns.[78] Each NH should work with their local fire marshals to ensure that installation of these dispensers is consistent with local, state, and national fire codes.

Challenges in promoting and implementing hand hygiene programs exist, and recently multimodal strategies have emerged as the best approach to improving compliance. Eight key components have been proposed for hand hygiene bundles: establishing ongoing monitoring and feedback on infection rates; establishing administrative leadership and support; establishing a multidisciplinary design and response team; providing ongoing education and training for staff, patients, families, and visitors; ensuring that hand hygiene resources are accessible facility wide and at the point of care; reinforcing hand hygiene behavior and accountability; providing reminders throughout the health care setting; and establishing and ongoing monitoring and feedback of hand hygiene compliance.[79] Although each individual component may improve outcomes, the greatest success occurs when all elements are applied together. A recent systematic review found bundled intervention strategies, including access to alcohol-based hand rub, administrative support, feedback, education, and reminders, were associated with an increase in hand hygiene compliance.[80] Additional high-quality studies are still needed to identify optimal hand hygiene bundles across all health care settings.

Device Care

Transitions of patients from acute care hospitals to NHs for subacute rehabilitation occur frequently. These transitions may increase the use of indwelling devices like urinary catheters, feeding tubes and peripherally inserted central catheters (PICC) in NHs. Inadequate care of these devices may contribute to MDRO transmission and infection. It is important to implement and periodically review policies and procedures used for the care of these devices.

UTIs are the most common infections among NH residents. The rates of UTIs are higher in residents with a urinary catheter compared with noncatheterized residents. A study reviewing data from the minimum data set reported that the presence of an indwelling urinary catheter was the primary predictor of whether a resident developed a UTI (adjusted incidence ratio = 3.35; $P<.001$).[81] The majority of residents with long-term indwelling urinary catheters have persistent asymptomatic bacteriuria, and they are more likely to have UTIs caused by MDROs than residents without catheters.[82] A national survey reported that even though there is a strong link between urinary catheter use and subsequent UTIs, no strategy was widely used to prevent hospital acquired UTI.[83] Several studies in acute care hospitals have demonstrated that automatic stop orders safely reduce the duration of inappropriate urinary catheter use in hospitalized patients, but did not reduce UTIs.[82,83] In 2008 the Association for Professionals in Infection Control and Epidemiology published the "Guide to the Elimination of Catheter-Associated Urinary Tract Infections (CAUTIs)",[84] and embraced the "Bladder Bundle" concept to prevent CAUTIs. A systematic review of CAUTI prevention bundles showed some evidence of success in the NH setting.[85] These bundles included strategies found in acute care bundles such as hand hygiene, strategies to avoid placement, prompt removal of catheters, and proper catheter insertion and maintenance, as well as interventions focused on chronic catheter needs, hydration, incontinence, and preemptive barrier precautions. A multimodal targeted infection prevention intervention, including preemptive barrier precautions, active surveillance for infections and MDROs, hand hygiene promotion, and a structured educational program for NH staff demonstrated a reduction in overall MDRO prevalence density, new MRSA acquisitions, and clinically defined CAUTI rates in high risk NH residents with indwelling devices.[86]

Beginning in 2013, the "AHRQ Safety Program in Long-Term Care: HAIs/CAUTI," by the Agency for Healthcare Research and Quality, will be implemented in 500 NHs in the United States to reduce indwelling urinary catheter use and CAUTIs. Building on the organization and lessons learned from the Targeted Infection Prevention study[86] and from an initiative in acute care hospitals "On the CUSP: STOP CAUTI",[87] this program will emphasize professional development in catheter utilization, catheter care and maintenance, antimicrobial stewardship, as well as promoting patient safety culture, team building, and leadership engagement. This approach integrates technical and socioadaptive principals and may serve as a model for other infection prevention and control program initiatives in NHs.

NHs are caring for an increasing number of residents with PICC lines, mostly for intravenous antibiotic administration.[88] PICCs have been associated with exit site and blood stream infections in 3% to 5% of hospitalized patients.[89,90] There is a paucity of similar studies in the NH setting. A recently published study was among the first to observe care practices and PICC use in NHs, and identified areas for improvement.[88] Nursing education and competencies for PICC care need to be addressed as it is likely that more patients with these devices will need NH care.

Multidrug-resistant Organism Prevention

A number of screening and intervention programs have been proven capable of limiting the impact of MDROs in health care settings. However, most such initiatives were not focused specifically on NHs, and many initiatives were targeted only on 1 or a few specific pathogens, notably MRSA. Thus, the major challenges for NHs in planning and implementing prevention initiatives are adapting effective strategies to the structure, workflow, and specific needs of their facility.

Bundled interventions show promise (**Table 4**). A very successful example of such a program is the MRSA reduction program implemented by the Department of Veterans Affairs. This nationwide initiative, encompassing acute and long-term care facilities, led to a 36% reduction in MRSA infections.[91] The program is centered on a bundle of strategies that included active surveillance, improved hand hygiene, and contact precautions. In addition to screening nearly 100% of patients and isolating carriers, the success of the program relied on careful evaluation of MRSA transmission opportunities and tracking each facilities' adherence to bundle components.

Differences between isolation practices in NHs and acute care hospitals have been described. NHs face unique challenges as they must prevent infection transmission while providing an environment focused on promoting the quality of life of each resident. Challenges in NHs include the presence of common living areas, rehabilitation areas, and shared bathrooms and showers. Access to alcohol-based hand rub dispensers and sinks, and disinfection of shared equipment are paramount to reducing transmission in these common areas. Moreover, NHs care for residents with more functional disability upon admission. Earlier new MRSA and vancomycin-resistant enterococci acquisition has been observed in NH residents with higher needs for nursing care, compared with residents with mild functional impairment.[17]

In NHs, each individual resident's clinical condition and the local prevalence of MDROs must be considered when deciding whether to implement or discontinue the use of contact precautions for residents colonized or infected with an MDRO.[92] Concerns about the lack of specificity of current clinical guidelines have been raised. In a recent qualitative study, variations in isolation practices and availability of resources between 10 NHs were reported.[93] Greater specificity of recommendations and a standardization of resources are required to achieve consistent infection prevention and control program practices in NHs.

Staff Education

Educational programs are recommended as means to inform all HCWs in appropriate infection prevention and control practices at the time of hire and regularly thereafter. A lack of understanding of key infection prevention concepts among NH staff has been reported.[93] To address this, programs should focus on disease transmission, hand hygiene practices, and standard and transmission-based precautions. Additional topics should be customized to specific NH needs according to local process and infection surveillance data. Specific emphasis on early symptom recognition should also be encouraged.

Nursing assistants provide the majority of direct resident care in NHs. Nursing assistants perceive language, knowledge, part-time status, workload demands, and accountability as barriers to using infection prevention and control practices. Strategies to overcome these barriers included translating in-services, hands-on training, on-the-spot training for part-time staff, increased staffing ratios, and inclusion and empowerment.[94]

Table 4
Studies based on controlled multicomponent interventions leading to decreased endemic rate of infection and/or colonization with MDROs

Reference and year	Location	VA NHs Included?	Interventions	Results
Mody et al,[86] 2015	MI	No	Multimodal intervention including preemptive barrier precautions, active surveillance for MDROs and infections, and NH staff education.	Decrease in overall MDRO prevalence density (rate ratio, 0.77). Decrease in first and overall CAUTI (hazard ratio, 0.54 and 0.69).
Evans et al,[91] 2014	US Nationwide	Yes	Multiple measures undertaken in 133 VA Nursing Homes.	Rate of MRSA health care-associated infections decreased by 36%.
Schora et al,[98] 2014	IL	No	Decolonization with nasal mupirocin and chlorhexidine bathing. Enhanced environmental cleaning every 4 mo.	MRSA colonization was reduced from 16.44% to 10.55%.
Ho et al,[99] 2012	Hong Kong	No	WHO multimodal strategy: ABHR racks, pull reels, hand hygiene posters and reminders, educational program, performance feedback.	Improved hand hygiene compliance. Reduction of respiratory outbreaks and MRSA infections requiring hospital admission.
Ho et al,[100] 2012	Hong Kong	No	Comprehensive infection control program established.	Decreased MRSA colonization of health care workers' hands, and contamination of enteral feed.
Makris et al,[101] 2000	NJ, PA	No	Educational program. Replaced all germicidal products with single-branded products.	Decrease of infection incidence density rate (from 6.33 to 4.15). Greatest reduction was in upper respiratory infections.
Silverblatt et al,[102] 2000	RI	Yes	Rectal VRE screening before transfer to nursing home, contact isolation, oral bacitracin to eliminate colonization.	VRE transfer between resident was eliminated.
Armstrong-Evans et al,[103] 1999	Ontario	No	Cohorting and restrictions of colonized residents. Gown and gloves. No equipment sharing; 2X daily cleaning of rooms, wheelchairs.	VRE colonization abated, with no new cases found within 9 mo of the intervention.

Abbreviations: ABHR, alcohol-based hand rub; CAUTI, catheter-associated urinary tract infection; MDRO, multidrug-resistant organism; MI, Michigan; MRSA, methicillin-resistant *Staphylococcus aureus*; NHs, nursing homes; VA, Department of Veterans Affairs; VRE, vancomycin-resistant enterococci; WHO, World Health Organization.

Data from Refs.[86,91,98–103]

NHs are mandated to have medical directors.[95] The role of the medical director in infection control is to advise on infection prevention and control program issues and approve specific policies and procedures to reduce infections.[96] Education of geriatric medicine fellows should incorporate topics related to medical directorship, because they are likely to be future medical directors in NHs. A recent study highlighted the importance of integrating infection prevention and control program into the first attempt at developing a curriculum for medical directors.[97] Creation of a national standardized program to train future NH medical directors according to current clinical guidelines is needed.

SUMMARY

NHs are a unique environment with challenges for infection prevention and control. Infection control practitioners are essential to enforce compliance with hand hygiene, device care and increase awareness of MDROs. Multimodal interventions including barrier precautions, active surveillance for MDROs and infections, and NH staff education have been proven to be effective. These interventions are being implemented at a national level with the goal of reducing CAUTIs. Continued efforts to standardize infection prevention and control in NHs encouraging use of currently available evidence-based guidelines are necessary in this setting.

REFERENCES

1. Aronow WS. Clinical causes of death of 2372 older persons in a nursing home during 15-year follow-up. J Am Med Dir Assoc 2000;1:95–6.
2. Strausbaugh LJ, Joseph CL. The burden of infection in long-term care. Infect Control Hosp Epidemiol 2000;21:674–9.
3. Benoit SR, Nsa W, Richards CL, et al. Factors associated with antimicrobial use in nursing homes: a multilevel model. J Am Geriatr Soc 2008;56:2039–44.
4. Gurwitz JH, Field TS, Avorn J, et al. Incidence and preventability of adverse drug events in nursing homes. Am J Med 2000;109:87–94.
5. Kahvecioglu D, Ramiah K, McMaughan D, et al. Multidrug-resistant organism infections in US nursing homes: a national study of prevalence, onset, and transmission across care settings, October 1, 2010-December 31, 2011. Infect Control Hosp Epidemiol 2014;35(Suppl 3):S48–55.
6. Crossley KB, Peterson PK. Infections in the elderly. Clin Infect Dis 1996;22:209–15.
7. McElhaney JE, Effros RB. Immunosenescence: what does it mean to health outcomes in older adults? Curr Opin Immunol 2009;21:418–24.
8. Nichol KL, Nordin JD, Nelson DB, et al. Effectiveness of influenza vaccine in the community-dwelling elderly. N Engl J Med 2007;357:1373–81.
9. Arens R, Remmerswaal EB, Bosch JA, et al. 5(th) International Workshop on CMV and Immunosenescence - a shadow of cytomegalovirus infection on immunological memory. Eur J Immunol 2015;45:954–7.
10. Man AL, Gicheva N, Nicoletti C. The impact of ageing on the intestinal epithelial barrier and immune system. Cell Immunol 2014;289:112–8.
11. Biniek K, Levi K, Dauskardt RH. Solar UV radiation reduces the barrier function of human skin. Proc Natl Acad Sci U S A 2012;109:17111–6.
12. Tseng CW, Kyme PA, Arruda A, et al. Innate immune dysfunctions in aged mice facilitate the systemic dissemination of methicillin-resistant S. aureus. PLoS One 2012;7:e41454.

13. Grishina I, Fenton A, Sankaran-Walters S. Gender differences, aging and hormonal status in mucosal injury and repair. Aging Dis 2014;5:160–9.

14. Fujita K, Sayama T, Abe S, et al. Age-dependent aminoglycoside nephrotoxicity. J Urol 1985;134:596–7.

15. Mouton CP, Bazaldua OV, Pierce B, et al. Common infections in older adults. Am Fam Physician 2001;63:257–68.

16. Lawton MP, Brody EM. Assessment of older people: self-maintaining and instrumental activities of daily living. Gerontologist 1969;9:179–86.

17. Min L, Galecki A, Mody L. Functional disability and nursing resource use are predictive of antimicrobial resistance in nursing homes. J Am Geriatr Soc 2015;63:659–66.

18. Chen TY, Anderson DJ, Chopra T, et al. Poor functional status is an independent predictor of surgical site infections due to methicillin-resistant Staphylococcus aureus in older adults. J Am Geriatr Soc 2010;58:527–32.

19. McNulty CA, Bowen J, Foy C, et al. Urinary catheterization in care homes for older people: self-reported questionnaire audit of catheter management by care home staff. J Hosp Infect 2006;62:29–36.

20. Daneman N, Bronskill SE, Gruneir A, et al. Variability in antibiotic use across nursing homes and the risk of antibiotic-related adverse outcomes for individual residents. JAMA Intern Med 2015;175:1331–9.

21. Mody L, Crnich C. Effects of excessive antibiotic use in nursing homes. JAMA Intern Med 2015;175:1339–41.

22. Strausbaugh LJ, Jacobson C, Sewell DL, et al. Antimicrobial therapy for methicillin-resistant Staphylococcus aureus colonization in residents and staff of a Veterans Affairs nursing home care unit. Infect Control Hosp Epidemiol 1992;13:151–9.

23. McKinnell JA, Miller LG, Eells SJ, et al. A systematic literature review and meta-analysis of factors associated with methicillin-resistant Staphylococcus aureus colonization at time of hospital or intensive care unit admission. Infect Control Hosp Epidemiol 2013;34:1077–86.

24. Kindschuh W, Russo D, Kariolis I, et al. Comparison of a hospital-wide antibiogram with that of an associated long-term care facility. J Am Geriatr Soc 2012; 60:798–800.

25. Troillet N, Carmeli Y, Samore MH, et al. Carriage of methicillin-resistant Staphylococcus aureus at hospital admission. Infect Control Hosp Epidemiol 1998;19: 181–5.

26. Latour K, Catry B, Broex E, et al. Indications for antimicrobial prescribing in European nursing homes: results from a point prevalence survey. Pharmacoepidemiol Drug Saf 2012;21:937–44.

27. Loeb M, Bentley DW, Bradley S, et al. Development of minimum criteria for the initiation of antibiotics in residents of long-term-care facilities: results of a consensus conference. Infect Control Hosp Epidemiol 2001;22:120–4.

28. Monette J, Miller MA, Monette M, et al. Effect of an educational intervention on optimizing antibiotic prescribing in long-term care facilities. J Am Geriatr Soc 2007;55:1231–5.

29. Dwyer LL, Harris-Kojetin LD, Valverde RH, et al. Infections in long-term care populations in the United States. J Am Geriatr Soc 2013;61:342–9.

30. Stevenson KB, Moore J, Colwell H, et al. Standardized infection surveillance in long-term care: interfacility comparisons from a regional cohort of facilities. Infect Control Hosp Epidemiol 2005;26:231–8.

31. Koch AM, Eriksen HM, Elstrøm P, et al. Severe consequences of healthcare-associated infections among residents of nursing homes: a cohort study. J Hosp Infect 2009;71:269–74.

32. Wang L, Lansing B, Symons K, et al. Infection rate and colonization with antibiotic-resistant organisms in skilled nursing facility residents with indwelling devices. Eur J Clin Microbiol Infect Dis 2012;31:1797–804.

33. Teresi JA, Holmes D, Bloom HG, et al. Factors differentiating hospital transfers from long-term care facilities with high and low transfer rates. Gerontologist 1991;31:795–806.

34. Strausbaugh LJ. Emerging health care-associated infections in the geriatric population. Emerg Infect Dis 2001;7:268–71.

35. Dosa D. Should I hospitalize my resident with nursing home-acquired pneumonia? J Am Med Dir Assoc 2005;6:327–33.

36. Nicolle LE, Strausbaugh LJ, Garibaldi RA. Infections and antibiotic resistance in nursing homes. Clin Microbiol Rev 1996;9:1–17.

37. Jones SR, Parker DF, Liebow ES, et al. Appropriateness of antibiotic therapy in long-term care facilities. Am J Med 1987;83:499–502.

38. Dommeti P, Wang L, Flannery EL, et al. Patterns of ciprofloxacin-resistant gram-negative bacteria colonization in nursing home residents. Infect Control Hosp Epidemiol 2011;32:177–80.

39. Nace DA, Drinka PJ, Crnich CJ. Clinical uncertainties in the approach to long term care residents with possible urinary tract infection. J Am Med Dir Assoc 2014;15:133–9.

40. Hooton TM, Bradley SF, Cardenas DD, et al. Diagnosis, prevention, and treatment of catheter-associated urinary tract infection in adults: 2009 international clinical practice guidelines from the Infectious Diseases Society of America. Clin Infect Dis 2010;50:625–63.

41. O'Fallon E, Gautam S, D'Agata EM. Colonization with multidrug-resistant gram-negative bacteria: prolonged duration and frequent cocolonization. Clin Infect Dis 2009;48:1375–81.

42. Fisch J, Lansing B, Wang L, et al. New acquisition of antibiotic-resistant organisms in skilled nursing facilities. J Clin Microbiol 2012;50:1698–703.

43. De Vecchi E, Sitia S, Romanò CL, et al. Aetiology and antibiotic resistance patterns of urinary tract infections in the elderly: a 6-month study. J Med Microbiol 2013;62:859–63.

44. European Centre for Disease Prevention and Control. Point prevalence survey of healthcare-associated infections and antimicrobial use in European long-term care facilities. April-May 2013. Stockholm (Sweden): ECDC; 2014.

45. Marik PE, Kaplan D. Aspiration pneumonia and dysphagia in the elderly. Chest 2003;124:328–36.

46. Bohte R, van Furth R, van den Broek PJ. Aetiology of community-acquired pneumonia: a prospective study among adults requiring admission to hospital. Thorax 1995;50:543–7.

47. Ma HM, Ip M, Hui E, et al. Role of atypical pathogens in nursing home-acquired pneumonia. J Am Med Dir Assoc 2013;14:109–13.

48. Carman WF, Elder AG, Wallace LA, et al. Effects of influenza vaccination of health-care workers on mortality of elderly people in long-term care: a randomised controlled trial. Lancet 2000;355:93–7.

49. Mody L, Kauffman CA, Donabedian S, et al. Epidemiology of Staphylococcus aureus colonization in nursing home residents. Clin Infect Dis 2008;46:1368–73.

50. Mody L, Bradley SF, Galecki A, et al. Conceptual model for reducing infections and antimicrobial resistance in skilled nursing facilities: focusing on residents with indwelling devices. Clin Infect Dis 2011;52:654–61.

51. Murphy S, Denman S, Bennett RG, et al. Methicillin-resistant Staphylococcus aureus colonization in a long-term-care facility. J Am Geriatr Soc 1992;40:213–7.

52. Hudson LO, Reynolds C, Spratt BG, et al. Diversity of methicillin-resistant Staphylococcus aureus strains isolated from residents of 26 nursing homes in Orange County, California. J Clin Microbiol 2013;51:3788–95.

53. Crnich CJ, Duster M, Hess T, et al. Antibiotic resistance in non-major metropolitan skilled nursing facilities: prevalence and interfacility variation. Infect Control Hosp Epidemiol 2012;33:1172–4.

54. Furuno JP, Shurland SM, Zhan M, et al. Comparison of the methicillin-resistant Staphylococcus aureus acquisition among rehabilitation and nursing home residents. Infect Control Hosp Epidemiol 2011;32:244–9.

55. McGeer A, Campbell B, Emori TG, et al. Definitions of infection for surveillance in long-term care facilities. Am J Infect Control 1991;19:1–7.

56. Stone ND, Ashraf MS, Calder J, et al. Surveillance definitions of infections in long-term care facilities: revisiting the McGeer criteria. Infect Control Hosp Epidemiol 2012;33:965–77.

57. Olsho LE, Bertrand RM, Edwards AS, et al. Does adherence to the Loeb minimum criteria reduce antibiotic prescribing rates in nursing homes? J Am Med Dir Assoc 2013;14:309.e1–7.

58. Crnich CJ, Jump R, Trautner B, et al. Optimizing antibiotic stewardship in nursing homes: a narrative review and recommendations for improvement. Drugs Aging 2015;32:699–716.

59. Smith PW, Bennett G, Bradley S, et al. SHEA/APIC guideline: infection prevention and control in the long-term care facility. Am J Infect Control 2008;36:504–35.

60. American Medical Directors Association (AMDA). Common infections in the long-term care setting. Columbia (MD): American Medical Directors Association (AMDA); 2011. p. 46.

61. Schweon S, Burdsall D, Hanchett M, et al. Infection preventionist's guide to long term care. Washington DC: Association for Professionals in Infection Control and Epidemiology (APIC); 2013.

62. Roup BJ, Scaletta JM. How Maryland increased infection prevention and control activity in long-term care facilities, 2003-2008. Am J Infect Control 2011;39:292–5.

63. Mody L, Langa KM, Saint S, et al. Preventing infections in nursing homes: a survey of infection control practices in southeast Michigan. Am J Infect Control 2005;33:489–92.

64. Stone PW, Herzig CT, Pogorzelska-Maziarz M, et al. Understanding infection prevention and control in nursing homes: a qualitative study. Geriatr Nurs 2015;36:267–72.

65. Murphy DM, Hanchett M, Olmsted RN, et al. Competency in infection prevention: a conceptual approach to guide current and future practice. Am J Infect Control 2012;40:296–303.

66. Interim Guidance for Influenza Outbreak Management in Long Term Care Facilities. Centers for Disease Control and Prevention (online). Available at: www.cdc.gov/flu/professionals/infectioncontrol/ltc-facility-guidance.htm. Accessed November 1, 2015.

67. Pop-Vicas A, Mitchell SL, Kandel R, et al. Multidrug-resistant gram-negative bacteria in a long-term care facility: prevalence and risk factors. J Am Geriatr Soc 2008;56:1276–80.

68. Siegel JD, Rhinehart E, Jackson M, et al. 2007 Guideline for isolation precautions: preventing transmission of infectious agents in health care settings. Am J Infect Control 2007;35(10 Suppl 2):S65–164.

69. Bardenheier BH, Shefer AM, Lu PJ, et al. Are standing order programs associated with influenza vaccination? - NNHS, 2004. J Am Med Dir Assoc 2010;11: 654–61.

70. Centers for Disease Control and Prevention. Immunization of health-care personnel: recommendations of the advisory committee on immunization practices (ACIP). MMWR Morb Mortal Wkly Rep 2011;60(RR07):1–45. Available at: http:// www.cdc.gov/mmwr/preview/mmwrhtml/rr6007a1.htm. Accessed November 1, 2015.

71. Rutala WA, Weber DJ. Guideline for disinfection and sterilization of prion-contaminated medical instruments. Infect Control Hosp Epidemiol 2010;31: 107–17.

72. Kilpatrick C, Pittet D. WHO SAVE LIVES: Clean Your Hands global annual campaign. A call for action: 5 May 2011. Infection 2011;39:93–5.

73. Hocine MN, Temime L. Impact of hand hygiene on the infectious risk in nursing home residents: a systematic review. Am J Infect Control 2015. http://dx.doi.org/ 10.1016/j.ajic.2015.05.043.

74. Boyce JM, Pittet D. Guideline for hand Hygiene in health-care settings: recommendations of the healthcare infection control practices advisory committee and the HICPAC/SHEA/APIC/IDSA Hand Hygiene Task Force. Infect Control Hosp Epidemiol 2002;23:S3–40.

75. Mody L, McNeil SA, Sun R, et al. Introduction of a waterless alcohol-based hand rub in a long-term-care facility. Infect Control Hosp Epidemiol 2003;24:165–71.

76. Schweon SJ, Edmonds SL, Kirk J, et al. Effectiveness of a comprehensive hand hygiene program for reduction of infection rates in a long-term care facility. Am J Infect Control 2013;41:39–44.

77. Centers for Medicare and Medicaid Services (CMS), HHS. Medicare and Medicaid programs; fire safety requirements for certain health care facilities; amendment. Final rule. Fed Regist 2006;71:55326–41.

78. Pincock T, Bernstein P, Warthman S, et al. Bundling hand hygiene interventions and measurement to decrease health care-associated infections. Am J Infect Control 2012;40:S18–27.

79. Schweizer ML, Reisinger HS, Ohl M, et al. Searching for an optimal hand hygiene bundle: a meta-analysis. Clin Infect Dis 2014;58:248–59.

80. Castle N, Engberg JB, Wagner LM, et al. Resident and facility factors associated with the incidence of urinary tract infections identified in the nursing home minimum data set. J Appl Gerontol 2015 [pii:0733464815584666; Epub ahead of print].

81. Terpenning MS, Bradley SF, Wan JY, et al. Colonization and infection with antibiotic-resistant bacteria in a long-term care facility. J Am Geriatr Soc 1994; 42:1062–9.

82. Saint S, Kowalski CP, Kaufman SR, et al. Preventing hospital-acquired urinary tract infection in the United States: a national study. Clin Infect Dis 2008;46: 243–50.

83. Meddings J, Rogers MA, Krein SL, et al. Reducing unnecessary urinary catheter use and other strategies to prevent catheter-associated urinary tract infection: an integrative review. BMJ Qual Saf 2014;23:277–89.

84. Rebmann T, Greene LR. Preventing catheter-associated urinary tract infections: an executive summary of the Association for Professionals in Infection Control and Epidemiology, Inc, elimination guide. Am J Infect Control 2010;38:644–6.

85. Meddings J, Rogers MA, Macy M, et al. Systematic review and meta-analysis: reminder systems to reduce catheter-associated urinary tract infections and urinary catheter use in hospitalized patients. Clin Infect Dis 2010;51:550–60.

86. Mody L, Krein SL, Saint S, et al. A targeted infection prevention intervention in nursing home residents with indwelling devices: a randomized clinical trial. JAMA Intern Med 2015;175:714–23.

87. Fakih MG, George C, Edson BS, et al. Implementing a national program to reduce catheter-associated urinary tract infection: a quality improvement collaboration of state hospital associations, academic medical centers, professional societies, and governmental agencies. Infect Control Hosp Epidemiol 2013; 34:1048–54.

88. Chopra V, Montoya A, Joshi D, et al. Peripherally inserted central catheter use in skilled nursing facilities: a pilot study. J Am Geriatr Soc 2015;63:1894–9.

89. Chopra V, O'Horo JC, Rogers MA, et al. The risk of bloodstream infection associated with peripherally inserted central catheters compared with central venous catheters in adults: a systematic review and meta-analysis. Infect Control Hosp Epidemiol 2013;34:908–18.

90. Bouzad C, Duron S, Bousquet A, et al. Peripherally inserted central catheter-related infections in a cohort of hospitalized adult patients. Cardiovasc Intervent Radiol 2016;39(3):385–93.

91. Evans ME, Kralovic SM, Simbartl LA, et al. Nationwide reduction of health care-associated methicillin-resistant Staphylococcus aureus infections in Veterans Affairs long-term care facilities. Am J Infect Control 2014;42:60–2.

92. Strausbaugh LJ, Siegel JD, Weinstein RA. Preventing transmission of multidrug-resistant bacteria in health care settings: a tale of 2 guidelines. Clin Infect Dis 2006;42:828–35.

93. Cohen CC, Pogorzelska-Maziarz M, Herzig CT, et al. Infection prevention and control in nursing homes: a qualitative study of decision-making regarding isolation-based practices. BMJ Qual Saf 2015;24:630–6.

94. Travers J, Herzig CT, Pogorzelska-Maziarz M, et al. Perceived barriers to infection prevention and control for nursing home certified nursing assistants: a qualitative study. Geriatr Nurs 2015;36:355–60.

95. Schnelle JF, Ouslander JG. CMS guidelines and improving continence care in nursing homes: the role of the medical director. J Am Med Dir Assoc 2006;7: 131–2.

96. American Medical Directors Association. Roles and responsibilities of the medical director in the nursing home: position statement A03. J Am Med Dir Assoc 2005;6:411–2.

97. Higuchi M, Wen A, Masaki K. Developing future nursing home medical directors: a curriculum for geriatric medicine fellows. J Am Med Dir Assoc 2013;14: 157–60.

98. Schora DM, Boehm S, Das S, et al. Impact of detection, education, research and decolonization without isolation in long-term care (DERAIL) on methicillin-resistant Staphylococcus aureus colonization and transmission at 3 long-term care facilities. Am J Infect Control 2014;42:S269–73.

99. Ho ML, Seto WH, Wong LC, et al. Effectiveness of multifaceted hand hygiene interventions in long-term care facilities in Hong Kong: a cluster-randomized controlled trial. Infect Control Hosp Epidemiol 2012;33:761–7.
100. Ho SS, Tse MM, Boost MV. Effect of an infection control programme on bacterial contamination of enteral feed in nursing homes. J Hosp Infect 2012;82:49–55.
101. Makris AT, Morgan L, Gaber DJ, et al. Effect of a comprehensive infection control program on the incidence of infections in long-term care facilities. Am J Infect Control 2000;28:3–7.
102. Silverblatt FJ, Tibert C, Mikolich D, et al. Preventing the spread of vancomycin-resistant enterococci in a long-term care facility. J Am Geriatr Soc 2000;48:1211–5.
103. Armstrong-Evans M, Litt M, McArthur MA, et al. Control of transmission of vancomycin-resistant Enterococcus faecium in a long-term-care facility. Infect Control Hosp Epidemiol 1999;20:312–7.

Vaccinations for the Older Adult

Gowrishankar Gnanasekaran, MD, MPH[a], Rex Biedenbender, MD, MPH[b],
Harley Edward Davidson, PharmD, MPH[c], Stefan Gravenstein, MD, MPH[a,d],*

KEYWORDS

- Vaccine • Tetanus • Diphtheria • Influenza • Pneumococcus • Immune senescence
- Pertussis • Conjugate

KEY POINTS

- Influenza vaccines reduce clinical influenza in outpatient elderly adults, more so after vaccination with the high-dose vaccine.
- Standard-dose vaccines that are well matched to circulating influenza also reduce hospitalization risk in older adults compared with those who are not vaccinated.
- The 13-valent pneumococcal conjugate vaccine reduces both vaccine-specific invasive disease and pneumonia in older adults as well as nasal colonization and, hence, reduced transmissibility.
- The increase in pertussis prevalence over the last 50 years has led to its recommendation as part of the vaccine schedule for elderly patients.

INTRODUCTION

Four major vaccine-preventable diseases affect older adults in the United States, including influenza, herpes zoster, pneumococcal disease, and pertussis, based on their incidence and consequent health care cost (**Table 1**). This article focuses on

Funding source: Grant support from Sanofi Pasteur (G. Gnanasekaran, H.E. Davidson, S. Gravenstein); no funding (R. Biedenbender).

Conflict of interest: No disclosures (G. Gnanasekaran, R. Biedenbender); grant support from Sanofi Pasteur (H.E. Davidson); consultant or speakers bureau for Merck, Novartis, Novavax, Pfizer, Sanofi Pasteur in the last year. Grant support from Sanofi Pasteur (S. Gravenstein).

[a] Department of Medicine-Geriatrics, University Hospitals, Case Medical Center, Case Western Reserve University, 11100 Euclid Avenue, Cleveland, OH 44106, USA; [b] Jencare Neighborhood Medical Center, 5516 Virginia Beach Boulevard, Virginia Beach, VA 23462, USA; [c] Department of Clinical Internal Medicine, Eastern Virginia Medical School, Insight Therapeutics, LLC, 142 West York Street, Suite 605, Norfolk, VA 23510, USA; [d] Health Services Policy and Practice, Warren Alpert Medical School, Brown University, Providence, RI, USA

* Corresponding author. Department of Medicine-Geriatrics, Center for Geriatrics and Palliative Care, University Hospitals, Case Medical Center, Case Western Reserve University, 11100 Euclid Avenue, Cleveland, OH 44106.

E-mail address: Sgravensteinwork@gmail.com

Table 1
Estimated incidence and cost of major vaccine-preventable disease in adults 65 years old and older in the United States in 2013

Disease	Incidence N (%)	Cost ($)
Influenza	4.0 M (77%)	8.3 B (54%)
Herpes zoster	0.6 M (11%)	3.0 B (20%)
Pneumococcal disease	0.4 M (8%)	3.8 B (25%)
Pertussis	0.2 M (4%)	2.1 M (1%)

Abbreviations: B, billion; M, million.

Data from McLaughlin JM, McGinnis JJ, Tan L, et al. Estimated human and economic burden of four major adult vaccine-preventable diseases in the United States, 2013. J Prim Prev 2015;36(4):264.

these diseases, with the exception of herpes zoster, which is covered elsewhere in this issue (See Schmader K: Herpes Zoster, in this issue), as well as diphtheria and tetanus, as these conditions are important globally. Diphtheria and tetanus incidence in the United States is low because of high prevailing underlying immunity from past vaccinations. Hepatitis and hepatitis vaccine are not covered, as it is not a universally recommended vaccination because of limited data in older adults.

The need for vaccination and booster vaccination with advancing age relates to 2 primary concepts. One concerns normal anatomic and physiologic changes with aging that result in more serious disease as people get older. For example, elderly persons with a respiratory illness already have increased residual lung volume, reduced mucociliary escalator efficiency, and reduced force of cough. All of these affect pathogen clearance from the respiratory tract.[1] Secondly, from an immunologic perspective,[2,3] individuals produce less antibody in response to disease and infection with age—less so because of B-cell failure and more so because of thymic involution and reduced T-cell help to drive B-cell activity. The rate of cytokine increase, total amplitude, and rate of decrease on recovery is also tempered with age.

Consequently, cytokines that drive fever, for example, (interleukin-6 among others) do not elevate the temperature as efficiently and, therefore, do not inhibit temperature-sensitive replication of pathogens. Also, some symptoms, including anorexia and malaise associated with specific cytokines, such as tumor necrosis factor-alpha, may be delayed or less prominent in older adults. So with aging, the presentation of disease can be altered, making diagnosis and early intervention more challenging, even to experienced practitioners (See Norman DC: Clinical Features of Infection in Older Adults, in this issue). Vaccines may also attenuate other important clinical symptoms or illness severity, if not prevent disease altogether.

Primary prevention remains the core approach for vaccine-preventable diseases. Vaccines are relatively cost-effective strategies for older adults, especially our oldest and most frail patients. Vaccines may also attenuate other important clinical symptoms or illness severity. For these and other reasons, vaccines have an increasingly important role for older adults.

INFLUENZA AND INFLUENZA VACCINATION
Influenza Epidemiology

Influenza and pneumonia remain the leading cause of infectious morbidity and mortality for older adults. Influenza accounts for more than three-quarters of incident vaccine-preventable disease in people 65 years of age and older, some 4 million cases each year in the United States.[4] It also is responsible for half the health care costs for vaccine-preventable disease (see **Table 1**). More than 90% of influenza deaths occur in patients 65 years of age and older,[5] and the likelihood of dying increases incrementally beginning around 50 years of age.[6] Individuals with underlying circulatory or respiratory disease are at a much higher risk of influenza-related mortality and complications. Additionally, studies have shown that influenza infection is also associated with an increased risk of heart attacks and stroke.[7]

Nichol and colleagues[8] reported on a population of nearly 150,000 veterans, 60% of whom had been vaccinated, and noted a reduced incidence of pneumonia by 29%, cardiac disease by 19%, and cerebrovascular disease by 23% among the vaccinated population. Some have criticized this study, suggesting that the vaccinated cohort was healthier than the comparison group, but other studies around the world have substantiated these findings. For example, a 2011 study followed a subset of 439 patients with a mean age of 66 years and mostly male, who were admitted to the hospital for acute coronary syndrome. Within 8 weeks of admission, half were randomly assigned to receive influenza vaccination and the other half to routine care that did not include vaccination. The primary end point, combined cardiovascular events, showed a similar effect size as that of Nichol and colleagues.[8] The vaccinated group had about a 30% reduction in major cardiovascular events (**Table 2**).[9] Nevertheless, controversy remains regarding influenza vaccine's effectiveness in reducing influenza and its complications in older adults.[10,11]

Traditional influenza vaccines have greater effectiveness in younger adults, presumably because of the attenuated antibody response.[12] Efforts to produce more immunogenic influenza vaccines for older adults, therefore, continues, using several strategies, including adjuvants, varied delivery methods, and dosing adjustments. One such vaccine was introduced into the European market several years ago and contains a monophoryl lipid A adjuvant. Another, licensed in the United States by the Food and Drug Administration (FDA) in 2009 for adults older than 65 years (Fluzone High Dose, Sanofi Pasteur), contains 4 times more antigen than the standard-dose trivalent influenza vaccine (**Table 3**). Both vaccines produce more antibody than their standard-dose counterparts.[13–15]

In 2014, DiazGranados and colleagues[16] reported on a randomized controlled trial of 31,989 outpatient elderly patients aged 65 years and older that ran from 2011 to 2013. In this intent-to-treat study, half the population received high-dose vaccine, whereas the other half received standard-dose vaccine. The high-dose group had higher influenza antibody titers as well as 24.2% less laboratory-confirmed clinical influenza than the standard-dose group. Izurieta and colleagues[17] subsequently published results from a metadata-type comparative effectiveness study, comparing high-dose and standard-dose vaccines in an elderly population. They found a similar effect size (22%) in both groups for treated influenzalike illnesses and hospitalizations.

High-dose influenza vaccine retains superior immunogenicity in the long-term care population,[14] a finding that could translate into improved protection and fewer hospitalizations. A trial is currently underway to evaluate this outcome.[18] The FDA approved an adjuvanted trivalent influenza vaccine for adults aged 65 years and older in November 2015. The adjuvanted vaccine was shown to elicit higher antibody titers than nonadjuvanted TIV.[19,20] Despite recent studies showing that high-dose vaccines provide better outcomes in the elderly population than do standard-dose vaccines, the Advisory Committee on Immunization Practices (ACIP) has not given any influenza vaccine preferential status for elderly individuals as of this writing.

Table 2
Effects of influenza vaccine on major cardiovascular events

End Points	Vaccine (n = 221)	Control (n = 218)	Unadjusted HR (95% CI)	P Value (Unadjusted HR)	Adjusted HR (95% CI)	P Value (Adjusted HR)
MACE, n (%)	21 (9.5)	42 (19.3)	0.70 (0.75–0.86)	.004	0.67 (0.51–0.86)	.005
Death, n (%)	6 (2.7)	12 (5.5)	0.73 (0.50–1.03)	.113	0.62 (0.34–1.12)	.113
Hospitalization for ACS, n (%)	10 (4.5)	23 (10.6)	0.73 (0.55–0.91)	.032	0.68 (0.47–0.98)	.039
Hospitalization for HF, n (%)	4 (1.8)	10 (4.6)	0.69 (0.49–1.01)	.111	0.62 (0.19–2.04)	.136
Hospitalization for stroke, n (%)	1 (0.5)	0	—	1.0	—	—

Hazard ratios were adjusted for age, sex, serum creatinine, treatment with angiotensin-converting enzyme inhibitors, and coronary revascularization.
Abbreviations: ACS, acute coronary symptoms; CI, confidence interval; HF, heart failure; HR, hazard ratio; MACE, major adverse cardiovascular events.
From Phrommintikul A, Kuanprasert S, Wongcharoen W, et al. Influenza vaccination reduces cardiovascular events in patients with acute coronary syndrome. Eur Heart J 2011;32:1733; with permission.

Table 3
Influenza vaccines licensed for use in individuals 65 years old and older

Source	Number of Antigens in the Vaccines	Dose (mcg of Antigen)	Special Considerations
Egg grown	Trivalent[a]	15	This dose is considered the standard dose.
	Trivalent[b]	60	The high-dose vaccine is more immunogenic than standard-dose vaccines.
	Quadrivalent[c]	9	It contains an additional B antigen that is not present in trivalent vaccines; lower dose of antigen provides adequate immunogenicity.
	Trivalent[d]	15	The adjuvanted vaccine is more immunogenic than standard-dose vaccines.
Recombinant	Trivalent[a]	15	There is no contraindication with egg allergy.

[a] Trivalent egg-grown vaccines available by brand name include Afluria, Fluvirin, Fluzone, and one cell-culture-based vaccine by brand name FlucelVax. One trivalent recombinant vaccine is available by brand name Flublok.
[b] One high-dose influenza vaccine is available by brand name Fluzone High-Dose.
[c] Quadrivalent vaccines available by brand name include Fluarix Quadrivalent, FluLaval Quadrivalent, and Fluzone Quadrivalent. Quadrivalent vaccines include the 3 virus strains in the trivalent vaccine and an additional influenza B virus strain.
[d] One adjuvanted influenza vaccine is available by brand name Fluad.
Data from PL detail document, flu vaccines for 2015-2016. Pharmacist's letter/prescriber's letter. September 2015.

INFLUENZA VACCINES AND VACCINE ADMINISTRATION

Over the last few years, the FDA approved several new influenza vaccines for use in the United States. These vaccines include a recombinant egg-free manufacturing process for one of the influenza vaccines, so an egg allergy need no longer be a concern for those receiving the influenza vaccine; quadrivalent influenza vaccines, which are replacing trivalent vaccines and include an additional influenza B virus antigen; cell-culture-based influenza vaccine; high-dose influenza vaccine; and adjuvanted trivalent influenza vaccine.[21] (see **Table 3**).

The decision to include an extra influenza B antigen in the quadrivalent vaccine, in addition to the combination of 2 A strains and 1 B strain in the trivalent vaccine, was based on the recognition that circulating influenza B in each year was largely of 2 lineages. Such a simple solution is not available for influenza A strains, which are more subject to antigenic change through antigenic drift and the less frequent shifts that produce pandemics.

All the vaccines available for older adults in the United States are administered intramuscularly; none contain live virus. Although vaccine efficacy is established, many vaccines do not have randomized controlled trials with subjects aged 65 years and older.[22] Annual influenza vaccination is recommended for everyone aged 6 months and older without contraindications. The optimal timing is before influenza onset (usually October, in the Northern Hemisphere) if possible or during routine health care visits and hospitalizations as opportunities present themselves. Providers should continue to offer vaccines until influenza virus is no longer circulating, usually between March and May in the Northern Hemisphere.[23]

INFLUENZA VACCINATION OF HEALTH CARE WORKERS

A separate issue of note to health care personnel (HCP) is that they themselves should receive the annual influenza vaccine. All paid and unpaid individuals working in a health care setting who have the potential for exposure to patients should be considered HCP. For HCP younger than 65 years of age, there are more vaccine options available, including both an intranasal and intradermal quadrivalent vaccine.[24] HCP immunization is recommended to prevent the spread of infection, especially to individuals at high risk for complications, such as frail elders. HCP may come into contact with those infected with influenza and expose other patients and coworkers, even if they themselves do not feel sick.

The Healthy People 2020 goal for influenza vaccination of HCP is 90%.[25] The immunization rate for HCP in long-term care settings was 63% for the 2013 to 2014 season, the lowest of any health care setting.[26] Hospitals that mandate HCP vaccination as a condition of employment have the highest vaccination rates. An ongoing debate regarding personal rights versus the patient benefit has delayed a universal approach to mandatory HCP vaccination. Workers' rights to choose whether or not to be vaccinated have been typically defended by unions. Nevertheless, the weight of the evidence to date favors universal HCP vaccination as a means to protect patients.[27,28] One such study of HCP vaccination on influenza incidence, respiratory tract infections, and death in long-term care hospitals found that HCP vaccination is associated with reduced elderly mortality (10% vs 17%) in hospitals with high staff vaccination versus low staff vaccination, respectively.[29]

Although settling the debate over mandatory HCP vaccination is beyond the authors' scope here, evidence suggests that HCP vaccination directly benefits health care workers and their employers. For this reason alone, and not just to reduce patient risk, maximizing HCP vaccination should be part of every employer's goals. In 2013, the National Vaccine Advisory Committee published recommendations on strategies to achieve Healthy People 2020 annual influenza vaccination goals.[30] Their tiered recommendations, which can be applied to most health care settings, include a comprehensive influenza infection prevention program with HCP education as a key component, the integration of influenza vaccination programs into existing infection prevention or occupational health programs, and employer vaccination requirements if other strategies have been unsuccessful. Additional strategies include

- Articulated policy favoring universal health care worker vaccination
- Free on-site vaccination at multiple times, locations, and days
- A system enabling review and update of an individual employee's vaccination status
- Rewards or recognition for receiving the vaccine (such as buttons or stickers that vaccinated workers can wear to promote the benefit on behalf of patients, eg, perhaps declaring: I got shot for you)
- Negative consequences for those without a medical reason to avoid vaccination, such as lost employment (if dictated by policy), required declination forms in which employees describe reason for refusing, mask requirements for working while influenza is circulating, or mandatory sick leave for unvaccinated employees with mild respiratory tract symptoms

Vaccination policies should be reviewed and updated annually, and influenza vaccine should be ordered early in the year so there is plenty available for staff at the beginning of the influenza season.

PNEUMOCOCCAL DISEASE AND PNEUMOCOCCAL VACCINATION
Epidemiology of Pneumococcal Disease

Pneumococcal pneumonia, which may occur after influenza, has a mortality rate higher than any other vaccine-preventable disease, with an estimated 40,000 deaths annually.[31] Although pneumococcal pneumonia is the most common clinical presentation of pneumococcal disease in adults, serious complications, such as meningitis and bacteremia, are more likely in older adults, children, and those living with chronic diseases.[5] Further, antibiotic resistance is a continuing problem worldwide and complicates treatment.[32]

Several factors contribute to the incidence and severity of pneumococcal disease. Some 20% of adults who develop pneumococcal disease have underlying medical conditions. In a recent meta-analysis of risk factors for pneumococcal disease in adults 65 years of age or older, 26.4% had at least one at-risk condition, 9.5% had 2, and 3.1% had 3 or more. The most common conditions were coronary heart disease (52%), diabetes mellitus (50%), and chronic obstructive pulmonary disease (COPD) (20%).[33] Another important factor that contributes to disease severity is the pneumococcal pathogen serotype. The clinical impact of serotypes may vary, with some increasing the risk of meningitis, bacteremia (also referred to as *invasive pneumococcal disease* [IPD]), and antibiotic resistance.[34]

IPD results in as many as 12,000 annual pneumococcal bacteremia hospitalizations, with a 20% mortality (60% of which is in the elderly population), and up to 6000 cases of meningitis, with a 22% mortality in adults (compared with 8% in children). Noninvasive disease, which includes pneumonia and acute otitis media, is no less important. Up to 36% of adult community-acquired pneumonia (CAP) is due to *Streptococcus pneumoniae*, accounting for 100,000 to 400,000 hospitalizations annually. CAP also carries an overall 5% to 7% mortality, which is higher in the elderly.[5]

An additional factor that complicates disease severity is that disease-causing pneumococcal serotypes change over time due to bacterial, host, and environmental factors.[35] Of the more than 83 polysaccharide serotypes of S pneumoniae, most disease is caused by bacteria with one of 30 serotypes. Of the 2 pneumococcal vaccines licensed in the United States, one is a 23-valent vaccine (polysaccharide pneumococcal [PPSV]-23) and the other a 13-valent conjugate vaccine (pneumococcal conjugate vaccine [PCV]-13), addressing 23 and 13 of the most common serotypes, respectively. One of the challenges with evaluating the efficacy of pneumococcal vaccines is that we do not have a direct immune measure of protection. The level of antibodies that correlates with protection against pneumococcal disease (ie, a serologic correlate of protection) is not clearly defined for adults.[35]

The rate of pneumococcal vaccination in older adults has remained near the 64% reported in Healthy People 2010, with a Healthy People 2020 target of 90% coverage. Compared with the influenza vaccine, fewer adults get the pneumococcal vaccine. The PPSV-23 has been available since 1983; though vaccination rates have increased over time, it has not been optimal, with uptake remaining lowest in minority groups.[36] It was noted that African Americans had pneumococcal vaccine coverage of 48.7%, Asians 45.3%, and Hispanics has 39.2% coverage compared with 63.6% for whites aged 65 years and older.[36]

POLYSACCHARIDE PNEUMOCOCCAL VACCINE

The 23 antigens in PPSV-23 represent the strains most commonly associated with both noninvasive and invasive pneumococcal disease. The vaccine seems to reduce vaccine-strain bacteremia, but its effectiveness has been less adequate for other types of pneumococcal disease. This ineffectiveness led to the development of a new-generation conjugate vaccine (PCV)[5] and to dual recommendations for immunization with the new PCV-13 as well as PPSV-23 to maximize coverage across strains and immunity. Unlike the conjugate vaccines, the first version of which became available in 2000, immunization with PPSV-23 does not induce robust mucosal immunity and, thus, does not result in reduced nasal colonization or provide herd immunity. PPSV-23 is recommended for adults 65 years and older as well as those with chronic medical conditions or tobacco use. PPSV-23 induces a B-cell-dependent immune response and is found to be 60% to 70% effective against IPD but with less efficacy against pneumococcal pneumonia.[5]

CONJUGATED PNEUMOCOCCAL VACCINES

In 2000, the PCV with 7 antigens (PCV-7) was licensed for use in children. It was shown to generate a memory response by both B and T cells. Immunization of children with the conjugate vaccine induces antibodies that clear nasopharyngeal carriage, and this presumably has led to clearance of localized and nonbacteremic infections like otitis media by strains included in the vaccine.[37]

PCV-7 reduces IPD by 97%; it also reduces episodes of radiograph-confirmed pneumonia, acute otitis media, placement of tympanostomy tubes, and nasopharyngeal carriage.[37] By 2007, IPD in children decreased from 80 cases to 1 case per 100,000 persons (**Fig. 1**A).[38] Coincidentally, even though PCV-7 was not given to older adults, they still experienced a substantial decrease in PCV-7 serotype IPD, and evidence of replacement of non-PCV-7 serotypes causing IPD (including the pathogenic 19A serotype, see **Fig. 1**B). In 2010, the PCV-13 (which replaced PCV-7) included all 7 serotypes of PCV-7 and 6 additional ones, including 19A. PCV-13 was found efficacious against all 13 serotypes, leading to a 93% reduction in IPD by 2013.[39] In adults, IPD overall decreased by 12% to 32% and PCV-13/PCV-7 serotype-IPD decreased by 58% to 72% (depending on age), adding up to 30,000 cases of IPD and 3000 deaths prevented.[39] In comparison with PCV-7, IPD in children younger than 5 years declined by an additional 64%.[39] Notably, there was also a coincident reduction in penicillin resistance.[38]

But the study to prove direct effectiveness in older adults had yet to be done. This point was addressed by the Community-Acquired Pneumonia immunization Trial in Adults (CAPiTA), based in the Netherlands where, notably, children were not yet routinely receiving a conjugate vaccine and there was no underlying reduction in IPD related to population vaccination effects. The CAPiTA trial studied the PCV-13 vaccine in 84,496 adults 65 years and older in a double-blind randomized control trial. It demonstrated (1) a primary end point reduction of 45.5% (*P*<.0001) in vaccine-type strains (VT) of CAP; (2) a secondary end point reduction of 45% (*P*<.001) in nonbacteremic, non-VT CAP; and (3) a reduction of 75% in VT IPD.[40] The evaluation of this pivotal trial led ACIP to add PCV-13 to the vaccine schedule for older adults. ACIP did not remove the PPSV-23 vaccine, as it covers yet an additional 10 serotypes (**Fig. 2**); the recommended vaccination schedule, therefore, contains both PCV-13 and PPSV-23, as discussed later.

PNEUMOCOCCAL VACCINE ADMINISTRATION RECOMMENDATIONS

One dose of PCV-13 vaccine is recommended for all adults 65 years of age and older who have not previously received a pneumococcal vaccine. A dose of PPSV-23 is recommended 6 to 12 months later. People who have already received PPSV-23 vaccine before reaching their 65th birthday should receive one dose of PCV-13 at least 1 year after receiving their most recent PPSV-23. After at least a 6-month interval following PCV-13 and at least after 5 years after the first dose of PPSV-23 vaccine, another dose of PPSV-23 vaccine is recommended. If PCV-13 was administered before 65 years of age, no additional doses of PCV-13 are recommended. Please refer to the

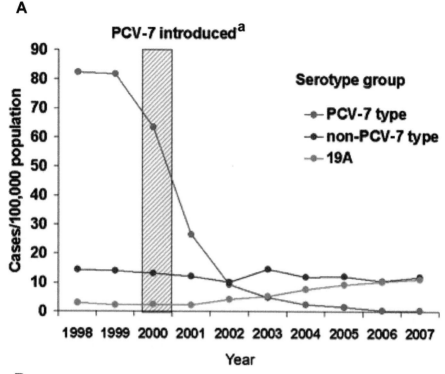

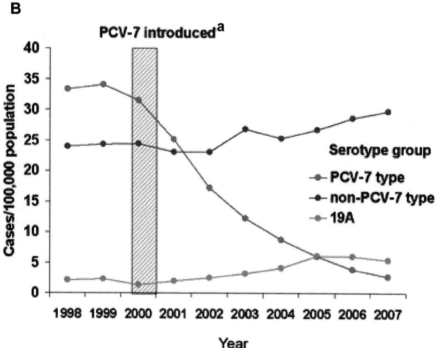

Fig. 1. (A) Declining invasive disease in children younger than 5 years and (B) older adults at least 65 years old after PCV-7 introduction in 2000. [a] PCV7 was introduced in the United States for routine use among young children and infants in the second half of 2000. (*From* Pilishvili T, Lexau C, Farley MM, et al. Sustained reductions in invasive pneumococcal disease in the era of conjugate vaccine. J Infect Dis 2010:201:36; with permission.)

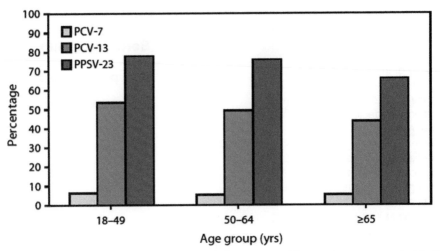

Fig. 2. Percentage of invasive pneumococcal disease caused by serotypes represented in 3 pneumococcal vaccines. (*From* Centers for Disease Control and Prevention. Updated recommendations for prevention of invasive pneumococcal disease among adults using the 23-valent pneumococcal polysaccharide vaccine (PPSV23). MMWR Morb Mortal Wkly Rep 2010;59:1102–6; and Centers for Disease Control and Prevention. Combined Tdap vaccine. 2014. Available at: http://www.cdc.gov/vaccines/vpd-vac/combo-vaccines/DTaP-Td-DT/tdap. htm. Accessed October 19, 2015.)

Centers for Disease Control and Prevention (CDC) Web site for recommendations for children and younger adults without chronic conditions.[24] Most healthy adults develop immunity within 2 to 3 weeks following vaccination. Serologic response may be diminished and delayed in some individuals, particularly frail elderly or those with chronic medical illness.

INDIVIDUALS WITH CHRONIC DISEASE AND IMMUNOCOMPROMISED STATES

The recommendation for those with chronic conditions (heart disease except hypertension, lung disease including asthma, liver disease including cirrhosis, diabetes, and alcoholism) and residents of long-term care facilities mirror those of older adults, with the age restriction starting at 19 years of age.[24]

For people with immunocompromised states (including human immunodeficiency virus infection), chronic renal failure, nephritic syndrome, or asplenia, a PCV-13 vaccine followed at an 8-week interval by a PPSV-23 vaccine and a second PPSV-23 at a 5-year interval is recommended. For people with cerebrospinal leaks or cochlear implants, a PCV-13 vaccine followed at an 8-week interval by a PPSV-23 vaccine is recommended.[24]

TETANUS, DIPHTHERIA, AND PERTUSSIS
Tetanus

Although tetanus incidence remains low in the United States, it continues to cause serious health problems, principally for older adults. Caused by the toxin produced by *Clostridium tetani* spores, tetanus occurs almost exclusively in people with no or little antibody to tetanus toxin. Clinical manifestations follow inoculation via puncture or laceration. Classic signs include prolonged spasms of the flexor and extensor muscle groups. Progression to generalized flexion contractures and masseter muscle spasm (lockjaw) occurs in advanced cases. Involvement of the respiratory muscles leads to death by suffocation. Patients seeking medical care for a puncture wound or laceration need their tetanus vaccination status assessed to determine if tetanus toxoid or immune globulin is indicated.

The risk of tetanus infection doubles in those 60 years old and older, compared with those aged 20 to 59 years. The mortality risk also increases with age, as elderly adults experience declining serum antibody levels to the tetanus extracellular neurotoxin, tetanospasmin. For individuals with tetanus, mortality risk was higher in those aged 65 years or older compared with those who were younger (relative risk = 5.1; 95% confidence interval, 2.1–12.2).[41] A US population survey showed prevalent immunity in around 30% of those aged 70 years or older, as compared with about 70% in younger individuals.[42] An unknown history, or a history of receiving fewer than 2 doses of tetanus toxoid, predicts nonprotective titer levels. Vaccination remains an effective strategy to limit the incidence of tetanus.

DIPHTHERIA

Diphtheria is caused by *Corynebacterium diphtheriae*. Although diphtheria still occurs around the world, it is rare in the United States, with only a few cases reported per year. Widespread use of diphtheria toxoid limits annual incidence, with most cases occurring in unimmunized or inadequately immunized individuals.[5] Vaccination remains an effective strategy to limit the incidence of diphtheria.

PERTUSSIS

Pertussis, or whooping cough, is caused by the bacterium *Bordetella pertussis*. It can cause uncontrollable, violent coughing that makes it hard to breath and is often

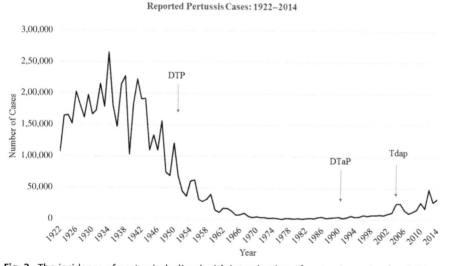

Fig. 3. The incidence of pertussis declined with introduction of pertussis vaccine for children (DTP, then DTaP) and again with the introduction of vaccine for adults, a reservoir for pertussis (Tdap). (*From* Centers for Disease Control and Prevention. Pertussis (whooping cough) surveillance and reporting. Available at: http://www.cdc.gov/pertussis/surv-reporting.html. Accessed October 19, 2015.)

Table 4
Summary of vaccination recommendations for adults aged 65 years and older

Vaccine	Dosing
Universal Recommendations for Adults Aged 65 y and Older	
Influenza	1 dose annually, standard or high-dose, preferably by October of each year (in North America)
Tetanus, diphtheria, pertussis (Td/Tdap)	Substitute 1-time dose of Tdap for Td booster, then boost with Td every 10 y
PPSV-23	• 1 dose after 65 y • 1 dose 5 years after the previous dose, if original dose of PPSV-23 was given when the individual was younger than 65 y. • Dosing must consider PCV-13, see later discussion
PCV-13	• 1-time dose (when both PCV-13 and PPV-23 indicated, PCV-13 administered first, but not administered during the same visit) • *For individuals who have not received PCV-13 or PPSV-23:* administer PCV-13 followed by PPSV-23 in 6–12 mo • *For individuals who have not received PCV-13 but have received a dose of PPSV-23 at 65 y of age or older:* administer PCV-13 at least 1 y after the dose of PPSV-23 • *For individuals who have not received PCV-13 but have received 1 or more doses of PPSV-23 before 65 y:* administer PCV-13 at least 1 y after the most recent dose of PPSV-23; administer a dose of PPSV-23 6–12 mo after PCV-13 (or as soon as possible if this time window has passed) and at least 5 y after the most recent dose of PPSV-23 • *For individuals who have had PCV-13 but not PPSV-23 before 65 y:* administer PPSV-23 6–12 mo after PCV-13 or as soon as possible if this time window has passed • *For individuals who have received PCV-13 and 1 or more doses of PPSV-23 before 65 y:* administer PPSV-23 6–12 mo after PCV-13 (or as soon as possible if this time window has passed) and at least 5 y after the most recent dose of PPSV-23

Herpes zoster	1 dose after 60 y
Varicella (for adults without evidence of immunity to varicella)	2 doses at least 4 wk apart

Recommendations for Adults Aged 65 y or Older with Additional Risk Factors (see current CDC Recommended Adult Immunization Schedule for description of risk factors)

Hepatitis B	• 3-dose schedule: second dose at least 1 mo after first dose and third dose at least 2 mo after the second dose (and at least 4 mo after the first dose) • 3- or 4-dose schedule if combined hepatitis A and hepatitis B vaccine is used: 3 doses at 0, 1, and 6 mo; alternatively 4 doses at days 0, 7, and 21–30 followed by a booster dose at 12 mo
Hepatitis A	• 2- dose schedule of single antigen vaccine at either 0 and 6–12 mo or 0 and 6–18 mo • 3- or 4-dose schedule if combined hepatitis A and hepatitis B vaccine is used: 3 doses at 0, 1, and 6 mo; alternatively 4 doses at days 0, 7, and 21–30 followed by a booster dose at 12 mo
Meningococcal	1 or more doses depending on individual risk factors and age

From Centers for Disease Control and Prevention. Recommended adult immunization schedule, United States, 2015. Available at: www.cdc.gov/vaccines/schedules/downloads/adult/adult-combined-schedule.pdf. Accessed October 21, 2015.

accompanied by the need to take deep breaths resulting in the characteristic whooping sound. Pertussis can be contracted by persons of all ages but is especially serious for infants. It is a disease that only occurs in people who serve as the reservoir for the bacteria. The introduction of pertussis vaccine first for children, and then later for adults, dramatically reduced the incidence of pertussis (**Fig. 3**). However, pertussis cases began gradually increasing in the 1980s; the United States saw more than 48,000 cases in 2012[5] and 32,000 cases in 2014.[43]

Previously, infants more frequently contracted the disease from adults; now infants and young children most often contract the disease from siblings, but other family members or caregivers are still a source of infection. Therefore, those who are in close contact with children are advised to stay current on their vaccination.[44,45] From 2000 to 2010, an average of 318 pertussis cases (range: 71–719 cases) were reported each year in adults aged 65 years and older, although ACIP puts the likely actual burden of pertussis in adults aged 65 years and older as at least 100 times greater than what is reported. Vaccination of adults remains an effective strategy to limit the incidence of pertussis and to cocoon infants and children from adult carriers.[46]

TETANUS TOXOID, REDUCED DIPHTHERIA TOXOID, AND ACELLULAR PERTUSSIS VACCINATION

Tetanus-diphtheria toxoids and acellular pertussis are among the most immunogenic vaccines approved for older adults. They are considered 100% effective for immuno-competent persons with up-to-date vaccination status. Natural immunity to tetanus does not occur, and natural immunity to diphtheria and pertussis occurs in only a subset of cases. Primary vaccination with tetanus toxoid provides 10 or more years of protection. Reemergence of pertussis in the United States and of diphtheria in Sweden and elsewhere has heightened awareness that a combined strategy for keeping adults current on the tetanus toxoid, reduced diphtheria toxoid, and acellular pertussis (Tdap) vaccine is important, not just for personal protection from the disease but also for cocooning protection of infants. In the last decade, the recommendations for Tdap vaccination have become more inclusive of adults. In October 2005, ACIP voted to recommend routine use of a single dose of Tdap for adults aged 19 to 64 years and for those who have close contact with infants younger than 1 year. In 2010, ACIP relaxed the recommendation to give the Tdap regardless of the interval from the prior tetanus- or diphtheria-containing vaccine and included certain adults older than 65 years. In 2011, grandparents and others who anticipated or who had close contact with infants less than a year old were recommended to receive a single dose of Tdap if they had not previously received it. Ideally, Tdap would be given at least 2 weeks before beginning close contact. In February 2012, ACIP went further, recommending vaccination with Tdap in all adults aged 65 years and older.[46]

In summary, adults who have not been immunized against tetanus, diphtheria, and pertussis should be vaccinated. For adults with no prior vaccination, the initial primary series should be given (earlier doses do not need to be repeated if the schedule is delayed). Those who did not complete the primary series should finish it with combined tetanus-diphtheria toxoid (Td) or Tdap vaccine and receive revaccination with Td every 10 years thereafter. A booster dose even years after the primary vaccination still provides protection.

Being up to date on the Tdap vaccination is especially important if travel to developing countries is anticipated. Td prophylaxis is recommended for clean, minor wounds if the primary series is incomplete or the last booster vaccination was more than 10 years ago. Serious wounds require added passive immunization with tetanus immune globulin.[5]

The available Tdap vaccines by brand name include Boostrix and Adacel Tdap. Although only Boostrix is approved for those aged 65 years and older, the CDC recommends administration of whichever vaccine is available; both are considered immunogenic.[5]

SUMMARY

The number and variety of vaccines available and recommended for older adults is increasing, as are the vaccination schedules, creating a challenge for providers to keep their patients up to date with the correct dosing and schedule (**Table 4**). In general, intramuscular vaccines cause local reactions, including mild local pain and erythema, usually lasting only a few days. Typically, the more immunogenic vaccines have slightly more local reactogenicity; but severe reactions are equally uncommon among the current recommended group of vaccines.

In terms of risk of specific adverse events, the influenza vaccine deserves special mention because of the concerns regarding Guillain-Barré and egg allergies. Only the 1976 influenza vaccine was significantly associated with Guillain-Barré and only at a frequency of less than 1 in a million vaccinated, far lower than the number of deaths the vaccine likely prevented. As for eggs and influenza vaccine, a recombinant egg-free formulation is now available, which removes concerns about egg allergies.

In terms of all vaccines and the presence of adjuvants and concern for an outcome of autism, no such concern exists for older adults and no credible scientific evidence supports such concern even for young patients, so it should not cause hesitation or delay in administering vaccines to older adults.

REFERENCES

1. Kale SS, Ahuja N, Yende S, et al. In: Newman AB, Cauley JA, editors. The epidemiology of aging. Dordecht (Netherlands): Springer; 2012. p. 237–53.
2. Taub DD, Longo DL. Insights into thymic aging and regeneration. Immunol Rev 2005;205:72–93.
3. Lambert ND, Ovsyannikova IG, Pankratz VS, et al. Understanding the immune response to seasonal influenza vaccination in older adults: a systems biology approach. Expert Rev Vaccines 2012;11:985–94.
4. McLaughlin JM, McGinnis JJ, Tan L, et al. Estimated human and economic burden of four major adult vaccine-preventable diseases in the United States, 2013. J Prim Prev 2015;36(4):259–73.
5. Centers for Disease Control and Prevention. Epidemiology and prevention of vaccine-preventable diseases. In: Hamborsky J, Kroger A, Wolfe S, editors. 13th edition. Washington, DC: Public Health Foundation; 2015. p. 12.
6. Thompson WW, Comanor L, Shay DK. Epidemiology of seasonal influenza: use of surveillance data and statistical models to estimate the burden of disease. J Infect Dis 2006;194(Suppl 2):S82–91.
7. Smeeth L, Thomas SL, Hall AJ, et al. Risk of myocardial infarction and stroke after acute infection or vaccination. N Engl J Med 2004;351:2611–8.
8. Nichol KL, Nordin J, Mullooly J, et al. Influenza vaccination and reduction in hospitalizations for cardiac disease and stroke among the elderly. N Engl J Med 2003;348:1322–32.
9. Phrommintikul A, Kuanprasert S, Wongcharoen W, et al. Influenza vaccination reduces cardiovascular events in patients with acute coronary syndrome. Eur Heart J 2011;32:1730–5.

10. Clar C, Oseni Z, Flowers N, et al. Influenza vaccines for preventing cardiovascular disease. Cochrane Database Syst Rev 2015;(5):CD005050.

11. Jefferson T, Di Pietrantonj C, Al-Ansary LA, et al. Vaccines for preventing influenza in the elderly. Cochrane Database Syst Rev 2010;(2):CD004876.

12. Goodwin K, Viboud C, Simonsen L. Antibody response to influenza vaccination in the elderly: a quantitative review. Vaccine 2006;24:1159–69.

13. Keitel WA, Atmar RL, Cate TR, et al. Safety of high doses of influenza vaccine and effect on antibody responses in elderly persons. Arch Intern Med 2006;166: 1121–7.

14. Nace DA, Len CJ, Ross TM, et al. Randomized, controlled trial of high-dose influenza vaccine among frail residents of long-term care facilities. J Infect Dis 2015; 211:1915–24.

15. DiazGranados CA, Dunning AJ, Jordanov E, et al. High-dose trivalent influenza vaccine compared to standard dose vaccine in elderly adults: safety, immunogenicity and relative efficacy during the 2009–2010 season. Vaccine 2013;31: 861–6.

16. DiazGranados CA, Dunning AJ, Kimmel M, et al. Efficacy of high-dose versus standard-dose influenza vaccine in older adults. N Engl J Med 2014;371:635–45.

17. Izurieta HS, Thadani N, Shay DK, et al. Comparative effectiveness of high-dose versus standard-dose influenza vaccines in US residents aged 65 years and older from 2012 to 2013 using Medicare data: a retrospective cohort analysis. Lancet Infect Dis 2015;15:293–300.

18. ClinicalTrials.gov Registration: NCT01815268.

19. FLUAD [package insert]. Cambridge, MA: Novartis Vaccines and Diagnostics, Inc.; 2015.

20. Della Cioppa G, Nicolay U, Lindert K, et al. Superior immunogenicity of seasonal influenza vaccines containing full dose of MF59 ((R)) adjuvant: results from a dose-finding clinical trial in older adults. Human Vaccines & Immunotherapeutics 2012;8:216–27.

21. Centers for Disease Control and Prevention. Influenza (flu). 2015. Available at: www.cdc.gov/flu/protect/vaccine/vaccines.htm. Accessed September 18, 2015.

22. Osterholm MT, Kelley NS, Sommer A, et al. Efficacy and effectiveness of influenza vaccines: a systematic review and meta-analysis. Lancet Infect Dis 2012;12: 36–44.

23. Grohskopf LA, Sokolow LZ, Olsen SJ, et al. Prevention and control of influenza with vaccines: recommendations of the advisory committee on immunization practices, United States, 2015-16 influenza season. MMWR Morb Mortal Wkly Rep 2015;64:818–25.

24. Centers for Disease Control and Prevention. Adult immunization schedules. United States, 2015. Available at: http://www.cdc.gov/vaccines/schedules/hcp/adult.html. Accessed September 15, 2015.

25. Office of Disease Prevention and Health Promotion. Increase the percentage of health care personnel who are vaccinated annually against seasonal influenza. 2013. Available at: https://www.healthypeople.gov/node/6361/data_details#revision_history_header. Accessed October 21, 2015.

26. Black CL, Yue X, Ball SW, et al. Influenza vaccination coverage among health care personnel – United States, 2013-14 influenza season. MMWR Morb Mortal Wkly Rep 2014;63:805–11.

27. Ahmed F, Lindley MC, Allred N, et al. Effect of influenza vaccination of healthcare personnel on morbidity and mortality among patients: systematic review and grading of evidence. Clin Infect Dis 2014;58:50–7.

28. Griffin MR. Influenza vaccination of healthcare workers: making the grade for action. Clin Infect Dis 2014;58:58–60.
29. Potter J, Stott DJ, Roberts MA, et al. Influenza vaccination of health care workers in long-term-care hospitals reduces the mortality of elderly patients. J Infect Dis 1997;175:1–6.
30. National Vaccine Advisory Committee. Strategies to achieve the Healthy People 2020 annual influenza vaccine coverage goal for health-care personnel: recommendations from the National Vaccine Advisory Committee. Public Health Rep 2013;128:7–25.
31. Centers for Disease Control and Prevention. National Center for Health Statistics. Health, United States, 2009: with special feature on medical technology. Hyattsville (MD): Department of Health and Human Services; 2010.
32. World Health Organization. 23-valent pneumococcal polysaccharide vaccine: WHO position paper. Wkly Epidemiol Rec 2008;83:373–84.
33. Curcio D, Cane A, Isturiz R. Redefining risk categories for pneumococcal disease in adults: critical analysis of the evidence. Int J Infect Dis 2015;37:30–5.
34. Moberley S, Holden J, Tatham DP, et al. Vaccines for preventing pneumococcal infection in adults. Cochrane Database Syst Rev 2013;(1):CD000422.
35. Musher DM. Editorial commentary: should 13-valent protein-conjugate pneumococcal vaccine be used routinely in adults? Clin Infect Dis 2012;55:265–7.
36. Williams WW, Lu PJ, O'Halloran A, et al. Vaccination coverage among adults, excluding influenza vaccination – United States, 2013. MMWR Morb Mortal Wkly Rep 2015;64:95–102.
37. Pletz MW, Maus U, Krug N, et al. Pneumococcal vaccines: mechanism of action, impact on epidemiology and adaption of the species. Int J Antimicrob Agents 2008;32:199–206.
38. Centers for Disease Control and Prevention. Manual for the surveillance of vaccine-preventable diseases. Atlanta (GA): Centers for Disease Control and Prevention; 2012.
39. Moore MR, Link-Gelles R, Schaffner W, et al. Effect of use of 13-valent pneumococcal conjugate vaccine in children on invasive pneumococcal disease in children and adults in the USA: analysis of multisite, population-based surveillance. Lancet Infect Dis 2015;15:301–9.
40. Bonten MJ, Huijts SM, Bolkenbaas M, et al. Polysaccharide conjugate vaccine against pneumococcal pneumonia in adults. N Engl J Med 2015;372:1114–25.
41. Centers for Disease Control and Prevention. Tetanus surveillance-United States, 2001-2008. MMWR Morb Mortal Wkly Rep 2011;60:365–9.
42. McQuillan GM, Kruszon-Moran D, Deforest A, et al. Serologic immunity to diphtheria and tetanus in the United States. Ann Intern Med 2002;136:660–6.
43. Centers for Disease Control and Prevention. Pertussis (whooping cough) surveillance and reporting. Available at: http://www.cdc.gov/pertussis/surv-reporting.html. Accessed October 19, 2015.
44. Skoff TH, Kenyon C, Cocoros N, et al. Sources of infant pertussis infections in the United States. Pediatrics 2015;136:635–41.
45. Grizas AP, Camenga D, Vázquez M. Cocooning: a concept to protect young children from infectious diseases. Curr Opin Pediatr 2012;24:92–7.
46. Centers for Disease Control and Prevention. Combined Tdap vaccine. 2014. Available at: http://www.cdc.gov/vaccines/vpd-vac/combo-vaccines/DTaP-Td-DT/tdap.htm. Accessed October 19, 2015.

Index

Note: Page numbers of article titles are in **boldface** type.

Clin Geriatr Med 32 (2016) 627–633
http://dx.doi.org/10.1016/S0749-0690(16)30042-8
0749-0690/16/$ – see front matter

geriatric.theclinics.com

Moving?

Make sure your subscription moves with you!

To notify us of your new address, find your **Clinics Account Number** (located on your mailing label above your name), and contact customer service at:

Email: journalscustomerservice-usa@elsevier.com

800-654-2452 (subscribers in the U.S. & Canada)
314-447-8871 (subscribers outside of the U.S. & Canada)

Fax number: 314-447-8029

Elsevier Health Sciences Division
Subscription Customer Service
3251 Riverport Lane
Maryland Heights, MO 63043

*To ensure uninterrupted delivery of your subscription, please notify us at least 4 weeks in advance of move.

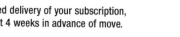